$49.95   11.421

Oxford American Handbook of
Hospice and
Palliative Medicine

St. Joseph Medical Center
The Otto C. Brantigan Medical Library
7601 Osler Drive
Towson, Maryland 21204

D0840358

About the Oxford American Handbooks in Medicine

The Oxford American Handbooks are pocket clinical books, providing practical guidance in quick reference, note form. Titles cover major medical specialties or cross-specialty topics and are aimed at students, residents, internists, family physicians, and practicing physicians within specific disciplines.

Their reputation is built on including the best clinical information, complemented by hints, tips, and advice from the authors. Each one is carefully reviewed by senior subject experts, residents, and students to ensure that content reflects the reality of day-to-day medical practice.

Key series features

- Written in short chunks, each topic is covered in a two-page spread to enable readers to find information quickly. They are also perfect for test preparation and gaining a quick overview of a subject without scanning through unnecessary pages.
- Content is evidence based and complemented by the expertise and judgment of experienced authors.
- The Handbooks provide a humanistic approach to medicine—it's more than just treatment by numbers.
- A "friend in your pocket," the Handbooks offer honest, reliable guidance about the difficulties of practicing medicine and provide coverage of both the practice and art of medicine.
- For quick reference, useful "everyday" information is included on the inside covers.

Published and Forthcoming Oxford American Handbooks

Oxford American Handbook of Clinical Medicine
Oxford American Handbook of Anesthesiology
Oxford American Handbook of Cardiology
Oxford American Handbook of Clinical Dentistry
Oxford American Handbook of Clinical Diagnosis
Oxford American Handbook of Clinical Examination and Practical Skills
Oxford American Handbook of Clinical Pharmacy
Oxford American Handbook of Critical Care
Oxford American Handbook of Emergency Medicine
Oxford American Handbook of Endocrinology and Diabetes
Oxford American Handbook of Gastroenterology and Hepatology
Oxford American Handbook of Geriatric Medicine
Oxford American Handbook of Hospice and Palliative Medicine
Oxford American Handbook of Nephrology and Hypertension
Oxford American Handbook of Neurology
Oxford American Handbook of Obstetrics and Gynecology
Oxford American Handbook of Oncology
Oxford American Handbook of Ophthalmology
Oxford American Handbook of Otolaryngology
Oxford American Handbook of Pediatrics
Oxford American Handbook of Physical Medicine and Rehabilitation
Oxford American Handbook of Psychiatry
Oxford American Handbook of Pulmonary Medicine
Oxford American Handbook of Rheumatology
Oxford American Handbook of Sports Medicine
Oxford American Handbook of Surgery
Oxford American Handbook of Urology

Oxford American Handbook of
Hospice and Palliative Medicine

Edited by

Sriram Yennurajalingam, MD

Assistant Professor
Department of Palliative Care & Rehabilitation Medicine
The University of Texas MD Anderson Cancer Center
Houston, Texas

Eduardo Bruera, MD

Professor and Chair
Department of Palliative Care & Rehabilitation Medicine
The University of Texas MD Anderson Cancer Center
Houston, Texas

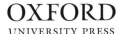

OXFORD
UNIVERSITY PRESS

OXFORD
UNIVERSITY PRESS

Oxford University Press, Inc. publishes works that further
Oxford University's objective of excellence
in research, scholarship and education.

Oxford New York

Auckland Cape Town Dar es Salaam Hong Kong Karachi
Kuala Lumpur Madrid Melbourne Mexico City Nairobi
New Delhi Shanghai Taipei Toronto

With offices in

Argentina Austria Brazil Chile Czech Republic France Greece
Guatemala Hungary Italy Japan Poland Portugal
Singapore South Korea Switzerland Thailand Turkey Ukraine Vietnam

Copyright © 2011 by Oxford University Press, Inc.

Published by Oxford University Press Inc.
198 Madison Avenue, New York, New York 10016

www.oup.com

Oxford is a registered trademark of Oxford University Press

All rights reserved. No part of this publication may be reproduced,
stored in a retrieval system, or transmitted, in any form or by any means,
electronic, mechanical, photocopying, recording, or otherwise,
without the prior permission of Oxford University Press.

Library of Congress Cataloging-in-Publication Data

Oxford American handbook of hospice and palliative medicine / edited by Eduardo
Bruera, Sriram Yennurajalingam.
p. ; cm. — (Oxford American handbooks in medicine)
Handbook of hospice and palliative medicine
Includes bibliographical references and index.
ISBN 978-0-19-538015-6
1. Palliative treatment–Handbooks, manuals, etc. 2. Hospice care–Handbooks,
manuals, etc. I. Bruera, Eduardo. II. Yennurajalingam, Sriram. III. Title: Handbook
of hospice and palliative medicine. IV. Series: Oxford American handbooks.
[DNLM: 1. Palliative Care–Handbooks. 2. Hospices–Handbooks. WB 39]
R726.8.O94 2011
362.17′56–dc22   2011012546

10 9 8 7 6 5 4 3 2 1
Printed in China
on acid-free paper
through Asia Pacific Offset

This material is not intended to be, and should not be considered, a substitute for medical or other professional advice. Treatment for the conditions described in this material is highly dependent on the individual circumstances. And, while this material is designed to offer accurate information with respect to the subject matter covered and to be current as of the time it was written, research and knowledge about medical and health issues is constantly evolving and dose schedules for medications are being revised continually, with new side effects recognized and accounted for regularly. Readers must therefore always check the product information and clinical procedures with the most up-to-date published product information and data sheets provided by the manufacturers and the most recent codes of conduct and safety regulation. Oxford University Press and the authors make no representations or warranties to readers, express or implied, as to the accuracy or completeness of this material, including without limitation that they make no representation or warranties as to the accuracy or efficacy of the drug dosages mentioned in the material. The authors and the publishers do not accept, and expressly disclaim, any responsibility for any liability, loss, or risk that may be claimed or incurred as a consequence of the use and/or application of any of the contents of this material.

Preface

In the United States, hospice and palliative medicine has emerged as a new subspecialty recently recognized by the American Board of Medical Specialties. During the last 10 years, there has been a very significant increase in the number of inpatient and outpatient palliative care programs as well as a major increase in the number of patients who access hospice for end-of-life care.

Unfortunately, educational efforts are lagging behind, and the vast majority of medical students, residents, and even fellows receive minimal palliative medicine education in the United States. However, these junior physicians along with a number of busy clinical specialists are exposed to patients with progressive incurable illnesses and their families on a daily basis.

The purpose of this Handbook is to provide up-to-date, practical, and concise information to health-care professionals delivering care to patients requiring hospice and palliative care in the United States. This includes physicians, nurse practitioners, fellows, residents, and students.

All the chapters are aimed primarily at the clinical and administrative arrangements within the American health-care system, including the hospice Medicare benefit.

We believe this book will provide rapid access to most of the daily bedside clinical and administrative needs, and we hope it will help our colleagues in the delivery of excellent palliative and hospice care.

We would like to acknowledge the authors of each of the chapters for having committed their time and effort to our joint project. We would also like to acknowledge the commitment to excellence by Oxford University Press and in particular Andrea Seils, our Senior Editor, for the excellent work in coordinating our book. Finally, we would like to acknowledge the daily effort of health-care professionals who have contributed by their daily clinical work, education, and research to the development of the extraordinary body of knowledge that we have had the privilege to synthesize in this book.

Sriram Yennu, MD
Eduardo Bruera, MD
Houston, March 2011

Preface

Contents

Contributors

Elizabeth A. Barnes, MD, FRCPC
Department of Radiation Oncology
Toronto Sunnybrook Regional Cancer Centre
Toronto, Ontario, Canada

Shirley H. Bush, MBBS, MRCGP, FAChPM
Division of Palliative Care, University of Ottawa
Clinical Scientist, Élisabeth Bruyère Research Institute (ÉBRI)
Palliative Care Physician, The Ottawa Hospital/Bruyère Continuing Care
Ottawa, Ontario, Canada

J. Randall Curtis, MD, MPH
Harborview Medical Center
Seattle, Washington

Shalini Dalal, MD
Palliative Care and Rehabilitation Medicine
The University of Texas MD Anderson Cancer Center
Houston, Texas

Sara Davison, MD, MSc, FRCPC
Associate Professor of Medicine
Division of Nephrology and Immunology
University of Alberta Faculty of Medicine
Edmonton, Alberta, Canada

Egidio Del Fabbro, MD
Palliative Care and Rehabilitation Medicine
The University of Texas MD Anderson Cancer Center
Houston, Texas

Marvin Omar Delgado Guay, MD
The University of Texas Medical School at Houston
Lyndon B. Johnson General Hospital
Houston, Texas

Rony Dev, DO
Palliative Care and Rehabilitation Medicine
The University of Texas MD Anderson Cancer Center
Houston, Texas

Deborah Dudgeon, MD
Director, Palliative Care Program
Queen's University Department of Medicine
Kingston, Ontario, Canada

James D. Duffy, MD, FAAHPM, FANPA
Professor of Psychiatry
The University of Texas MD Anderson Cancer Center
Houston, Texas

Ahmed Elsayem, MD
Palliative Care and Rehabilitation Medicine
The University of Texas MD Anderson Cancer Center
Houston, Texas

Nada Fadul, MD
Palliative Care and Rehabilitation Medicine
The University of Texas MD Anderson Cancer Center
Houston, Texas

Betty Ferrell, PhD, RN, FAAN
Professor, Nursing Research and Education
City of Hope
Duarte, California

Jaime S. Gomez MD, FACC, FSCAI
Spring, Texas

Sandra P. Gomez, MD, FAAHPM
Memorial Hermann The Hospital
Spring, Texas

Joan K. Harrold, MD, MPH
Medical Director
Vice President, Medical Services
Hospice of Lancaster County
Lancaster, Pennsylvania

David Hui, MD
Palliative Care and Rehabilitation Medicine
The University of Texas MD Anderson Cancer Center
Houston, Texas

Margaret Isaac, MD
Harborview Medical Center
Seattle, Washington

Meiko Kuriya, MD
Palliative Care and Rehabilitation Medicine
The University of Texas MD Anderson Cancer Center
Houston, Texas

Ana Leech, MD
Palliative Care and Rehabilitation Medicine
The University of Texas Health Science Center
Houston Medical School
Houston, Texas

Gabriel Lopez, MD
Palliative Care and Rehabilitation Medicine
The University of Texas MD Anderson Cancer Center
Houston, Texas

Mary Lynn Mcpherson, Pharm D, BCPS, CDE
Department of Pharmacy Practice and Science
University of Maryland School of Pharmacy
Baltimore, Maryland

Valentina Medici, MD
Division of Gastroenterology and Hepatology
University of California Davis Medical Center
Sacramento, California

Frederick J. Meyers, MD, MACP
Executive Associate Dean
Department of Internal Medicine
University of California Davis Medical Center
Sacramento, California

Jeff Myers, MD
Palliative Care Consult Team
Odette Cancer Centre
Sunnybrook Health Sciences
Toronto, Ontario, Canada

Zohra Nooruddin, MD
Palliative Care and Rehabilitation Medicine
The University of Texas MD Anderson Cancer Center
Houston, Texas

Edward O'Donnell, MA
Adjunct Assistant Professor
Clinical Management and Leadership
School of Health Sciences
The George Washington University
Washington, DC

Henrique A. Parsons, MD
Palliative Care and Rehabilitation Medicine
The University of Texas MD Anderson Cancer Center
Houston, Texas

V.S. Periyakoil, MD
Clinical Associate Professor, Medicine
Stanford School of Medicine
Stanford, California

Christina M. Puchalski, MD, FACP

Executive Director
George Washington Institute for Spirituality and Health
Professor of Medicine and Health Sciences
George Washington University School of Medicine
Washington, DC

Suresh K. Reddy, MD

Palliative Care and Rehabilitation Medicine
The University of Texas MD Anderson Cancer Center
Houston, Texas

Christine S. Ritchie, MD, MSPH

Division of Gerontology and Geriatric Medicine
Department of Medicine
The University of Alabama at Birmingham
Birmingham, Alabama

Rhonda Robert, PhD

Associate Professor, Pediatrics – Patient Care
The University of Texas MD Anderson Cancer Center
Houston, Texas

Lorenzo Rossaro, MD, FACP

Chief of Gastroenterology and Hepatology
University of California Davis Medical Center
Sacramento, California

Mary L.S. Vachon, RN, PHD

Research Scientist and Senior Mental Health Consultant
Clarke Institute of Psychiatry
Toronto, Ontario, Canada

Charles F. von Gunten, MD, PhD

Provost, Center for Palliative Studies
San Diego Hospice and Institute for Palliative Medicine
San Diego, California

Tobias Walbert, MD, PhD, MPH

Department of Neuro-oncology
The University of Texas MD Anderson Cancer Center
Houston, Texas

Paul W. Walker, MD

Palliative Care and Rehabilitation Medicine
The University of Texas MD Anderson Cancer Center
Houston, Texas

Kirsten Wentlandt, MD

Princess Margaret Hospital
The University Health Network
Toronto, Ontario, Canada

Donna S. Zhukovsky, MD, FACP
Palliative Care and Rehabilitation Medicine
The University of Texas MD Anderson Cancer Center
Houston, Texas

Camilla Zimmermann, FRCPC, MD, MSc
Princess Margaret Hospital
The University Health Network
Toronto, Ontario, Canada

Chapter 1

Definitions and key elements in palliative care

Sriram Yennurajalingam, MD
Eduardo Bruera, MD

Introduction

The aim of palliative care, derived from a Latin word meaning "to cloak," is to relieve suffering and improve quality of life in patients and their family and caregiver(s).[1] The term *palliative care* is commonly used for palliative care in a hospital setting.

The word *hospice*, derived from a Latin root, "hospes," refers to both to guests and hosts. The term *supportive care* refers to care that helps the care that helps the patient and family to cope with cancer and treatment of it.

Terminal care usually refers to management of patients during their last few days, weeks, or months of life from the point when it is clear that the patient is in a state of progressive decline.

The World Health Organization (WHO) definition of palliative care and the *Clinical Practice Guidelines for Quality Palliative Care* consensus definition of palliative care are those definitions commonly accepted. Following are the definitions as described at http://www.who.int/cancer/palliative/definition/en/ (WHO definition) and http://www.nationalconsensusproject.org (NCP definition) (taken verbatim to retain their original meaning).

WHO definition of palliative care*

The WHO defines *palliative care* as "an approach that improves the quality of life of patients and their families facing the problem associated with life-threatening illness, through the prevention and relief of suffering by means of early identification and impeccable assessment and treatment of pain and other problems, physical, psychosocial and spiritual."[2] In addition, the WHO defines the key elements of palliative care:

- Provide relief from pain and other distressing symptoms
- Affirm life and regard dying as a normal process
- Intend neither to hasten nor postpone death
- Integrate the psychological and spiritual aspects of patient care
- Offer a support system to help patients live as actively as possible until death
- Offer a support system to help the family cope during the patient's illness and in their own bereavement
- Use a team approach to address the needs of patients and their families, including bereavement counseling, if indicated
- Enhance quality of life, and may also positively influence the course of illness
- Is applicable early in the course of illness, in conjunction with other therapies that are intended to prolong life, such as chemotherapy or radiation therapy, and includes those investigations needed to better understand and manage distressing clinical complications

*Reprinted with permission from WHO Definition of Palliative Care. Available at http://www.who.int/cancer/palliative/definition/en.

Quality practice guidelines

The National Consensus Project (NCP) was formed to meet the need for standardization of palliative care, with a goal to improve palliative care in the United States. The NCP for Quality Palliative Care Consortium mainly consists of 1) the American Academy of Hospice and Palliative Medicine (AAHPM), 2) the Center of Advanced Palliative Care (CAPC), 3) the Hospice and Palliative Nurses Association (HPNA), and 4) the National Hospice and Palliative Care Organization (NHPCO).

In late 2006 the National Quality Forum, a national leader in health care quality, accepted and adopted the clinical practice guidelines for quality palliative care by NCP within the document "A National Framework for Palliative and Hospice Care."

Consensus definition of palliative care*

The NCP defines palliative care as follows[3]: "The goal of palliative care is to prevent and relieve suffering and to support the best possible quality of life for patients and their families, regardless of the stage of the disease or the need for other therapies.

Palliative care is both a philosophy of care and an organized, highly structured system for delivering care. Palliative care expands traditional disease-model medical treatments to include the goals of enhancing quality of life for patient and family, optimizing function, helping with decision making, and providing opportunities for personal growth. As such, it can be delivered concurrently with life-prolonging care or as the main focus of care (Fig. 1.1).

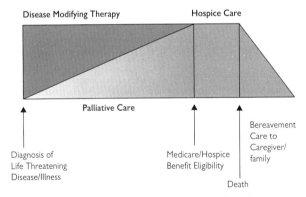

Fig 1.1 Delivery of palliative care during the life-threatening illness disease trajectory. *Source:* National Consensus Project for Quality Palliative Care.

*Reprinted with permission from the *National Consensus Project. Clinical Practice Guidelines for Quality Palliative Care, Second Edition.* 2009, p. 6.

Palliative care is operationalized through effective management of pain and other distressing symptoms, while incorporating psychosocial and spiritual care with consideration of patient and family needs, preferences, values, beliefs, and culture. Evaluation and treatment should be comprehensive and patient-centered with a focus on the central role of the family unit in decision making.

Palliative care affirms life by supporting the patient and family's goals for the future, including their hopes for cure or life-prolongation, as well as their hopes for peace and dignity throughout the course of illness, the dying process, and death. Palliative care aims to guide and assist the patient and family in making decisions that enable them to work toward their goals during whatever time they have remaining.

Comprehensive palliative care services often require the expertise of various providers to adequately assess and treat the complex needs of seriously ill patients and their families. Leadership, collaboration, coordination, and communication are key elements for effective integration of these disciplines and services (NCP, 2004)."[3]

The NCP's key elements of palliative care are described below.*

Patient population

The population served includes patients of all ages experiencing a debilitating chronic or life-threatening illness, condition, or injury.

Patient and family centered care

The uniqueness of each patient and family is respected, and the patient and family constitute the unit of care. The family is defined by the patient or, in the case of minors or those without decision-making capacity, by their surrogates.

In this context, family members may be related or unrelated to the patient; they are individuals who provide support and with whom the patient has a significant relationship.

The care plan is determined by the goals and preferences of the patient and family, with support and guidance in decision-making from the healthcare team.

Timing of palliative care

Palliative care ideally begins at the time of diagnosis of a life-threatening or debilitating condition and continues through cure or until death and into the family's bereavement period.

Comprehensive care

Palliative care employs a multidimensional assessment to identify and relieve suffering through the prevention or alleviation of physical, psychological, social, and spiritual distress.

Care providers should regularly assist patients and their families to understand changes in the patient's condition and the implications of these changes as they relate to ongoing and future care and goals of treatment.

---

* Reprinted with permission from the National Consensus Project (2009). *Clinical Practice Guidelines for Quality Palliative Care, Second edition.* pp. 9–10.

Palliative care requires the regular and formal clinical process of patient-appropriate assessment, diagnosis, planning, interventions, monitoring, and follow-up.

Interdisciplinary team

Palliative care presupposes indications for, and provision of, interdisciplinary team evaluation and treatment in selected cases. The palliative-care team must be skilled in care of the patient population to be served.

Palliative-care teams may be expanded to include a range of professionals based on the services needed. They include a core group of professionals from medicine, nursing, and social work, and may include some combination of volunteer coordinators, bereavement coordinators, chaplains, psychologists, pharmacists, nursing assistants and home attendants, dietitians, speech and language pathologists, physical, occupational, art, play, music, and child-life therapists, case managers, and trained volunteers.

Attention to relief of suffering

The primary goal of palliative care is to prevent and relieve the many and various burdens imposed by diseases and their treatments and consequent suffering, including pain and other symptoms and psychological distress.

Communication skills

Effective communication skills are requisite in palliative care. These include developmentally appropriate and effective sharing of information, active listening, determination of goals and preferences, assistance with medical decision-making, and effective communication with all individuals involved in the care of patients and their families.

Skill in care of the dying and the bereaved

Palliative care specialist teams must be knowledgeable about prognostication, signs and symptoms of imminent death, and the associated care and support needs of patients and their families before and after the death, including age-specific physical and psychological syndromes, opportunities for growth, normal and aberrant grief, and bereavement processes.

Continuity of care across settings

Palliative care is integral to all health-care delivery system settings (hospital, emergency department, nursing home, home care, assisted living facilities, outpatient, and nontraditional environments, such as schools).

The palliative care team collaborates with professional and informal caregivers in each of these settings to ensure coordination, communication, and continuity of palliative care across institutional and home care settings.

Proactive management to prevent crises and unnecessary transfer are important outcomes of palliative care.

Equitable access

Palliative care teams should work toward equitable access to palliative care across all ages and patient populations, all diagnostic categories, all health-care settings, including rural communities, and regardless of race, ethnicity, sexual preference, or ability to pay.

Table 1.1 National Consensus Project's domains of quality palliative care

Domain 1: Structure and processes of care
Domain 2: Physical aspects of care
Domain 3: Psychological and psychiatric aspects of care
Domain 4: Social aspects of care
Domain 5: Spiritual religious existential aspects of care
Domain 6: Cultural aspects of care
Domain 7: Care of imminently dying patient
Domain 8: Ethical and legal aspects of care

Reprinted with permission from the National Consensus Project (2009). *Clinical Practice Guidelines for Quality Palliative Care, Second Edition.* p. 13.

Quality assessment and performance improvement
Palliative care services should be committed to the pursuit of excellence and high quality of care. Determination of quality requires the development, implementation, and maintenance of an effective quality assessment and performance improvement program.

This requires regular and systematic assessment and evaluation of the processes of care and measurement of outcomes using validated instruments for data collection.

The Institute of Medicine has identified six aims for quality health-care delivery. They include the following:
- Timely—delivered to the right patient at the right time
- Patient-centered—based on the goals and preferences of the patient and the family
- Beneficial and/or effective—demonstrably influencing important patient outcomes or processes of care linked to desirable outcomes
- Accessible and equitable—available to all who are in need and who could benefit
- Knowledge- and evidence-based
- Efficient and designed to meet the actual needs of the patient and not wasteful of resources

The NCP has identified eight domains as the framework for specific clinical practice guidelines regarding professional behavior and service delivery (see Table 1.1). Each domain is followed by
1. Specific clinical practice guidelines regarding professional behavior and service delivery
2. Justifications, supporting and clarifying statements, and suggested criteria for assessing whether the identified expectation has been met
3. References that support these recommendations
4. Case examples to illustrate the operationalization of the domains into practice

While most of the key aspects are discussed in Chapter 21 (Spiritual issues in palliative care, p. 233), a more comprehensive resource is available at www.nationalconsensusproject.org.

References

1. O'Neill B, Fallon M (1997). ABC of palliative care: principles of palliative care and pain control. *BMJ* 315:801–804.
2. World Health Organization (n.d.). WHO definition of palliative care. Retrieved November 18, 2009, from http://www.who.int/cancer/palliative/definition/en/
3. National Consensus Project for Quality Palliative Care (NCP) (2009). *Clinical Practice Guidelines for Quality Palliative Care, Second Edition.* Retrieved November 18, 2009, from www.nationalconsensusproject.org

Symptom assessment

Marvin Omar Delgado Guay, MD
Sriram Yennurajalingam, MD

Introduction

Symptom assessment is very important because symptoms directly affect patients' distress level, quality of life (QOL), and survival.[1] Symptoms can be related to the disease itself, its treatment, and comorbid illnesses.[1]

Multiple physical, psychological, and spiritually distressing factors affect QOL, a multidimensional construct with specific emotional, physical, and social aspects[2] (Fig. 2.1).

The early stages of cancer are associated with considerable symptoms. The symptoms and their interference with life increase with increasing cancer stage, possibly reflecting tumor burden and treatment complications.[3] This symptom burden decreases patients' QOL.[2] Symptoms affect but do not necessarily determine patients' QOL.[1]

In clinical practice, patients present with multiple symptoms that require simultaneous assessment and management. Clinicians must have an effective assessment strategy that respects the treatment goals and the patient's wishes.

This chapter describes some of the instruments used to assess symptoms and certain conditions, such as delirium, in patients with advanced cancer who require palliative care.

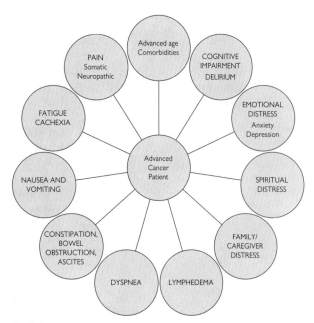

Fig. 2.1 Factors associated with quality of life in patients with advanced cancer.

Symptom assessment

There is no gold standard for assessing symptoms in palliative care patients.[1,4] Assessment tools enable clinicians to identify many more symptoms than those found with simple unstructured evaluations.[4]

Symptom assessment instruments used in the clinical setting include the Edmonton Symptom Assessment Scale (ESAS), the Memorial Symptom Assessment Scale (MSAS), and the Symptom Distress Scale (SDS).

The ESAS is used to assess 10 common symptoms (pain, fatigue, nausea, depression, anxiety, drowsiness, shortness of breath, appetite, feeling of well-being and other symptoms [e.g. sleep disturbances]) and feeling of well-being experienced over the past 24 hours by cancer patients or patients with other chronic illnesses.[5] Using the ESAS, patients rate the intensity of their symptoms on a scale of 0 to 10, with 0 representing "no symptom" and 10 representing the "worst possible symptom" (Fig. 2.2a).

The ESAS, which is widely used in palliative care, is reliable in assessing cancer patients and has internal consistency, criterion validity, and concurrent validity.[5] Patients complete the ESAS in about 5 minutes.[5] Its ease of use and visual representation make the ESAS an effective and practical bedside tool that allows health-care providers to track patients' symptoms over time in terms of intensity, duration, and therapy response[5] (Fig. 2.2b).

With the MSAS, patients rate the frequency, severity, and distress associated with 32 physical and psychological symptoms.[6] Because it takes longer to complete than other assessment tools, the MSAS is mostly used for research purposes.

The short-form version of the MSAS, the MSAS-SF, captures the patient-rated distress associated with 26 physical symptoms and the frequency of 4 psychological symptoms.[7] The condensed MSAS (CMSAS), which provides QOL and survival information that is approximately equivalent to that of the original MSAS, can be completed in 2 to 4 minutes.[8]

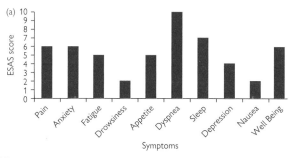

Fig. 2.2a Edmonton Symptom Assessment Scale (ESAS) scores of a patient with advanced cancer and severe dyspnea secondary to lung metastasis and pleural effusion. The patient also had associated moderate pain and anxiety and other physically and emotionally distressing symptoms.

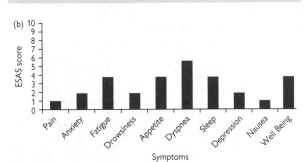

Fig. 2.2b ESAS scores of the same patient 24 hours after assessment and multiple interventions. Note the improvement of the physical and emotional symptoms.

The SDS is an assessment instrument that patients use to rate the intensity, frequency, and level of distress associated with nine physical and two psychological symptoms.[9]

Many larger, more complex symptom assessment tools have been developed for clinical research use. Research instruments may differ from those used in clinical practice.[8] Regardless of the type of scale used, a good symptom assessment precedes effective symptom treatment.

Instruments for the assessment of prognosis and function

Functional status, an independent predictor of survival, must be considered when planning patient care at a hospice, hospital, or home.[10] The most frequently used performance status assessment scales in oncology treatment and research are the Karnofsky Performance Status (KPS) score and the Eastern Co-operative Oncology Group (ECOG) score. Each tool has reliable prognostic value.[4,11]

The Karnofsky Performance Status (KPS) score enables physicians to classify patients according to their functional impairment. This classification can be used to compare the effectiveness of different therapies and to assess prognosis in individual patients. For many patients with serious illnesses, a lower Karnofsky score indicates lower survival.[12] The Palliative Performance Scale (PPS) is a prognostic tool used in palliative care patients, which correlates with KPS. See Chapter 25 (Prognostication in palliative care, p. 299) for details.

The ECOG score measures the intensity with which cancer affects patients' daily living abilities.[13] The ECOG scale ranges from 0 (fully active, no restrictions) to 5 (dead).

Physiotherapists and trained nurses use the Edmonton Functional Assessment Tool to determine functional performance and evaluate other factors that contribute to functional impairment in patients with advanced cancer, such as communication ability, mental status, pain level, and dyspnea intensity.[14]

The Functional Independence Measure can be used in research settings to assess the functional status of patients with advanced cancer.[15] The Functional Independence Measure includes 18 items that are used to evaluate patients' sphincter control, self-care, mobility, locomotion, communication, and social cognition.

Activities of daily living (ADL) scales are used to evaluate patients' level of physical impairment. Specifically, the Katz index of ADL assesses such activities as eating, bathing, dressing, toileting, transfer (e.g., bed to chair) and continence.[4]

The Instrumental Activities of Daily Living (IADL) questionnaire assesses how well patients perform complex life activities, such as light housework, laundry, meal preparation, transportation, grocery shopping, telephone use, medication management, and money management.[4] The IADL questionnaire helps physicians identify cognitive impairment, physical limitations, distressing symptoms, and related clinical problems in patients with advanced cancer.

Assessment of physical symptoms and complications

Pain

Clinicians should comprehensively assess all patients with advanced cancer who present with pain and related symptoms (such as fatigue, depression, sleep disturbance) (Table 2.1). When clinicians take the histories of cancer patients who present with pain, they should ask for the location, characteristics, and intensity of the pain; about any variation in the pain with

Table 2.1 Comprehensive palliative care assessment of advanced cancer patients with pain and other symptoms

Dimension	Assessment tool
History	• Cancer stage • Recent chemotherapy and/or radiotherapy • Vertical, horizontal, and faces self-rated pain scales • Characteristics, intensity, location, and aggravating factors of pain and other symptoms
Performance status	Karnofsky Performance Scale or Eastern Co-operative Oncologic Group Scale scores
Activities of daily living (ADL)	ADL assessment (bathing; dressing and undressing; eating; transferring from bed to chair and back; controlling urinary and fecal discharge; using the toilet; walking)
Instrumental activities of daily living (IADL)	IADL assessment (light housework, preparing meals, taking medications, shopping for groceries or clothes, using the telephone, managing money).
Physical symptoms related to pain (fatigue, anorexia, nausea, dyspnea, insomnia, drowsiness, constipation)	• Edmonton Symptom Assessment System (ESAS) • Abdominal radiography to assess constipation and/or bowel obstruction (consider abdominal computed tomography)
Psychosocial symptoms (anxiety and/or depression)	Anxiety and/or depression (ESAS)
Family/caregiver's distress	Assessment for family/caregiver distress during the interview
Delirium	• Memorial Delirium Assessment Scale (MDAS) • Mini-Mental State Examination (MMSE) • Confusion Assessment Method (CAM)
Spiritual distress	• SPIRITual history • FICA • Identification of spiritual distress during interview
Chemical coping	CAGE questionnaire
Medication history and polypharmacy	
Physical exam	Focused physical examination

change of movement or time of the day; how the pain affects the patients' ADLs; and the possible cause(s) of the pain.[16] Using the ESAS, clinicians can identify several potential underlying symptoms and better understand the causes of the patient's pain.

The CAGE questionnaire can be used to screen patients with advanced illnesses and pain for alcohol abuse.[17] The CAGE questionnaire consists of four questions: 1) Have you ever felt that you should **C**ut down on your drinking; 2) Have you been **A**nnoyed by people criticizing your drinking; 3) Have you ever felt bad or **G**uilty about your drinking; and 4) Have you ever had a drink to get rid of a hangover, i.e., an **E**ye-opener?

A positive score, defined as positive answers to two or more of the four questions, has been shown to have prognostic value in opioid management in cancer patients who experience pain.

The CAGE questionnaire helps physicians identify patients who are at high risk of developing chemical coping, opioid dose escalation, and opioid-induced toxicity. Approximately 20% of cancer patients have a positive CAGE questionnaire result.[17]

Fatigue

Fatigue, a multidimensional syndrome defined as a "decrement in performance of either physical or psychological tasks,"[18] often has multiple contributing causes. Clinicians can assess patients' fatigue by characterizing its severity and temporal features (onset, course, duration, and daily pattern) and by evaluating its exacerbating, contributing, and relieving factors; its effect on patients' daily lives; and its associated distress.[18]

In palliative patients, fatigue and other symptoms such as pain and depression can be assessed with the ESAS as detailed above. Physical and/or psychological symptoms such as pain, depression, and anxiety correlate significantly with fatigue.[19]

In research settings, fatigue can be evaluated with the Functional Assessment of Chronic Illness Therapy–Fatigue (FACIT-F) subscale[20] and the Brief Fatigue Inventory, which has been validated as a measure of fatigue in cancer patients.[21]

Cachexia

Cachexia, a complex metabolic syndrome characterized by a profound loss of lean body mass, occurs in up to 80% of patients with advanced cancer.[18] Clinical assessment for cachexia should include a physical examination and a thorough history that focuses on nutritional issues.

Secondary causes of cachexia, including nausea, vomiting, constipation, ascites, swallowing problems, oral candidiasis, taste alteration, early satiety, and deconditioning, should be investigated.[18] Any loss of appetite (anorexia) expressed by the patient can be assessed with a numerical rating scale such as the ESAS or other symptom evaluation tools. Body weight should also be evaluated.

Measuring the circumference of the patient's mid-upper arm may also have prognostic value.[22] In a research setting, the 12-item Functional Assessment of Anorexia/Cachexia Therapy (FAACT) symptom-specific subscale, in addition to FACIT-F, can be used to measure patients' concerns about their anorexia and/or cachexia during the past 7 days.[21]

Nausea and constipation

Nausea is a subjective symptom, frequently multifactorial. Nausea is commonly accompanied by pain, insomnia, anorexia, fatigue, anxiety, and/or depression. Because these symptoms can contribute to or worsen nausea (thereby increasing distress in patients and their families), physicians should assess patients for all these symptoms.

To record intensity and frequency of nausea, physicians should use a validated tool such as the ESAS not only at the initial evaluation but also at regular intervals to evaluate patients' response to nausea treatment.[4]

Constipation is difficult to assess and treat because of the wide variety of presenting symptoms.[4] Because patients with advanced disease have a greater risk for severe constipation than those with early cancer, physicians should obtain complete clinical histories of patients' bowel habits, including their bowel patterns and stool characteristics.

The Rome Criteria (romecriteria.org) can be used to help assess constipation but do not consider QOL.[4,16]

Abdominal radiography can be used to help assess bowel gas patterns and rule out ileus or bowel obstruction. In addition, an abdominal X-ray film can be divided into four quadrants by drawing an "X" across the film.

Each quadrant is assigned a score of 0 to 3, with 0 indicating no stool in the lumen, 1 indicating stool occupancy of <50%, 2 indicating >50% occupancy, and 3 indicating complete stool occupancy of the lumen. The cumulative "constipation score" can range from 0 to 12. A score of 7 or more indicates severe constipation.[4]

Malignant bowel obstruction

In cases of malignant bowel obstruction, a common and distressing occurrence, particularly in patients with gastrointestinal and/or gynecologic cancer,[23] it is important to carefully assess the patient and the possible causes of the obstruction to ensure that the patient does not require emergent surgery.[23] Computed tomography (CT) can be used to help physicians decide whether a surgical or medical approach would be more effective to relieve bowel obstruction.[23]

Dyspnea

Dyspnea is defined as difficult, labored, or uncomfortable breathing as experienced by the patient.[24] The gold standard for diagnosing dyspnea is the patient's self-report, because dyspnea is a subjective symptom that has multiple potential causes, and the tachypnea and degree of oxygen saturation and other arterial blood gas results might not reflect the distress that dyspnea causes.

Dyspnea can be assessed using numeric, oral, or visual analog scales. Instruments used to assess the intensity of dyspnea include the Support Team Assessment Scale[25] and the ESAS.

However, no single scale can accurately reflect the far-reaching effects of breathlessness on patients and their family or caregivers. Patients with high dyspnea scores have a poorer QOL than patients with low dyspnea scores as assessed by 0–10 severity scale (e.g., ESAS-dyspnea scale).

Delirium

The main features of delirium, a transient and potentially reversible disorder of cognition and attention, are a fluctuating course of acute-onset reduced sensorium, attention deficit, and cognitive or perceptual disturbances.[26] In patients with advanced cancer, delirium causes significant distress and frequently complicates end-of-life care.[26]

Assessment instruments with adequate psychometric properties, such as the Mini-Mental State Examination (MMSE; originally used for the diagnoses of dementia), the Confusion Assessment Method (CAM), and the Memorial Delirium Assessment Scale (MDAS), facilitate the diagnosis of delirium and impose relatively little burden on patients.[27–29]

The MDAS, a validated tool used in palliative care, measures the severity of delirium and therefore captures behavioral manifestations as well as cognitive deficits.[29] The MDAS measures relative impairment in awareness, orientation, short-term memory, digit span, attention capacity, organizational thinking, perceptual disturbance, delusions, psychomotor activity, and sleep–wake cycle. Items on the MDAS are rated from 0 (none) to 3 (severe), with a maximum possible score of 30.

A total MDAS score of 7 yields the highest sensitivity (98%) and specificity (96%) for delirium diagnosis.[29]

Assessment of sleep disturbance

Sleep disturbance (SD) negatively affects QOL.[30] Sleep deprivation, an underreported problem among patients with advanced cancer, heightens physical, psychological, social, and existential suffering; diminishes coping capacity; and exacerbates symptoms such as pain and discomfort by increasing the perceived level of illness severity.[30]

Several tools have been used to evaluate SD in non-cancer settings; however, there is no validated single item screening scale to identify SD in palliative population.

The Pittsburgh Sleep Quality Index (PSQI), which measures sleep quality and patterns, can be used in the research or clinical setting.[31] The PSQI differentiates "poor" from "good" sleep by measuring seven areas: subjective sleep quality, sleep latency, sleep duration, habitual sleep efficiency, sleep disturbances, use of sleeping medication, and daytime dysfunction over the previous month. Patients rate each of these seven areas on a 0 to 3 scale; the maximum combined score is 21.

A combined score of 5 or more indicates a "poor" sleeper (i.e., a patient who experiences sleep disturbance). The PSQI can be used to provide an initial assessment and/or ongoing comparative measurements in all healthcare settings. PSQI has high validity, reliability, and internal consistency.[31]

Assessment of emotional and spiritual distress

Assessment of anxiety and depression

Although mood disorders such as depression and anxiety are among the most prevalent psychiatric illnesses experienced by patients with advanced cancer, mood disorders often remain underdiagnosed and thus undertreated.[32] However, several easy-to-administer self-reporting assessment tools have been created to improve the accuracy of screening for anxiety and depression.[33]

The Hospital Anxiety and Depression Scale (HADS) is a brief, self-administered screening tool used to measure patients' psychological distress.[34] The HADS is sensitive to change, both during the course of disease and in response to medical and psychological interventions. The HADS consists of two subscales comprising 14 items (7 for anxiety and 7 for depression). Patients use a 4-point scale to rate the degree of distress they experienced during the previous week.

The two subscales are then scored separately. A score of 7 or less indicates non-cases of anxiety and/or depression; 8–10 indicates doubtful cases; and 11–21 indicates definite cases. Also, it has been proposed that scores of 14 or 15 or more indicate severe disorders.

The HADS has good reliability and validity in assessing symptom severity, anxiety disorders, and depression in somatic, psychiatric, and primary care patients as well as the general population.[34]

Assessment of spirituality and religiousness

Spirituality and religiousness, which can influence coping strategies and QOL, must be considered when evaluating terminally ill patients. Spiritual pain can occur in patients with chronic or acute pain and with other physical and psychological symptoms. The line between assessment and intervention is blurred.

There is no widely accepted measure of spirituality. Although simply inquiring about patients' religious or spiritual coping may provide the patient with an opening for further exploration and validation, assessment tools can also be used to examine patients' spiritual history, engage patients in dialogue, identify possible areas of concern, and investigate the need for providing resources such as referral to a chaplain or support group.

For example, Puchalski's and Romer's Faith, Importance/Influence, Community, and Address (FICA) assessment tool can be used to evaluate patients' spirituality and religiousness.[35] The FICA questionnaire includes questions that explore each of these areas (e.g., What is your faith? How important is it? Are you part of a religious community? How would you like me as your provider to address these issues in your care?).

Although originally developed to assess primary care patients' spiritual history, the FICA can be used in any patient population. The relative simplicity of the approach has led to its adoption by many clinicians (see Chapter 21 for further details).

Another spirituality assessment tool, the SPIRITual History questionnaire, explores six domains: the patient's **S**piritual belief system, **P**ersonal spirituality, **I**ntegration within a spiritual community, **R**itualized practices and restrictions, **I**mplications for medical care, and **T**erminal events planning.[35] These six domains include 22 items that may all be covered in as little as 10 or 15 minutes or integrated into several interviews.

Assessment of family distress and caregiver burden

The Zarit Burden Interview is the most widely referenced scale in studies of caregiver burden. "Caregiver burden" is an all-encompassing term used to describe the physical, emotional, and financial toll of providing care for patients with advanced illnesses. The Zarit Burden Interview has high internal consistency (Cronbach's A = 0.94).[36]

The Brief Symptom Inventory (BSI), an 18-item self-reported symptom inventory designed to reflect the psychological symptom patterns of psychiatric and medical patients and caregivers, provides an overview of a caregiver's symptoms and their intensity at a specific point in time.[37]

The BSI reports profiles of nine primary symptom dimensions and three global indices of distress. Each item is rated on a 5-point distress scale that ranges from 0 ("not at all") to 4 ("extremely").

The depression and anxiety subscales of the BSI are well established. The approximate completion time for these items is 5 minutes. The internal consistency estimates of these two subscales are 0.85 (depression) and 0.81 (anxiety). Estimates of the construct validity of these subscales also are satisfactory.[37]

Conclusion

Caring for patients with advanced illnesses involves relieving distressing physical, psychosocial, and spiritual problems and empowering patients and their families to retain control while balancing the benefits and risks of treatments.

Recognizing these patients' distressing symptoms as multidimensional complexes and using appropriate and validated assessment tools help physicians manage these symptoms to improve patients' QOL and decrease caregiver burden.

Clinical pearls

- Multiple distressing symptoms directly affect patients' level of distress, QOL, and survival.
- Patients receiving palliative care present with multiple symptoms that require simultaneous assessment of these symptoms and management.
- Patients should be assessed not only for physical symptoms that cause physical distress but also for symptoms that cause emotional and spiritual distress.

References

1. Kirkova J, Davis M, Walsh D. et al. (2006). Cancer symptom assessment instruments: a systematic review. *J ClinOncol* 24:1459–1473.
2. Cleeland C, Reyes-Gibby C (2002). When is it justified" to treat symptoms? Measuring symptom burden. *Oncology* 16:64–70.
3. Corner J, Hopkinson J, Fitzsimmons D, et al. (2005). Is late diagnosis of lung cancer inevitable? Interview study of patients' recollections of symptoms before diagnosis. *Thorax* 60:314–319.
4. Dalal S, Del Fabbro E, Bruera E (2006). Symptom control in palliative care–part 1: oncology as a paradigmatic example. *J Palliat Med* 9:391–408.
5. Bruera E, Kuehn N, Miller M.J, Selmser P, Macmillan K (1991). The Edmonton Symptom Assessment System (ESAS): a simple method for the assessment of palliative care patients. *J Palliat Care* 7:6–9.

6. Portenoy R, Thaler H, Kornblith A, et al. (1994). The Memorial Symptom Assessment Scale: an instrument for the evaluation of symptom prevalence, characteristics and distress. *Eur J Cancer* 30A:1326–1336.
7. Chang V, Hwang S, Feuerman M, Kasimis B, Thaler H (2000). The Memorial Symptom Assessment Scale Short Form (MSAS-SF). Validity and reliability. *Cancer* 89:1163–1171.
8. Chang V, Hwang S, Kasimis B, Thaler H (2004) Shorter symptom assessment instruments: the Condensed Memorial Symptom Assessment Scale (CMSAS). *Cancer Invest* 22:526–536.
9. McCorkle R, Young K (1978). Development of a symptom distress scale. *Cancer Nurs* 1:373–378.
10. Viganó A, Dorgan M, Buckingham J, Bruera E, Suarez-Almazor M (2000). Survival prediction in terminal cancer patients: a systematic review of the medical literature. *Palliat Med* 14:363–374.11. Schag C, Heinrich R, Ganz P (1984). Karnofsky Performance Status revisited: reliability validity and guidelines. *J ClinOncol* 2:187–193.
12. Mor V, Laliberte L, Morris J.N, Wiemann M (1984). The Karnofsky Performance Status Scale. An examination of its reliability and validity in a research setting. *Cancer* 53 (9):2002–2007.
13. Oken MM, Creech RH, Tormey DC, et al. (1982). Toxicity and response criteria of the Eastern Cooperative Oncology Group. *Am J ClinOncol* 5:649–655.
14. Kaasa T, Weesel J (2001). The Edmonton Functional Assessment Tool: further development and validation for use in palliative care. *J Palliat Care* 17:5–11.
15. Marcianiak C, Sliwa J, Spill G, Heinemann A, Semik P (2004). Functional outcome following rehabilitation of the cancer patient. *Arch Phys Med Rehab* 77:54–57.
16. Delgado-Guay MO, Bruera E (2008) Management of pain in the older person with cancer. Part 1. *Oncology* 22:56–61.
17. Bruera E, Moyano J, Seifert L, et al (1995). The frequency of alcoholism among patients with pain due to terminal cancer. *J Pain Symptom Manage* 10:599–603.
18. Yennurajalingam S, Bruera E (2007). Palliative management of fatigue at the close of life "It feels like my body is just worn out". *JAMA* 297:295–304.
19. Del Fabbro E, Dalal S, Bruera E (2006). Symptom control in palliative care—part II: cachexia/anorexia and fatigue. *J Palliat Med* 9:409–421.
20. Cella D (1997). *Manual of the Functional Assessment of Chronic Illness Therapy (FACIT) measurement system.* Center on Outcomes, Research and Education (CORE). Evanston, Northwestern Healthcare and Northwestern education. Version 4, 1997.
21. Mendoza T, Wang X, Cleeland C, et al (1999). The rapid assessment of fatigue severity in cancer patients. *Cancer* 85:1186–1196.
22. Mantovani G, Maccio A, Madeddu C, Massa A (2003). Cancer-related cachexia and oxidative stress: beyond current therapeutic options. *Expert Rev Anticancer Ther* 3:381–392.
23. Ripamonti CI, Eason A, Gerdes H. (2008) Management of malignant bowel obstruction. *Eur J Cancer* 44(8):1105–1115.
24. Del Fabro E, Dalal S, Bruera E (2006). Symptom control in palliative care. Part III. Dyspnea and delirium. *J Palliat Med* 9:422–436.
25. Bausewein C, Farquhar M, Booth S, Gysels M, Higginson I (2007). Measurement of breathlessness in advanced disease: a systematic review. *Respir Med* 101:399–410.
26. Lawlor P, Fainsinger R, Bruera E (2000). Delirium at the end of life. Critical issues in clinical practice and research. *JAMA* 284:2427–2429.
27. Folstein MF, Folstein SE, McHugh PR (1975). Mini-Mental State: a practical method for grading the cognitive state of patients for the clinician. *J Psychiatr Res* 12:189–198.
28. Inouye SK, van Dyck CH, Alessi CA, et al. (1990). Clarifying confusion: the Confusion Assessment Method: a new method for detection of delirium. *Ann Intern Med* 113:941–948.
29. Lawlor P, Nekolaichuk C, Gagnon B, et al. (2000). Clinical utility, factor analysis, and further validation of the Memorial Delirium Assessment Scale in patients with advanced cancer. *Cancer* 88:2859–2867.
30. Fortner B, Stepanski E, Wang S, Kasprowicz S, Durence H (2002). Sleep and quality of life in breast cancer patients. *J Pain Symptom Manage.* 24:471–480.
31. Buysse DJ, Reynolds CF, Monk TH, Berman SR (1989). Pittsburgh Sleep Quality Index: a new instrument for psychiatric practice and research. *Psychiatr Res* 28(2):192–213.
32. Massie MJ (2004). Prevalence of depression in patients with cancer. *J Natl Cancer Inst Monogr,* 32:57–71.
33. Lloyd-Williams M, Dennis M, Taylor F (2004). A prospective study to determine the association between physical symptoms and depression in patients with advanced cancer. *Palliat Med* 18:558–563.

34. Bjelland I, Dahl AA, Haug TT, Neckelmann D (2002). The validity of the Hospital Anxiety and Depression Scale: an updated literature review. *J Psychosom Res* 52:69–77.

35. Puchalski C, Romer A (2000). Taking a spiritual history allows clinicians to understand patients more fully. *J Palliat Med* 3:129–137.

36. Zarit S, Reever K, Bach-Peterson J (1980). Relatives of the impaired elderly: correlates of feelings of burden. *Gerontologist*, 20:649–655.

37. Derogatis LR, Melisaratos N (1983). The Brief Symptom Inventory: an introductory report. *Psychol Med* 13:595–605.

Clinical decision making

Henrique A. Parsons, MD
Eduardo Bruera, MD

Definition

Clinical decision making is the process used by health care providers to make clinical judgments and treatment decisions.[1] The way in which decisions in health care are made has been a field of study for more than 35 years, with an extensive body of knowledge.

Decision making in health care is a process that involves different reasoning processes occurring at the same time, ranging from the most intuitive and informal to the most formal and analytical ones.[2] The art of decision making in medicine lies in the correct balance between formal and informal decision-making strategies.

The aim of health-care decisions in general is to determine which conduct will yield the most favorable outcome in a specific situation. The process of decision making includes two basic phases: (1) determining the possible outcomes for the possible alternative conducts, and (2) analyzing the desirability of each outcome.[3]

Palliative care specificities

In patients receiving palliative care, decisions regarding the introduction of new treatments or withdrawal of already established therapies are almost equally frequent. As with every medical decision, palliative care decisions must reflect the ethical principles of beneficence, nonmaleficence, distributive justice, and patient autonomy.[4]

In particular, patient goals need to be taken into consideration, and that is why they need to be elicited very early in the relationship. For example, discussions regarding advance directives, which can significantly alter the desirability of certain outcomes, must be undertaken as early as possible in the course of life-threatening diseases, irrespective of the proximity of the end of life.

Evidence-based medicine

Defined as "the conscientious, explicit, and judicious use of current best evidence in making decisions about the care of individual patients,"[5] the practice of evidence-based medicine actually means the integration of the clinical expertise with the best available evidence from clinically relevant research conducted using solid methodology. It is not, therefore, the practice of "ivory tower" medicine, with strict and unchangeable guidelines, and it certainly does not exclude one professional's expertise.

The quality of the formal evidence from systematic research can be evaluated by applying a criterion of levels of evidence. A summary of the levels of evidence can be found in Table 3.1.

The recommendation for or against an intervention can also be classified in levels, using the "grades of recommendation" shown in Table 3.2. Interventions with grade of recommendation A have good evidence for recommendation, whereas those with grade D are not really backed up by solid, well-conducted research.

In the process of decision making, benefits, harms, and costs must be identified. An evidence-based approach is fundamental in this first step, in which possible alternative conducts are pondered and the determination of their possible outcomes takes place.

Table 3.1 Summary of the levels of evidence

Level 1

a. Systematic review (SR) of randomized controlled trials (RCTs) with homogeneity*

b. Single RCT with narrow confidence interval

Level 2

a. Systematic review of cohort studies

b. Single cohort studies

c. Low-quality RCTs

d. Outcomes research

Level 3

a. Systematic review of case–control studies

b. Single case–control study

Level 4

a. Case series

b. Poor-quality case–control studies

Level 5

Expert opinion

*Homogeneity = SR free of worrisome variations among the RCT results.

†The Agency for Healthcare Research and Quality defines *outcomes research* as that which "seeks to understand the end results of particular health care practices and interventions." End results might be a change in the ability to function, a change in quality of life, or mortality, for example.[6]

Source: Centre for Evidence Based Medicine (CEBM), Department of Primary Care, University of Oxford (2009). Levels of evidence (March 2009). Available at www.cebm.net.

Table 3.2 Grades of recommendation

Grade	Definition
A	Consistent level 1 studies
B	Consistent level 2 or 3 studies or extrapolations* from level 1 studies
C	Level 4 studies or extrapolations from level 2 or 3 studies
D	Level 5 evidence or troublingly inconsistent or inconclusive studies of any level

* Extrapolations = data used in a situation that has potentially clinically important differences from the original study situation.

Source: Centre for Evidence Based Medicine (CEBM), Department of Primary Care, University of Oxford (2009). Levels of evidence (March 2009). Available at www.cebm.net.

High-quality evidence is not present for every single clinical problem. Different degrees of clinical reasoning almost always have to take place in order to determine the most suitable procedure.

Clinical reasoning

Clinical reasoning is the actual thought process that takes place in medical decision making. It comprises the combined use of evidence-based medicine and other sources of medical information, such as the physician's expertise.

For a description of several models of clinical reasoning, refer to Box 3.1.[7] All clinical reasoning models might be appropriate in different situations.

Box 3.1 Clinical reasoning models

- Hypotheticodeductive—inference based on preliminary findings and modified by subsequent findings
- Algorithmic—diagnostic or therapeutic pathway based on inflexible criteria
- Pattern recognition—combination of salient features determining a diagnosis
- Exaustive—time-consuming indiscriminate accumulation of facts
- Event driven—symptomatic treatment and frequent re-evaluations

Outcome desirability

The second basic step involved in medical decision making is the determination of the desirability of an outcome. This determination has to consider the following:

- The potential benefits vs. the potential harms of a given intervention. Taken into consideration are, for example, side effects, risks, costs, and individual preferences.
- The resource availability. When resources are limited, the size of an intervention's benefit has to be weighed against the costs involved. Sometimes, other interventions with lower cost will bring higher yield.

The five-step approach

Palliative care requires an extensive and structured assessment procedure, and a disciplined decision-making approach is advisable. However, every patient is unique, and the exact same issue might demand completely different management in different patients.

A practical approach[4] for decision making that takes into account the patient's specificities is presented in Table 3.3 and will be further described in the sections that follow.

Step 1: Issue identification and exploration

Patients present to palliative care with a multitude of issues that can in turn trigger new problems. For example, an infection might trigger or worsen nausea, delirium, pain, and other problems, or the presence of hypercalcemia might cause vomiting, sedation, and delirium.

The first step is tightly related with the need for structured clinical assessment in palliative care. The accurate determination of the issues that affect the patient precedes the identification of the effects of each of these issues on the patient's quality of life.

Several examples are identified in Table 3.4.

Table 3.3 The 5-step approach

Step	Activities
1	Identify issues and their effects on the patient.
2	Rank the degree of discomfort of each specific issue.
3	Identify potential problems associated with the intervention.
4	Balance the overall pros and cons of the intervention vs. no intervention.
5	Discuss care plan with the patient, family, and care team.

Table 3.4 Some examples of common palliative care situations

Issue	Potentially related problems and side effects
Infection	Pain, nausea, delirium, convulsions
Anemia	Fatigue, chest pain, shortness of breath, palpitations
Dehydration	Delirium, myoclonus, hallucinations, fatigue
Renal failure	Delirium, nausea, vomiting, fatigue, edema
Lymphedema	Pain, heaviness, inability to move
Constipation	Pain, nausea, vomiting, anorexia
Hypercalcemia	Sedation, confusion, delirium, nausea, vomiting
Pathological fracture	Inability to move, pain, thrombosis/embolism, respiratory infections due to being immobile

Step 2: Determination of the patient's discomfort

After identification of the issues that affect the patient, the patient's discomfort associated with each specific problem must be identified. This is especially important, because as the disease progresses, the impact of each symptom or problem on the patient's quality of life can change.

For example, if nausea caused extreme discomfort for a patient in the earlier stages of a cancer treatment, the same symptom might not generate the same discomfort in the presence of severe pain in the more advanced stages of the disease.

Step 3: Identification of problems associated with the treatment

Once issues to be tackled are indentified and ranked, it is fundamental to also identify all potential problems associated with the correction of the issue. Sometimes the side effects of the correction of a problem are more bothersome to a given patient than the problem itself.

Some examples are found in Box 3.2.

Box 3.2 Examples of situations in which treatment might be especially bothersome

- Hospital admission
- Intensive care unit (ICU) transfer
- Surgery risks and discomfort
- Inconvenience of multiple radiation sessions
- Side effects of chemotherapy
- Discomfort of maintaining an intravenous (IV) line
- Hassle involved with hospital in repetitive and long visits for dialysis

Step 4: Risk–benefit analysis

Once the issues affecting the patient, their potential side effects, their importance and rank according to the effect on the patient's quality of life, and the side effects of treatment are identified, the palliative care provider must undertake a risk–benefit analysis, weighting all the pros and cons of specific measures (Box 3.3).

Box 3.3 Important questions to be answered in the process of decision making

- What is the clinical problem?
- To what extent does the problem affect the patient?
- What are the patient's wishes and preferences?
- What are the potential effects of the problem correction (desired and undesired)?
- What will be the effect of withholding the problem correction?
- Is this decision supported by the best evidence available?
- Was the decision discussed with the patient and family? Do they understand and agree with the decision?
- What are the alternatives?

Step 5: Consensus

The course of action must be discussed with the patient (whenever possible), family, and the team in order to develop a consensus. Depending on the severity of the issues and the complexity of the relationships, family meetings or several encounters might be needed to ensure complete understanding and to reach consensus.

Flexibility on the side of the care team is needed; as conversations with the patient and family evolve, some of the previous steps may need to be re-evaluated.

Clinical pearls

- In palliative care, decision making regarding introduction of new treatments can be as frequent and important as withdrawal of current treatments.
- Always have in mind the ethical principles: beneficence, nonmaleficence, distributive justice, and autonomy.
- The practice of evidence-based medicine involves the integration of clinical expertise with the best available evidence from clinically relevant research.
- A structured approach for decision making in palliative care includes identification of issues, ranking of types of discomfort, determination of potential side effects, balance between intervention and non-intervention, and discussion with the patient, family, and team.

References

1. Encyclopædia Britannica (2009). Clinical decision making. Retrieved February 10, 2009, from http://www.britannica.com/EBchecked/topic/121745/clinical-decision-making
2. Croskerry, P (2005). The theory and practice of clinical decision-making. *Can J Anesth* 52(6):8.
3. Eddy DM (1990). Clinical decision making: from theory to practice. Anatomy of a decision. *JAMA* 263(3):441–443.
4. Driver LC, Bruera E (2000), Decision-making. In *The M. D. Anderson Palliative Care Handbook*, Houston, TX: University of Texas Health Science Printing, pp. 5–8.
5. Sackett DL, Rosenberg WM, Gray JA, Haynes RB, Richardson WS (1996). Evidence-based medicine: what it is and what it isn't. *BMJ* 312(7023):71–72.
6. Agency for Healthcare Research and Quality (2000). Outcomes research fact sheet. Available from: http://www.ahrq.gov/clinic/outfact.htm
7. Sandhu H, Carpenter C, Freeman K, Nabors SG, Olson A (2006). Clinical decision making: opening the black box of cognitive reasoning. *Ann Emerg Med* 48(6):713–719.

Chapter 4

Pain assessment and management

Gabriel Lopez, MD
Suresh K. Reddy, MD

Introduction

Pain is one of the main symptoms experienced by cancer patients, during both curative and palliative therapy, and often triggers the patient's initial medical evaluation prior to the diagnosis of malignancy. Numerous national and international surveys have found that 30% to 50% of cancer patients in active therapy and as many as 60% to 90% with advanced disease have pain.[1-5]

Pain, however, is undertreated. The reasons are many and include physician's lack of knowledge, lack of availability of opioid medication, governmental regulations, physicians' fear of regulations, diversion of medication, and fear of addiction.[6,7]

Malignant diseases, whether solid tumors such as lung or colon cancer or liquid tumors such as leukemias, can lead to pain symptoms. The pain may be due to the tumor itself, either by direct involvement (e.g., of the bone, nerves, or viscera) or by indirect effects (e.g., tumor release of inflammatory mediators), or to treatments aimed at cure or palliation (see Box 4.1). Pain associated with direct tumor involvement occurs in 65% to 85% of patients with advanced cancer.[1]

Cancer therapy accounts for pain in approximately 15% to 25% of patients receiving chemotherapy, surgery, or radiation therapy.[8] Pain syndromes commonly observed in the non-cancer population are present in 10–15% of cancer patients—for example, lower back pain secondary to degenerative disc disease.

Effective pain management involves an interdisciplinary approach using multimodal techniques, the goal being to relieve the patient's suffering. Precise assessment of pain and associated factors is crucial, as the objective of treatment is to treat the cause whenever possible.

In this chapter, the authors discuss the most practical aspects of pain management in patients receiving palliative care. While the focus here is on pain management in patients with cancer because cancer-related pain is common and often severe, the same principles of pain management apply to patients receiving palliative care for a variety of diseases.

Box 4.1 Causes of pain in cancer

- Related to direct tumor involvement: 60–65%
- Related to cancer treatment: 20–25%
- Unrelated to cancer: 10–15%

Definition

Cancer pain is pain as a result of cancer or its therapy. Pain is subjective and varies in expression from person to person, and these individual differences must be considered when developing a plan of symptom management (see Fig. 4.1).

A useful method of treating pain is to not only respond to the patient's current symptom constellation but also anticipate the patient's symptom-control needs based on the specific cancer diagnosis and sites of tumor involvement.

The participation of a palliative care specialist or team at a cancer center is vital to the successful management of cancer pain.

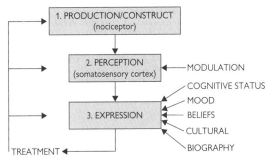

Fig. 4.1 Steps involved in the expression of pain in cancer patients. Numerous factors are believed to contribute to the overall expression of pain. Many of those factors are known and summarized in this figure. The bright gray lines indicate the factors that diminish pain intensity. Adapted from Bruera E, Kim HN (2003). Cancer pain. *JAMA* 290(18):2476–2479.

Mechanisms of pain and pathophysiology

The pathophysiological classification of pain forms the basis for therapeutic choices. Pain states may be broadly divided into those associated with ongoing tissue damage *(nociceptive)* and those resulting from nervous system dysfunction *(neuropathic)*, the latter of which may or may not be accompanied by tissue damage (see Boxes 4.2 and 4.3).

Nociceptive pain can be of the somatic or visceral type. *Somatic pain* results from the activation of nociceptors in cutaneous and deep tissues; it is described as well-localized aching, throbbing, and gnawing.

Visceral pain is caused by the activation of nociceptors resulting from distension, stretching, and inflammation of visceral organs; it is described as poorly localized deep aching, cramping, and pressure. Visceral pain may be referred—for example, pancreatic cancer pain in the abdomen with referral to the back.

Breakthrough pain is common in cancer patients and is defined as a "transitory exacerbation of pain that occurs on a background of otherwise stable persistent pain."[9] Breakthrough pain may be caused by activity or end-of-dose failure; it can also occur spontaneously.

It tends to be moderate to severe and, according to one study, lasts less than 3 minutes in 43% of pain cases. The typical frequency is 1 to 4 episodes per day. Breakthrough pain tends to be prognostic of poor response to pain treatment.[10]

In many cases, the etiology of cancer pain is multifactorial. Pain may be nociceptive in origin and related to direct tumor invasion of bone and soft tissue or related to perineural involvement, benign inflammation, or superimposed infection.

Pain may also be neuropathic in origin and secondary to peripheral or cranial nerve involvement or related to the sequelae of surgery or radiation therapy.

Clinical pearls

- Pain can be nociceptive (visceral or somatic) or neuropathic.
- Somatic nociceptive pain is localized throbbing, gnawing; visceral pain is poorly localized cramping or pressure and is associated with autonomic symptoms.

Box 4.2 Types of pain

Nociceptive
- Somatic: Sharp, localized, aching, throbbing, gnawing, e.g., pain in muscle, bone, soft tissues
- Visceral: Dull, poorly-localized, crampy, nauseous, squeezy, pressure, e.g., pain in the pancreas, liver, small bowel

Neuropathic
- Burning, tingling, shooting, stabbing, itching, electric-like, numb, e.g., peripheral neuropathy, plexopathy from tumors, postherpetic neuralgia

Box 4.3 Cancer pain syndromes

Acute
- Due to cancer or related disorders
- Due to diagnostic interventions
- Due to anticancer therapy

Chronic
Nociceptive somatic
- Bone pain
- Soft tissue
- Muscle
- Pleural pain
- Paraneoplastic syndromes

Nociceptive visceral
- Hepatic distension syndrome
- Midline retroperitoneal syndrome
- Chronic intestinal obstruction
- Peritoneal carcinomatosis
- Malignant perineal syndrome
- Adrenal pain syndrome
- Ureteric obstruction syndrome

Neuropathic
- Leptomeningeal metastases
- Painful cranial neuralgias (e.g., glossopharyngeal neuralgia)
- Painful radiculopathy
- Painful peripheral mononeuropathies
- Paraneoplastic peripheral neuropathy

- Neuropathic pain is described as numb, shooting, or electric-like.
- More than two types of pain occur commonly in cancer.
- Breakthrough pain can occur spontaneously or be caused by activity or end-of-dose failure.
- Cancer pain is multifactorial, requiring an interdisciplinary approach to treatment.
- A cancer pain syndrome includes acute or chronic pain or both.
- Acute pain may be due to procedures, cancer therapy, or pre-existing medical conditions.
- Chronic pain may be neuropathic, nociceptive somatic, or nociceptive visceral.
- Precise assessment of the type and cause of pain is the cornerstone of optimal pain treatment.
- Cancers have specific well-defined pain syndromes but patients may also present with pain that is not related to the cancer. One must differentiate between the two types of pain.

Assessment of pain

Intensity of pain assessment

It is crucial to assess and monitor the intensity of pain. Pain intensity can be measured by using simple visual analog, verbal, or numerical scales or more complex pain questionnaires[11] (see Box 4.4).

Most instruments and techniques are very reliable for assessing the intensity of pain. The assessment can be made more effective by a graphic ongoing display of pain and other symptoms in the patient's chart, along with other vital-sign monitoring. This establishes a baseline against which outcomes can be measured and helps the physician effectively administer appropriate care.

Current institutional pain management guidelines were established by the Joint Commission on Accreditation of Health Care Organizations (JCAHO) in 2000. On a 0 to 10 scale, mild pain can be defined as 0–3, moderate pain as 4–7, and severe pain as 8–10.

Pain assessment should always be done in the context of other cancer symptoms. In patients with a complex and evolving cancer history, visual representations of the patient's tumor sites and treatment can aid the physician in developing a tailored pain management strategy.

The Edmonton Labeled Visual Information System (ELVIS), validated in a randomized trial as a rapid and effective pictorial memorization tool, can prove useful to this end.[12]

Psychosocial assessment

Pain as a symptom cannot be adequately evaluated in isolation from a patient's total symptom burden. The Edmonton Symptom Assessment System (ESAS) is a validated and effective tool used for identifying symptoms commonly experienced by cancer patients.[11]

Box 4.4 Pain assessment tools

Behavioral
- CAGE: **C**ut down, **A**nnoyed, **G**uilty, **E**ye opener

Pain
- Brief Pain Inventory Short Form (SF) and Long Form (LF)
- Pain thermometer
- Wong–Baker FACES pain rating scale

Psychosocial
- Edmonton Symptom Assessment System (ESAS)
- Memorial Symptom Assessment Scale (MSAS) and MSAS–Short Form (MSAS-SF)

Cognitive
- Folstein Minimental Status Exam (MMSE)
- Memorial Delirium Assessment Scale (MDAS)

Assessment of a pain complaint is not valid unless a thorough psychosocial assessment is done. The clinician should evaluate psychosocial factors such as anxiety, depression, loss of independence, family challenges, financial difficulties, social isolation, and fear of death.

Cancer patients more often meet the diagnostic criteria for adjustment disorder with anxiety and depressed mood than the criteria for major depressive disorder.[13]

The effect of pain and other symptoms on functional status must be understood to establish treatment goals. Pain, when evaluated in conjunction with other distressing psychosocial symptoms, leads to the calculation of "total pain" or "suffering."

Clinical pearls

- Comprehensive assessment is vital for good symptom management (see Box 4.5).
- Prognostic factors and performance status need to be assessed.
- Delirium will complicate pain assessment and management. Beware of misinterpreting delirium as pain.
- Validated instruments are invaluable for measuring pain severity.
- Pain assessment must be done in the context of other symptoms contributing to the illness experience.
- Psychosocial factors affect pain reporting and expression.

Box 4.5 General pain management principles

- Respect and accept the complaint of pain as real.
- Treat pain appropriately.
- Treat underlying disorder(s).
- Address psychosocial issues.
- Use a multidisciplinary approach.

Pharmacotherapy

Management of cancer pain has made significant progress in recent years, partly because of Agency for Health Care Policy and Research (AHCPR) guidelines,[14] but mostly because of an international movement to optimize symptom management in the chronically ill and dying.

Cancer pain in particular can present a challenge, necessitating accurate diagnosis and appropriate intervention. Pharmacotherapy with analgesics remains the mainstay of treating cancer pain.

Most cancer pain syndromes present with moderate to severe pain and are associated with several comorbidities, requiring a multidisciplinary approach for optimal management.

The analgesics used to manage cancer-related pain can be divided into three categories:

- Non-opioid medications such as acetaminophen and nonsteroidal anti-inflammatory drugs (NSAIDs)
- Weak opioid medications such as codeine or strong opioids such as morphine
- Adjuvant medications such as tricyclic antidepressants (TCAs) and anti-epileptic drugs (AEDs)

WHO analgesic ladder

In 1984, the World Health Organization (WHO) proposed a simple analgesic "ladder" for the pharmacological management of cancer-related pain[15] (see Fig. 4.2). Experience applying this ladder in several countries has shown that the simple principle of escalating from nonopioid to strong opioid analgesics is safe and effective.

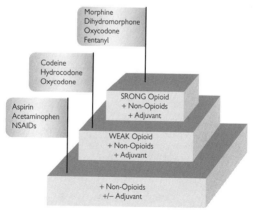

Fig. 4.2 The WHO pain ladder. Adapted by Yennurajalingam S, et al. (2005). Pain and terminal delirium research in the elderly. *Clin Geriatr Med* 21(1):93–119. Reprinted with permission from Elsevier.

Step 1

The first step of the analgesic ladder is to use a nonopioid analgesic, e.g., acetaminophen or an NSAID. Adjuvant drugs can be added to enhance analgesic efficacy, treat concurrent symptoms that exacerbate pain, and provide independent analgesic activity for specific types of pain. Adjuvant medications, such as TCAs, may be used at any step.

- Identify pain syndrome: identify
- Pain intensity: mild (0 to 3)
- Medications: acetaminophen, anti-inflammatory agents, TCAs, or AEDs
- Response: somatic and neuropathic pain syndromes respond mildly.

Step 2

If pain persists despite step 1 medications, then a mild low-potency opioid such as codeine should be added (not substituted). The pain syndrome is any or specific.

- Pain syndrome: identify
- Pain intensity: moderate (4–7)
- Medications: mild opioids, NSAIDs, TCAs, or AEDs
- Response: varies

Step 3

If the pain persists despite step 2 efforts, then strong (high-potency) opioids such as morphine are initiated in step 3. The dose of the stronger opioid can be titrated upward according to the patient's pain, as there is no ceiling dose for morphine.

Medications for persistent or continuous pain require an around-the-clock prescription, with an extra dose available in case the patient experiences breakthrough pain.

- Pain syndrome: identify
- Pain intensity: moderate to severe, 7–10/10
- Medications: strong opioid (morphine class), plus NSAIDs, AEDs, TCAs, or other agents
- Response: good, 80–90%

Opioids

Opioid medications form the basis for the management of cancer-related pain regardless of its pathophysiology. They are pharmacodynamically classified into pure agonists, mixed agonist–antagonists, and antagonists.

In clinical practice, only pure agonists are used. Mixed agonist-antagonists are not used because they exhibit a ceiling effect, at which point the benefit from agonist action on analgesia equals the side effects from antagonism, including the potential to precipitate symptoms of withdrawal.

Of the three classical opioid receptor types, mu, delta, and kappa, the mu receptor is most clinically relevant.

Low-potency (mild) opioids

The list of mild or low-potency opioids includes codeine, propoxyphene, hydrocodone, and dihydrocodeine, which have a potency of between one-tenth and one-fourth that of morphine sulfate.

Box 4.6 WHO approach to drug therapy of cancer pain

Five essential concepts

- *By the mouth:* The oral route is preferred for simplicity in management of nociceptive and neuropathic pain.
- *By the clock:* If the pain is persistent, then around-the-clock (atc) medication should be used, in addition to as-needed (prn) doses.
- *By the ladder:* This implies moving to the next step rather than sideways. (A next-step move would be from a nonopioid to an opioid; a sideways move would be from opioid to opioid, i.e., morphine to oxycodone.)
- *For the individual:* The dose varies from individual to individual. Hence, the right dose is the one that relieves pain without causing side effects.
- *With attention to detail:* Other factors (e.g., psychosocial distress, spiritual concerns) need to be assessed and dealt with in addition to pharmacotherapy, thereby treating total pain.

Indications for drugs from this group include mild to moderate pain not responsive to nonopioids. Examples include mild bone pain and early visceral pain.

These agents are also occasionally used for breakthrough pain in patients with constant pain who are receiving sustained-release opioids. This group of drugs is commonly formulated with acetaminophen, limiting dose escalation to the maximum allowable dose of acetaminophen. Formulations without acetaminophen can be prepared by some pharmacies.

Codeine

Codeine is commonly prescribed for both its analgesic properties and antitussive effect. It can be one of the most constipating of all drugs and is sometimes used to control diarrhea in opioid-tolerant cancer patients.

Codeine, with a plasma half-life of 2–3 hours, is metabolized by the liver to its active metabolite, morphine. Approximately 10% of the Caucasian population has mutations in the hepatic enzyme CYP2D6 and therefore cannot convert codeine to morphine, resulting in poor analgesic efficacy.

Tramadol

Codeine's synthetic analogue, tramadol, is not widely used in the treatment of cancer pain. It is a weak mu-receptor agonist most effective for the treatment of mild to moderate pain states.

With activity via blockade of presynaptic reuptake of serotonin and norepinephrine, there is evidence that it works in neuropathic pain states.[16] It is an effective step 2 medication in the appropriate clinical scenario.

Propoxyphene

Propoxyphene is a centrally acting narcotic analgesic agent with actions on opioid and *N*-methyl-D-aspartate (NMDA) receptors.

Dextropropoxyphene, a methadone derivative, has a duration of action of less than 4 hours, much shorter than that of its parent compound. It is available as a single agent or in combination with acetaminophen. It is metabolized by cytochrome CYP3A4 to its active metabolite, norpropoxyphene. The observed NMDA antagonistic activity makes it an attractive drug for use in neuropathic pain syndromes in cancer.

Limitations of propoxyphene use include norpropoxyphene accumulation in patients with renal insufficiency, leading to central nervous system side effects.

Caution must be exercised with its use in the elderly because of risk of precipitating confusion and delirium. Norpropoxyphene may also result in cardiac toxicity, with QRS interval prolongation on EKG proportional to dose.[17]*

No clear guidelines for its use in cancer pain have been established, pending much-needed evidence-based research.

Hydrocodone
Hydrocodone is currently the most widely used opioid in the United States and is commercially available in different concentrations. Oral formulations that include either acetaminophen or ibuprofen as a co-analgesic are available.

Hydrocodone is a mu-receptor agonist, with a half-life of 2–3 hours, perhaps acting through conversion to hydromorphone.

High-potency (strong) opioids
This class of drugs is used for all pain types and includes oxycodone, hydromorphone, meperidine, fentanyl, and methadone.

Morphine
Morphine is the most widely used and prototype drug of its class. It is a gold-standard drug available in all countries and is valued for its low cost, ease of use, and analgesic potency. It is converted to morphine-3-glucuronide and mophine-6-glucuronide (M3G and M6G, respectively) by UDP-glucuronyl transferase in the liver, acting on the mu receptor in the central nervous system.

Caution should be exercised when using morphine in patients with renal impairment, as these compounds are excreted by the kidney. Only M6G has been implicated in opioid activity and side effects (e.g., sedation) in animal studies. M3G has a very low affinity for opioid receptors and is largely ineffective as an analgesic. M3G may be responsible for morphine's observed neuroexcitatory toxicities.[18]

Morphine's duration of action is 2–4 hours; however, the sustained-release form can be administered as infrequently as every 8 to 12 hours. Morphine is available for oral, rectal, intramuscular (IM), intravenous (IV), and sublingual use as well as in epidural and intrathecal preparations.

Oxycodone
Once classified as a low-potency opioid when its dosage was limited by combination with acetaminophen or aspirin, oxycodone is now available as a stand-alone preparation. With a sustained-release as well as an immediate-release form, it has gained widespread popularity in the treatment of cancer pain.

---

* Due to the side effect profile, recently propoxyphene has been removed from market by the FDA.

Oxycodone is considered equipotent to, if not more potent than, morphine. It is available only in the oral form in the United States and has a higher oral bioavailability than that of morphine.

Oxymorphone

Oxymorphone (oxymorphone hydrochloride, or 14-hydroxydihydromorphinone) is a semisynthetic mu-opioid receptor agonist available in immediate- and extended-release formulations.[19] It is considered a more potent opioid than its parent compound, morphine.

Hydromorphone

Hydromorphone is a useful, short-acting opioid, 6–7 times more potent than morphine. It is available for administration via all routes, including neuraxial.

Hydromorphone is commonly used as a "rescue" agent in patients receiving longer-acting opioid preparations, since a sustained-release form is not commercially available in the United States. Long-acting formulations of hydromorphone available in Europe and North America have received favorable reviews.[20]

Meperidine

Meperidine is commonly used throughout the world as an opioid analgesic, although it is not used as often as morphine. It is predominantly a mu-opioid receptor agonist, available in oral and IV formulations. It undergoes hepatic metabolism to normeperidine and is excreted renally.

In the oral form, its potency is one-tenth that of morphine, which makes it less efficacious in most patients. Increased doses required to achieve morphine-equianalgesic levels are associated with the risk of normeperidine accumulation.

With the potential for increased central nervous system excitability and convulsions, it should be used with extreme caution in renally impaired and elderly patients.

Fentanyl

Fentanyl is a semisynthetic opioid available in parenteral, transdermal, and oral preparations. The prototype of a semisynthetic opioid, it is the only drug of this class available in parenteral form. Its rapid onset and relatively short duration of action make it a good choice for control of acute pain and for use in patient-controlled analgesia (PCA) pumps.

Unlike other opioids, a sustained-release form (transdermal) was developed long before its breakthrough nonparenteral counterpart, oral transmucosal fentanyl.[21–23] The sustained-release, transdermal form has been used successfully for stable pain.

Once applied, it forms a depot under the skin and is slowly released into the circulation. This limits its use in emergency situations, though, since it takes up to 18 hours to reach peak.[24] Each patch is changed every 72 hours, which is convenient in patients whose pain is stable. Its use is difficult, however, in patients requiring frequent dose titration.

Oral transmucosal fentanyl has been approved for use in cancer patients with breakthrough pain, based on its rapid absorption via the oral mucosa.[25]

A new oral preparation uses a novel effervescent drug delivery shown to enhance absorption across the buccal mucosa.[26]

Sufentanil

This synthetic derivative of fentanyl is 5–10 times more potent than fentanyl itself. Its use has been mostly limited to anesthetic purposes.

As clinical familiarity increases and more routes of administration become available (only an injectable form is available now), it is expected that the use of sufentanil will increase in patients with cancer pain, especially those who are highly tolerant to opioids. It has shown good results when used intravenously in PCAs and in subcutaneous (SC) infusions in the context of palliative care.[27]

According to one report, it can be used successfully for breakthrough pain when applied sublingually.[28] Neuraxial application of sufentanil is an option in select patients.

Methadone

Because of its low cost and well-understood pharmacological properties, methadone is now accepted as a second-line opioid for the treatment of cancer-related pain.

Methadone is tightly bound to α-1-acid-glycoprotein, shows high lipid solubility, and given its significant tissue distribution, sustains a steady level in plasma during chronic treatment. No active metabolites are currently known.

It is generally available as a racemic mixture containing both D and L isomers. Levo-methadone, with twice the potency of the racemic form, is available in some countries.

The frequently observed interindividual variation in methadone pharmacokinetics has been attributed to differences in metabolism by the cytochrome P450 hepatic enzyme family. At least four heterologously expressed P450 proteins have been shown to catalyze the N-demethylation of methadone, for which the P450 3A4 type appears to be the main enzyme.

Caution should be observed with the coadministration of other drugs that interact with the cytochrome P450 system. Cytochrome P450 inhibitors include certain antibiotics, antifungals, antivirals, and antidepressants. Induction of the P450 system may be caused by anticonvulsants, rifampin, and corticosteroids.

Despite a wide range in interindividual pharmacokinetic variations of methadone, there are two phases identified: a rapid and extensive distribution phase (half-life of 2–3 hours) followed by a slow elimination phase (half-life of 15–60 hours). This extended elimination phase is of particular clinical importance since it can result in accumulation and toxicity. Adverse effects include sedation, nausea, and respiratory depression.

One limitation with the use of methadone is how it is viewed by society. Methadone is stigmatized because of its traditional use in the management of opioid addiction. It was termed a "killer drug" by the *New York Times* because of an increase in use by recreational drug users and the associated rise in overdoses and subsequent deaths.[29]

Despite its questionable reputation, methadone has many advantages in palliative care. It can be administered orally, rectally, and intravenously and

Table 4.1 Method of rotation to methadone

	Morphine	Methadone dose*
Day 1–Day 3	Reduce the dose of morphine over the period of 3 days[†]	Increase the dose of methadone over the period of 3 days[†]
		4:1 morphine < 90 mg/day
		8:1 morphine 90–300 mg/day
		12:1 morphine> 300 mg/day
		Rescue [breakthrough] dose: one sixth of daily dose up to 3 allowed per day

*Methadone dose divided and administered every 8 hours. Ratio given is for morphine:methadone ratio.
Reprinted from Bruera E, Sweeney C (2002). Methadone use in cancer patients with pain: a review. *J Palliat Med* 5(1):127–138.
[†]Consider 50% on Day one, 30% on Day 2 and 20% on Day 3

is an effective alternative to morphine, hydromorphone, and fentanyl for treating cancer-related pain.

Finally, methadone is inexpensive and thus may be of particular interest for developing countries. It is also considered to be an NMDA receptor antagonist and may have a role in the management of opioid-resistant and neuropathic pain.

Methadone currently has two main indications in palliative care: (1) treatment of patients with opioid resistance and neuropathic pain and (2) as a second-line agent in opioid rotation.

An optimal conversion method, rotating commonly used opioids to methadone and vice versa, has not yet been established.

Patients usually benefit from rotations from a previous opioid to methadone over 3 days, progressively reducing the dose of the previous opioid and increasing the dose of methadone (PO doses). The usual ratio from methadone to morphine is 4:1 in patient's requiring < 90mg/day of morphine; 8:1 the ratio is 90-300mg/day, and 12:1 when the dose is > 300mg/day. See table 4.1.

This method was used in a prospective, multicenter study of 108 patients.[30] Although the multicenter study dealt mainly with the rotation from morphine to methadone, identical approaches have been used for rotation of other opioids to methadone.

Studies examining the frequency of administration, including every 8, 12, and 24 hours, have had different results. One prospective study rotated 52 patients receiving oral morphine to oral methadone every 8 hours using different dose ratios. Patients were switched because of poor analgesia or adverse effects related to morphine. Switching to methadone was considered effective in 42 (80%) of the patients. The average period after which results were achieved was 3.65 days.

Future prospective studies are needed to explore equianalgesic conversion ratios for rotation from opioids to methadone and vice versa, including the influence of methadone on neuropathic pain and fast-developing tolerance induced by other opioids.

Bruera et al. proposed the following considerations for the future development of equianalgesic tables:[31] first, methadone appears to be more potent than previously accepted; second, conversion ratios relative to methadone depend on the dose of the previously used opioid. Also, conversion ratios falter at extremes of doses.

In addition to an equianalgesic conversion factor, strong emphasis should be placed on the physician's clinical experience, the patient's clinical condition, the use of other interacting drugs, and use of other simultaneous interventions for pain relief, which may include radiation, surgery, chemotherapy, or a combination thereof, as well as the use of other analgesics.

After the administration of methadone, its side effects, in particular sedation and impaired cognition, should be monitored carefully. Monitoring should be continued for several days after successful rotation to another opioid because of potential accumulation of the drug and late toxicity.

For further details on pharmacological properties and the use of methadone in cancer patients, we refer the reader to some of the recent extensive reviews of methadone and international guidelines.[32–34]

Methadone's tendency to prolong the QTc interval, increasing the risk for conversion to torsades de pointes, has led to a black-box warning.[35]

Studies have shown a QTc increase between 9.5 ms and 20 ms on initiation of methadone therapy. This is of particular concern in patients with a history of cardiac conduction abnormalities, patients with a prolonged QTc (> 450 ms) at baseline, or patients receiving other commonly used medications that are cytochrome p450 inhibitors or known to prolong the QTc.

A recent study did not show QTc prolongation in patients given methadone in a palliative care setting.[36] Routine EKG screening of all patients in a palliative care setting may not be necessary; however, if circumstances permit, a routine EKG screening prior to initiation of methadone therapy is recommended.

Levorphanol

Levorphanol, a morphinian derivative, is available in oral, IV, and SC forms. It exerts its effects via mu, delta, and kappa opioid receptors; by inhibition of norepinephrine and serotonin uptake; and by NMDA receptor antagonism.[37]

Levorphanol is glucuronidated in the liver with its glucuronidated products renally excreted. Levorphanol's half-life of approximately 12–16 hours must be considered in patients with hepatic or renal dysfunction.

Clinical pearls

- Most pain can be satisfactorily controlled using relatively simple medication regimens.
- Personalized treatment goals should be discussed with patients and their families.
- The WHO ladder concept of escalating from nonopioid to strong opioid analgesics is safe and effective.
- Analgesics include nonopioids and opioids.
- Pure opioid formulations are preferred to combinations with low-potency analgesics, i.e., acetaminophen with oxycodone.

- Opioid medications form the basis of the management of cancer pain, regardless of the pathophysiology of the pain.
- Mu-opioid receptors are the most clinically relevant of the three classical opioid receptor types (mu, delta, and kappa).
- The pain regimen should be tailored to the type and intensity of pain.
- The clinician should schedule atc and adequate breakthrough dosing.
- Appropriate adjuvant analgesics should be considered.
- Antiemetics and laxatives should be prescribed proactively.
- Familiarization with opioid conversion principles is critical.
- Clinicians must recognize the signs and symptoms of opioid-induced delirium and overdose.
- Clinicians must use caution in prescribing benzodiazepines for anxiety-induced pain.
- Clinicians must identify and anticipate the potential for drug interactions and polypharmacy.
- Nonpharmacological approaches, i.e., anesthetic and neurosurgical procedures, should be considered where appropriate.
- Balanced analgesia is the key to good cancer pain management.
- Clinicians must be able to differentiate between tolerance and physical and psychological dependence.
- Clinicians should always consider the "total pain" concept and treat accordingly.

Steps to treating cancer pain

Pain severity, previous opioid use, dosing, and side effects, as well as any pre-existing conditions guide the principles of pain treatment.

Step 1

Assess pain severity

Pain severity serves as a guide in the decision-making process with regard to choosing a low-potency opioid vs. a high-potency drug like morphine. Most low-potency opioids are less suitable for severe pain because of their dose limitations and the presence of the ceiling effect.

Most cancer pain situations call for high-potency opioids. If a patient has an optimal trial with oral opioids, including rotation to a different opioid, or has experienced dose-limiting side effects, an alternative route such as IV or neuraxial may be tried.

Pain severity reported on a verbal numeric scale should be interpreted in the context of other psychosocial symptoms.

Step 2

Assess opioid history and side effects

Patient-to-patient variability in response to a specific opioid has been widely appreciated and documented.[38] Some patients may respond well to one opioid after other opioids fail or are intolerable.

This phenomenon is likely explained by the drugs' action on different receptors or genetic factors in opiate receptor constitution and will influence the selection of drugs within the same class.[38,39]

Step 3

Previous opioid dosing and pharmacokinetics

"Opioid-naïve" patients will require lower doses at least initially, reflecting the degree of tolerance. Opiate-tolerant patients are more likely to require longer-acting agents, while an as needed-only regimen is recommended for patients with incident pain syndromes.

Opioid-tolerant patients may require stronger and higher than conventional doses of opioids from the beginning.

Opioid medications exhibit a wide interindividual variation, possibly because of differences in intrinsic activity and action at different receptors and receptor subtypes.[38,39] Hence, opioid rotation is a worthwhile exercise when dose-limiting side effects are encountered.

The generally accepted method is to treat side effects before opioid switching. There is no general consensus on the number of opioid rotations, but in the authors' experience at least two or three opioid rotations, which should include methadone at some stage, need to be attempted.

Administration strategies

Around the clock (atc)

Atc administration is required in patients with continuous or frequent episodic pain. It is given to maintain a steady-state level and depends on the half-life of the drug chosen. Sustained-release oral preparations (morphine, oxycodone, oxymorphone) and transdermal patches (fentanyl) have gained popularity for their convenience.

Opioid-tolerant patients may require more frequent dosing regardless of the preparation used, to avoid end-of-dose failure.

Breakthrough (prn, or as needed)

Since fluctuations in the pain level occur in most patients on long-acting preparations, the need for shorter-acting agents is present in almost every case to provide coverage during surges. Rescue doses can be prescribed for as often as once every hour orally or even once every 15–20 minutes when the IV route is used.

Traditionally, 10–20% of the total opioid dose in a 24-hour period is given as a breakthrough dose. For patients experiencing less frequent episodic pain or pain related only to activity, only short-acting opioid medications are used, preferably on a preemptive basis.

Most of the short-acting opioids are not suitable for pain episodes lasting only a few minutes; however, transmucosal fentanyl preparations can be used for breakthrough cancer pain in these settings, with rapid onset and short clinical half-life.[40] High cost limits its use and accessibility.

Patient-controlled analgesia (PCA)

Delivery of opioids by PCA is occasionally indicated in refractory pain syndromes with acute exacerbations of pain. It is also used in patients unable to tolerate oral preparations. It can be delivered either intravenously or subcutaneously.

Although opioids are traditionally delivered intravenously in hospitalized patients, PCAs are available for use on an outpatient basis with appropriate supervision. In the outpatient or home setting, the SC route may be considered because of its convenience and ease of use.

The pharmacodynamics for both SC and IV delivery tends to be similar once steady state is achieved.

Presence of other symptoms

Sometimes symptoms of delirium, anxiety, and depression may be interpreted as physical pain, and opioid escalation is done with worsening of delirium. Hence, assessment of these symptoms is mandatory to avoid overdosing of opioids.

Step 4

Assess opioid side effects

A thorough knowledge of opioid side effects is necessary. While some side effects are common to all opioids, some patients may exhibit side effects unique to a specific drug and its metabolic end products.

Diminution or elimination of side effects is an important part of opioid therapy. Every effort should be made to treat side effects prophylactically, e.g., treat constipation with laxatives, and nausea with antiemetics. The opioid-switching phenomenon likely emerged in an effort to treat the side effects of opioids.

Whenever possible, dose readjustment should be the first measure in managing adverse reactions. Some common opioid side effects are described as follows (for a more detailed review of each symptom please refer to relevant chapters in this Handbook).

Sedation

Sedation is a commonly encountered side effect that often signifies excessive dosing. Downward titration of the dose to the level of analgesia is usually desirable. Drug combinations with opioids and other adjuvant medications may allow for an opioid-sparing effect, thereby minimizing sedation.

If sedation tends to be refractory to these maneuvers, the addition of a central nervous system stimulant (e.g., methylphenidate or dextroamphetamine) with upward titration could be helpful.[41] Methylphenidate (see Chapter 5, p. 73, for details) is started with an initial dose of 5 mg on wakening and 5 mg at noon, with upward titration to response.

The development of sedation following a period of adequate pain control may indicate improvement in or resolution of the original painful stimulus, i.e., decreased tumor burden after antineoplastic therapy. Downward titration of the opioid to the level of analgesia would again be recommended.

Tolerance

Tolerance is the second most common side effect and usually occurs within the first few days of opioid administration. It is defined as a reduction in the effectiveness of central or peripheral opioid activity, including analgesia, despite further attempts at dose escalation.

The dominant mechanism (central versus peripheral) should be determined in order to guide therapeutic choices (i.e., neuroleptics vs. motility agents, respectively).

Nausea and vomiting

Opioids can trigger nausea and vomiting directly by decreasing gastrointestinal (GI) motility and indirectly by inducing constipation. Patients with advanced malignancy can have decreased GI peristalsis secondary to circulating inflammatory mediators, with opioids compounding this effect.

Metoclopramide is frequently used to treat nausea and vomiting because it has multiple mechanisms of action that antagonize opioids, at both the central chemoreceptor trigger zone and the GI tract. Other agents include prochlorperazine, diphenhydramine, butyrophenones, benzodiazepines, steroids, and serotonin antagonists, such as ondansetron.

In patients who are receiving chemotherapy, a more aggressive approach should be used that is based on anticipated emetogenicity. This includes the use of aprepitant, a neurokinin-1 (NK_1) receptor antagonist.

Constipation

Constipation is one of the most common and easy-to-anticipate side effects. It often masquerades as other symptoms, presenting as intractable nausea and vomiting, increased abdominal pain, delirium, anorexia, or overflow diarrhea.

Since tolerance develops very slowly, if at all, patients will likely require regular laxative treatment from the inception and throughout the duration of opioid therapy. Dehydration, impaired mobility, autonomic dysfunction, and chemotherapy (e.g., vinca alkaloids) may compound the effects of opioid-induced constipation.

A bowel stimulant (e.g., senna) and a softening agent (e.g., docusate) is the most commonly used combination.[42] Multi-agent prophylaxis with gradual incremental dose increases may be necessary to reach the desired effect, based on patient subjective reports and clinical examination.

A kidney, ureters, and bladder (KUB) or flat-plate X-ray of the abdomen provides useful objective information regarding the degree of constipation when the clinical history or exam is inconclusive.[43]

Preparations such as polyethylene glycol (PEG) are tasteless, well tolerated, and useful as an adjunct to daily regular laxative therapy with senna and docusate. Resorting to an osmotic laxative such as lactulose or bowel preparations (magnesium citrate) is usually reserved for severe cases and could produce diarrhea.

As a backup measure, bowel lavage can be used in refractory cases until regular bowel movements are restored. A simple Fleet Enema, milk and molasses enema, or a manual maneuver may be the first remedies tried in these situations.

Caution should be used in patients whose constipation could be due to ileus, intestinal obstruction, or spinal cord compression, which is not uncommon in abdominopelvic malignancies and metastatic disease.

Neostigmine has been administered successfully in refractory cases, but caution should be exercised in cases of bowel obstruction and in patients with cardiac abnormalities. Oral naloxone has been used to manage severe cases of constipation.[44]

Recently, IV methylnaltrexone was approved for the management of refractory constipation in patients receiving opioid therapy. This drug has been shown to exert peripheral effects on the GI tract without reversing central analgesia.[45]

Important and commonly encountered considerations in patients undergoing active chemotherapy are neutropenia and thrombocytopenia. In patients with neutropenia (absolute neutrophil count <1000/μL blood), therapy is limited to the oral route, since rectal manipulation of any kind can lead to bacterial translocation and sepsis.

Thrombocytopenia (defined as <50,000 platelets/μL blood) also limits the physician to an oral route secondary to bleeding risks.

Cognitive impairment

Other causes of cognitive impairment should be aggressively sought before opioid medications are implicated. Impaired cognition presenting as delirium, hallucinations, agitation, or somnolence has been observed with sepsis, leptomeningeal disease, brain metastases, metabolic derangements (i.e., hypercalcemia), chemotherapy (e.g., ifosfamide-induced encephalopathy[46]), antifungal therapy (i.e., voriconazole), radiation (e.g., radiation-induced encephalopathy[47]), and hepatic encephalopathy.

Cancer patients often receive a variety of psychotropic medications for depression and other conditions, which alone or in conjunction with opioids may produce mental status changes. Benzodiazepines in combination with opioids and other psychotropic drugs can complicate matters.

When opioid-induced cognitive impairment is suspected, the initial step should be to lower the dose, which can also be diagnostic. It is highly recommended not to add another medication to treat agitation or other symptoms without this step.

If manipulation of the analgesic regimen, including opioid rotation, is ineffective, then haloperidol or a drug from the same class may be considered.

Urinary retention

Urinary retention is a relatively rare adverse reaction. It is usually observed in patients at extremes of age and is more likely to occur when medications with anticholinergic properties are administered concurrently with opioids.

It is commonly observed in patients receiving neuraxial opioids. Tolerance usually develops, but occasional patients may need temporary catheterization.

Myoclonus

Myoclonus is a dose-dependent phenomenon presumably related to opioid metabolites, more often those of morphine and meperidine. This phenomenon can occur with all opioids. It results from central motor excitability and could be a sign that a patient's level of tolerance has been overwhelmed.

A simple dose adjustment may abate the symptoms; however, rotating the opioid or temporarily adding a benzodiazepine may be necessary.

Respiratory depression

Respiratory depression is a rare occurrence in patients on chronic opioid therapy, as tolerance to this opioid action usually develops in a short time. However, accidental overdose or the addition of another sedative agent can trigger respiratory depression.

As long as respiratory function is not significantly impaired, temporary discontinuation and recommencement at a lower dose is recommended.

Opioids in combination with benzodiazepines are a common cause of respiratory depression. In cases where respiration is compromised leading to derangements in arterial blood gas values, the opioid antagonist naloxone can be titrated to response. It is given in 40 mcg increments rather than as a bolus to avoid acute opioid withdrawal.

Cases of tachyarrhythmias leading to myocardial compromise as well as pulmonary edema have been observed with bolus doses of 400 µg of naloxone.

Given the short half-life of naloxone, a continuous infusion of naloxone diluted in a liter of saline or dextrose solution may be required to prevent recurrence of respiratory depression.

Pruritis

The type of opioid medication and route of administration determine the likelihood of developing pruritis.[48]

For example, local administration of an opioid medication (i.e., SC or transdermal) can lead to a localized allergic wheal-and-flare reaction, whereas systemic administration (i.e., oral or IV) can lead to more generalized pruritis.

The mechanism behind opioid-induced pruritis is not completely understood. Peripheral and central pathways have been implicated, peripherally via histamine release and centrally via action of mu-opioid receptors.

Whereas histamine release can be treated with H2 antagonists such as diphenhydramine and ranitidine, centrally mediated pathways are more difficult to treat, requiring use of mu-opioid receptor antagonists such as naloxone for intractable pruritis. In less severe cases, opioid rotation in conjunction with antihistamines or ranitidine should be attempted prior to naloxone reversal.

Clinical pearls

- If the patient had an optimal trial with oral opioids, including rotation to a different opioid, or has experienced dose-limiting side effects, an alternative such as the IV or neuraxial route may be considered.
- Opioid escalation without identification of symptoms potentially augmenting pain expression can lead to worsening delirium.
- Common opioid side effects should be treated prophylactically, e.g., laxatives for constipation.
- Opioids trigger nausea and vomiting directly by decreasing gastrointestinal motility and indirectly through induction of constipation.
- Myoclonus is a dose-dependent phenomenon presumably related to opioid metabolites.
- Naloxone is used for opioid overdose and respiratory depression.
- Naloxone is given at 40 mcg increments rather than as a bolus to avoid acute opioid withdrawal.

Opioid rotation

Opioid rotation is the switch from one opioid to another when treatment-limiting toxicity results in poor responsiveness.[31,38,49] Opioid rotation is based on the concept of incomplete cross-tolerance between opioids: changing to an alternative drug may yield a far better balance between analgesia and side effects.

Guidelines for opioid rotation are intended to reduce the risk of relative overdosing or underdosing as one opioid is discontinued and another is administered (see Box 4.7). These guidelines require a working knowledge of an equianalgesic dose table (see Table 4.2).

The most common reasons for opioid rotation include cognitive failure, hallucinations, myoclonus, uncontrolled pain, and nausea.

Clinical scenarios and examples of opioid rotation

Case 1

A 56-year-old woman has mid-back pain from thoracic soft-tissue metastases from breast cancer. She is taking morphine sulfate immediate release (IR) 15 mg every 4 hours on an as-needed basis. She used 90 mg in the last 24 hours. She is being discharged home. If one needs to start sustained-release (SR) morphine, what will be the starting dose and what would be the breakthrough dose and frequency?

- *Step 1:* Take the total dose of short-acting morphine in 24 hours and divide it into two equal parts. Since the patient used 90 mg in the last 24 hours, the SR morphine dose would be 45 mg every 12 hours.
- *Step 2:* The breakthrough dose is 15–20% of the 24–hour morphine dose, or about 15 mg every hour as needed.

Box 4.7 Practical steps for opioid rotation

Five essential concepts

- Use the equianalgesic table to calculate the dose of the new opioid that is roughly equivalent to the dose of the current opioid.
- Determine the clinically relevant starting point. If switching to an opioid other than methadone or fentanyl, decrease the equianalgesic dose by 25–50%.
- Consider further dose adjustments based on medical condition and pain. If the patient is elderly or has significant organ failure, consider further dose reduction. If the patient has severe pain, consider a lesser dose reduction.
- If a rescue dose is to be used, calculate it as 15–20% of the total daily dose and administer at an appropriate interval. The exception is oral transmucosal fentanyl citrate, which should be started at a dose of 200 mcg or 400 mcg. Take into account simultaneous treatments that can potentially reduce pain, i.e., steroids, radiation, and surgery.
- Reassess and titrate the new opioids according to therapeutic response and side effects.

Table 4.2 Equianalgesic dose ratio table*

Opioid	From parenteral opioid to parenteral morphine	From same parenteral opioid to oral morphine	From oral opioid to oral morphine	From oral morphine to oral opioid
Morphine[†]	1	2.5	1	1
Hydromorphone	5	2	5	0.2
Meperidine	0.13	4	0.1	10
Levorphanol	5	2	5	0.2
Codeine	–	–	0.15	7
Oxycodone	–	–	1.5	0.7
Hydrocodone	–	–	0.15	7

* As per clinical guidelines in a comprehensive cancer center.
[†]Approximate: (a) Fentanyl patch in mcg/hour x 2 = daily morphine in mg orally. (b) Fentanyl parenteral 10 mcg = morphine 1 mg parenteral
Source: *MD Anderson Palliative Care Handbook*.

Case 2

A 66-year-old man with a history of squamous cell carcinoma of the lung has been receiving an IV morphine infusion of 2 mg/hour and also 5 mg IV/hour for breakthrough pain. He received 4 breakthrough doses in the last 24 hours. He is being discharged home and is able to take pills by mouth. What doses does he need for SR and for IR morphine?

- *Step 1:* Total morphine in 24 hours = (2 mg x 24 hours) + (5 mg x 4 doses) = 68 mg IV morphine, which is also 68 x 2.5 = 170 mg of oral morphine or approximately 90 mg of SR morphine every 12 hours.
- *Step 2:* Breakthrough dose is 15–20% of 170 mg or approximately 30 mg orally every hour as needed.

Case 2.1

If the above patient is unable to swallow pills, how do you convert to a transdermal fentanyl patch?

- *Step 1:* From the equianalgesic table, fentanyl patch x 2 = oral morphine PO. If the oral morphine equivalent daily dose (MEDD) is 170 mg, divide by 2. The fentanyl patch would therefore be 75 mcg/hour.
- *Step 2:* If incomplete tolerance is taken into account, then reduce the dose of fentanyl by 25–50%. The starting patch dose would therefore be 50 mcg/hour change every 72 hours.
- *Step 3:* For breakthrough dosing, try concentrated liquid morphine (20 mg:1 mL) at the same dose as above, 30 mg every hour as needed.

Case 3

A 46-year-old woman with history of gastric carcinoma is admitted with severe abdominal pain, myoclonus, sedation, and delirium. Her pain is currently treated with a fentanyl patch delivering 200 mcg/hour and with hydromorphone 8 mg oral every 2 hours as needed. She required 6 doses in the last 24 hours. The patient is being switched to PCA hydromorphone. What are the starting settings on PCA?

- *Step 1:* Convert fentanyl to hydromorphone. According to the conversion table, 200 mcg/hour patch of fentanyl is 400 mg oral morphine or 160 mg of IV morphine (400 mg divided by 2.5). This is equal to 30 mg of IV hydromorphone (160 mg IV morphine divided by 5). Reducing by 50% for incomplete tolerance, it will be 15 mg IV hydromorphone over 24 hours or 0.6 mg/hour of hydromorphone (15 mg divided by 24 hours).
- *Step 2:* Breakthrough dose: Calculate 15–20% of 15 mg, yielding a starting dose of 2 mg every hour as needed for breakthrough pain.

Case 4

A 52-year-old woman diagnosed with recurrent cervical carcinoma has been on SR morphine 120 mg orally every 12 hours and IR morphine 45 mg orally every 2 hours as needed for breakthrough pain. She received 8 doses of 45 mg within the last 24 hours. She had bilateral hydronephrosis with percutaneous nephrostomy tubes.

Her blood urea nitrogen (BUN) is 48 mg/dL and creatinine is 2.2 mg/dL. She presents with mental status changes and severe pain in the left lower extremity, radiating down the buttock into the little toe laterally. She is also on gabapentin 900 mg four times a day.

The spectrum of symptoms indicates a need for opioid rotation in the setting of opioid toxicity; methadone is chosen because the patient has renal insufficiency. How would you rotate from morphine to methadone?

- *Step 1:* Total morphine in 24 hours is 600 mg.
- *Step 2:* Because of incomplete tolerance, reduce the MEDD by 50%, yielding a new dose of 300 mg MEDD.
- *Step 3:* Conversion to methadone will be 15 mg orally every 12 hours. Calculation: (300 mg MEDD divided by 10) divided by 2 to obtain the dose given every 12 hours. Usually this is done over 3 days.
- *Step 4:* Breakthrough dose of morphine, if continued, would be 45–60 mg every hour as needed (or 15–20% of 300 mg MEDD).
- *Step 5:* Reduce the dose of gabapentin to account for altered renal function.

Case 5

A 44-year-old man with progressive metastatic sarcoma is transitioning to hospice care. He has been receiving IV PCA hydromorphone at a basal rate of 0.5 mg/hour, prn PCA demand dose of 0.5 mg every hour and a prn nursing bolus dose of 2 mg every hour for severe breakthrough pain. IV hydromorphone intake for the last 24 hours totaled 35 mg.

The referring doctor asks you to transition the patient to an appropriate regimen. The patient is able to tolerate liquids but cannot swallow tablets. What would you recommend?

- *Step 1:* Calculate the MEDD from 35 mg IV hydromorphone l 35 × 10, or MEDD of 350 mg.
- *Step 2:* Choose a regimen the patient will tolerate, taking into consideration his inability to swallow tablets. Consider a fentanyl patch

for basal pain control and high-concentration morphine (20 mg/mL) for prn dosing.

Step 3: Using prior 24-hour requirements (no dose reduction needed when converting to fentanyl patch*), fentanyl-patch dosing would be 350 MEDD divided by 2, or 175 mcg/hour. The prn dose would be 15–20% of MEDD, or 15% of 350, or 50 mg of morphine elixir (if 20 mg/mL, it would be 2.5 mL every 1 hour prn).

Opioid conversion exercises

a. PO morphine 300 mg. Convert to PO hydromorphone =
b. IV hydromorphone 50 mg. Convert to morphine PO =
c. PO morphine 100 mg over 24 hours (MEDD). Convert to transdermal fentanyl =
d. Fentanyl transdermal 100 mcg/hour. Convert to IV morphine =

ANSWERS: (a) 60 mg; (b) 500 mg; (c) 50 mcg/hour; (d) 80 mg.

Clinical pearls

- Opioid rotation should be considered when dose-limiting side effects are encountered.
- As general rule, treat side effects before opioid switching.
- Common side effects triggering rotation include cognitive impairment, hallucinations, and myoclonus.
- The rationale for opioid rotation is based on incomplete cross-tolerance between opioids.
- Working knowledge of an equianalgesic dose table is critical to successful opioid rotation.

As both clinical experience and survey data suggest, no reduction is needed for conversion to a transdermal fentanyl system (TFS). In addition, in the development of this formulation, conversion guidelines were developed that incorporated a safety factor, obviating the need for additional dose reductions in most patients.[49a]

*Approximate: (a) fentanyl patch in mcg/hour × 2 = daily morphine in mg orally. (b) Fentanyl parenteral 10 mcg = morphine 1 mg parenteral.

Analgesic adjuvants

Adjuvant analgesics are nonopioid medications with analgesic properties used for specific pain syndromes in conjunction with other medications, sometimes used as first-line agents in cancer pain management. They are recommended at every step of the WHO ladder. The main categories are TCAs and AEDs, but may include steroids and bisphosphonates.

Acetaminophen

Acetaminophen, or paracetamol, is an antipyretic analgesic with an unclear mechanism of action. It may inhibit cyclooxygenase (COX) in the central nervous system, with inhibitory effects on the serotonergic system.[50] It has little or no anti-inflammatory action and is usually combined with low-potency opioids.

Guidelines for the use of acetaminophen in cancer pain are empiric and based mostly on clinical experience.[51] The dose of acetaminophen varies widely between countries, with a dose of 0.5–1 g every 4 or 6 hours most commonly used. In the United States, given the concerns of liver toxicity, doses are limited to <4 g in a 24-hour period.

In a study by Stockler et al.[52] on the treatment of cancer pain, adding up to 6 g of acetaminophen to morphine for cancer pain can be safe.

In another study, volunteers taking acetaminophen alone or in combination with opioids had an increase in alanine aminotransferase up to three times the upper limit after 4 g of acetaminophen per day.[53] This study raises questions regarding the safety of acetaminophen use at higher doses.

The benefits of adding acetaminophen possibly outweigh the risks in countries where morphine availability continues to be a problem. Acetaminophen is freely available and affordable.

However, the use of acetaminophen should be individualized. It should be used with caution in chronic pain states, and liver function tests should be performed at regular intervals.

NSAIDs

NSAIDs are limited to the inhibitors of the enzyme cyclooxygenase (COX), inhibiting the synthesis of prostaglandins, which are mediators of pain and inflammation. This group is subdivided into nonspecific COX inhibitors and selective COX-2 inhibitors.

Nonselective inhibitors are medications like ibuprofen and naproxen. However, these drugs continue to cause concern about the integrity of gastric mucosa and alteration in renal function.

These medications are only useful as step 1 drugs or as adjuncts to opioid therapy in more advanced cases. They are very useful agents for treating bone pain and as adjuvants to opioid medications in a wide variety of pain syndromes.

In general, their use in cancer pain is limited because of the ceiling effect and the long-term side-effect profile. Their use is controversial in patients with thrombocytopenia, who constitute a large proportion of those receiving antineoplastic therapy.

Gastric and duodenal ulceration is another potential problem that could result from long-term use of aspirin and other nonselective NSAIDS. Other problems include salt and water retention and renal failure.

Ketorolac is formulated for parenteral administration and thus is considered unique, but there is concern over its effect on the integrity of the gastric mucosa.

COX-2 inhibitors

A more selective group of drugs, COX-2 inhibitors,[54] block the COX-2 enzyme with very little action on COX-1, thereby having minimal effect on the integrity of the gastric mucosa and platelet aggregation.

In clinical trials, these agents exhibited a safety profile comparable to that of placebo when compared to nonselective COX inhibitors. However, the efficacy remains the same as that of conventional NSAIDs. The COX-2 inhibitor drugs offer significant advantages in cancer patients undergoing chemotherapy.[55]

Controversy over increased cardiac events and strokes in patients taking the COX-2 inhibitor rofecoxib resulted in the U.S. Food and Drug Administration (FDA) withdrawing the drug from the market.[56]

TCAs (amitriptyline and nortriptyline)

TCAs are the main group of antidepressants used for the management of neuropathic pain syndromes. They have postulated action via serotonin and norepinephrine reuptake inhibition at nerve endings in the spinal cord and brain.

It is now widely accepted that the mechanism of action is independent of their mood-altering effects, resulting from an inherent influence over the nervous system or via modulation of opioid pathways.[57,58]

TCAs aren't universally tolerated, especially at the initiation of therapy, and often they have to be discontinued or their dosage decreased because of dose-limiting side effects, most commonly anticholinergic and sedative effects.

Amitriptyline and nortriptyline (with a lower cardiovascular side effect profile) are felt to be the most efficacious agents and are more often used.

The nonanalgesic properties of these agents are particularly useful in patients with depression and/or insomnia, symptoms frequently experienced by cancer patients. The tricyclic dose should be escalated gradually, with full benefit experienced in 3 to 4 weeks.

Anticonvulsants (antiepileptic drugs [AEDs])

Anticonvulsants are traditionally used with good results in the treatment of diabetic neuropathy, postherpetic neuralgia, trigeminal neuralgia, phantom pain, and similar syndromes,[58] all of which can coexist in cancer patients. Space-occupying lesions, due to new tumor growth or extension, may cause significant pain secondary to brachial and lumbosacral plexopathies.

Anticonvulsant agents are commonly used in the management of peripheral neuropathies resulting from chemotherapy (i.e., platinum agents, vinca alkaloids, and taxanes).

Traditional AEDs, e.g., phenytoin, valproate, and carbamazepine, have been used as anticonvulsants. Given the side effects and safety concerns, their use in pain control has been limited to neuropathic pain states.

Gabapentin has become the gold-standard, prototypical drug in this category to treat neuropathic pain.[59,60] With its wide therapeutic window, lack of need for blood monitoring, and comparable efficacy to that of other anticonvulsants, gabapentin is easier to manage than other drugs in its class. Sedation is a noted side effect that can be reduced by starting therapy at a low dose and titrating upward to the desired effect.

Newer AEDs are more widely used for non-cancer pain syndromes but have started to gain popularity in cancer pain situations. Such newer agents include pregabalin, oxcarbamazepine, and Lamictal (lamotrigine). Pregabalin has been studied in Indian patients with peripheral neuropathy and has shown favorable results.[61]

Miscellaneous

In refractory pain situations, drugs from other classes have the potential to achieve clinically meaningful responses. These alternative agents include psychotropic drugs,[62,63] benzodiazepines,[64] bisphosphonates,[65] steroids, lidocaine, ketamine, capsaicin, radiopharmaceuticals (strontium-89, samarium-153), and antibiotics for infection.

Pamidronate or zoledronic acid, both bisphosphonates, can be used routinely for pain control and hypercalcemia associated with metastatic bone disease, especially in patients with breast cancer or multiple myeloma.

Lidocaine

Analgesia can be achieved with systemic administration of lidocaine, presumably through its inhibitory action on sodium channels. Compared with other types of pain, more benefit has been observed in treatment of neuropathic pain and phantom pain syndromes with a predominance of central features.[66,67]

Low infusion rates have been used as third- or fourth-line treatment in opioid-tolerant patients at doses of 2.5–4 mg/kg. Incremental rate infusions over 20–30 minutes can be used as a therapeutic test before starting the oral form, mexiletine, especially in patients for whom anticonvulsants are not effective.

Cardiac monitoring is mandatory during IV therapy.

Ketamine

This anesthetic agent, an NMDA receptor antagonist, has well-documented analgesic properties; it is available in IV, oral, and rectal forms. Several reports have been published regarding its use in sub-anesthetic doses as an analgesic in cancer patients.[68,69]

Ketamine could be considered in cases of extreme opioid tolerance and may be used long term in palliative care situations. The recommended starting dose is 150 mg daily by SC infusion.

Capsaicin

Because of its high-toxicity profile, capsaicin is used only as a topical cream for management of neuropathic pain.[70] It acts by inhibiting substance P formation at the skin and is effective in only 50–60% of patients.

Clinical pearls

- Consider adjuvant medications where appropriate, e.g., AEDs for neuropathic pain.
- Avoid opioid combinations with acetaminophen as an analgesic adjuvant, as hepatotoxicity is a concern.
- Develop awareness of potential drug interactions and side-effect profiles of these groups of drugs.
- Avoid multiple adjuvant medications at the same time.
- Consider dose reductions in the setting of renal failure.

Spinal opioid therapy

Neurointerventional procedures such as neuraxial therapy have been increasingly used in the treatment of cancer pain,[71] especially for patients who develop pain refractory to opioid treatment. Spinal opioids work by binding to the mu receptor in the substantia gelatinosa and can be administered epidurally or intrathecally.

Options for delivering epidural or intrathecal opioids include percutaneous catheters, tunneled catheters, or implantable programmable pumps. Catheter obstruction and epidural fibrosis are more common with the epidural route.[72] Intrathecal administration has the advantage of being less affected by the presence of extensive epidural metastasis.[73]

A simple checklist can be followed prior to proceeding with neurointerventional procedures for cancer pain in patients with advanced cancer[74]:

- Is pain expression exclusively due to nociception? Initial pain assessment needs to rule out the presence of non-nociceptive factors capable of influencing pain expression, such as somatization related to depression or anxiety,[75] delirium with disinhibition of symptom expression,[76,77] and chemical coping.[78,79] If one of these factors is identified as a major contributor to the expression of pain, it needs to be treated prior to using an interventional approach to pain control.
- Does the patient have refractory pain? If patients have not had (1) adequate opioid titration, (2) trial of opioid rotation, or (3) consideration of adjuvant drugs, pain should not be considered refractory.
- Is the pain syndrome likely to respond to spinal opioids? To make this determination, physicians should rule out central deafferentation and the involvement of pain origination at higher anatomical locations that are less likely to benefit from spinal opioid treatment. Before permanent placement of an intrathecal opioid delivery system, an adequate response should be obtained with a trial administration of intrathecal spinal opioids.[80]
- Are there logistical problems? This consideration requires ensuring that patients are able to continue their treatment via a community hospice program. If such care is not available, the patient and family need to be informed that the patient may not be able to be discharged home, and this should be discussed prior to initiating the intervention.

Nonpharmacological treatment

Nerve blocks

The loss of normal sensory input, as occurs when a peripheral nerve is severed, may lead to a deafferentation pain. Some patients obtain relief from electrical stimulation, which augments non-nociceptive input.

Neurostimulation may be applied transcutaneously or via implanted devices to peripheral nerves, the spinal cord, or the brain. Carefully selected patients may benefit from surgical implantation of stimulation devices.[81,82]

Neuroablation, or destruction of nerve tissue, may be accomplished by chemical or surgical means. The goal of this technique is to isolate the site of somatic pain from the central nervous system. The efficacy of each procedure must be weighed against the risks.

A significant percentage of patients who fail to respond to oral therapy may be helped with appropriate nerve blocks. It is not known which patients might benefit from earlier procedures.[83,84]

Somatic nerve blocks may be diagnostic (i.e., to determine the indication for permanent neurolysis or somatic nerves), facilitative, prophylactic, or therapeutic. Visceral blocks (such as celiac plexus block) have been demonstrated to be effective for specific pain syndromes.[85]

Sympathetically maintained pain is suggested when signs of marked sympathetic dysfunction accompany typical diffuse burning or deep aching pain. Sympathetic blockade may then be diagnostic and therapeutic. In some cases of refractory generalized pain, pituitary adenolysis has been effective.

Some of the useful nerve blocks for head and neck pain include stellate ganglion block, trigeminal nerve block, mandibular block, maxillary nerve block, gasserian ganglion block, and glossopharyngeal nerve block. These blocks should be attempted using local anesthetic first, and then, based on a favorable risk–benefit ratio, a neurolytic agent like alcohol, phenol, or glycerine may be used.

Side effects to watch for following neurolytic blocks include brainstem anesthesia, convulsions (with volumes as low as 0.5 mL), hematoma, respiratory distress, recurrent laryngeal block, phrenic nerve block, pneumothorax, systemic toxicity, and unintended subarachnoid or epidural injection.

Evidence for the efficacy of nerve blocks in head and neck cancer is lacking. Most reports are based on anecdotal case reports or on clinical experience.

Somatic nerve blocks (root, brachial plexus, psoas compartment)

Somatic nerve blocks are effective for nociceptive somatic pain in the territory of root, plexus, or peripheral nerve. Blocks can be short lasting when a local anesthetic is employed.

These temporary blocks have a limited role in cancer pain management, but may act as a precursor to permanent neurolysis. Examples include root block, brachial plexus block, and psoas compartment block.

Neurolytic blocks

When taking into account their risk–benefit ratio, neurolytic blocks are generally favored in advanced-cancer patients with limited life expectancy. Sympathetic blocks such as celiac plexus block have been demonstrated to be effective for pancreatic cancer pain and other abdominal visceral pain syndromes.[86]

Contrary to an earlier study demonstrating improved survival,[87] Wong et al. showed that although pain was better controlled in the celiac plexus block group, there was no significant difference in survival or quality of life.[88]

Occasionally, a subarachnoid neurolytic block[89] or a neurolytic intercostal block may be employed. The risks of neurological deficits that may result from these blocks must be weighed against the possible benefits.

In a recent study by Smith et al.[90] randomizing patients to intrathecal opioid therapy vs. conservative management, the intrathecal group had improved survival; however, concerns were raised regarding the comprehensive medical management group.[91,92] Perhaps more studies with a better inception cohort are needed to confirm the findings.

Neurosurgical procedures

Surgical ablation

Surgical ablation[93] may be accomplished by rhizotomy (section of nerve root) or dorsal root entry-zone lesions. Spinal anterolateral tractotomy or cordotomy, mesencephalotomy, medullary tractotomy, and cingulotomy should be reserved for carefully selected cases. Vertebroplasty, which involves injecting cement into metastatic compression fractures, is gaining wide popularity.[94,95]

Percutaneous cordotomy employed for intractable pain of the lower extremity has been useful in select patients.[96] Radiofrequency lesioning of bone metastases has recently been shown to be another modality to treat bone pain.[97]

The loss of normal sensory input, as occurs when a peripheral nerve is severed, may lead to deafferentation pain. Some patients obtain relief from electrical stimulation, which augments non-nociceptive input. Neurostimulation may be applied transcutaneously or via implanted devices to peripheral nerves, the spinal cord, or the brain. Carefully selected patients may benefit from surgical implantation of stimulation devices.[98]

Neuroablation, or destruction of nerve tissue, may be accomplished by chemical or surgical means. The goal of this technique is to isolate the site of somatic pain from the central nervous system. The efficacy of each procedure must be weighed against the risks.

Ablative and neurointerventional procedures provide options for management of refractory cancer pain. However, prior to invasive procedures or placement of permanent pain pumps, a rigorous interdisciplinary team assessment and treatment of total pain (physical, psychological, spiritual, social, and practical) is recommended.

Psychological techniques for pain control

The following are brief descriptions of techniques that can enable a patient to accept the responsibility of managing their pain so they can begin to cope and function more effectively. These techniques include, but are not limited to, biofeedback, relaxation training, hypnosis, and cognitive and operant approaches.

Biofeedback

The aim of biofeedback techniques is to enable patients to bring involuntary physiological events into voluntary control using electronic equipment. Biofeedback can modify certain physiological processes that underlie pain disorders, e.g., electromyographic (EMG) feedback to treat muscle contraction headaches.

Affected physiological processes include the relaxation response (decreases in autonomic arousal will lead to reductions in pain) and self-regulation (patients become aware of their contribution to the pain experience and their ability to reduce it).

Biofeedback methods include EMG biofeedback, skin temperature or thermal biofeedback, alpha EEG, and cephalic blood volume pulse feedback.

Relaxation training

Relaxation training is used to control pain and increase body awareness. All techniques elicit the relaxation response, with the goal of achieving pain reduction and decreases in sympathetic activity, oxygen consumption, heart rate, and blood lactate concentration. Relaxation methods include progressive muscle relaxation, breathing therapy, and guided imagery.

Focused concentration reduces persistent intrusive thoughts, relaxes muscles, and reduces pain. In progressive muscle relaxation, the most common approach, patients are taught to tense and relax muscles that contribute to pain, techniques used in such activities as yoga.

Relaxation training is particularly useful in controlling migraines, muscle-contraction headaches, temporomandibular joint pain, chronic back pain, and myofascial pain.

Hypnosis

Hypnosis is a heightened state of responsiveness to suggestions and ideas. Pain relief may be dramatic in some cases and is not related to endorphin action. Hypnosis involves cognitive processes such as narrowing of attention, mental relaxation, and increased suggestibility.

Even though pain relief through hypnosis is of short duration and shows a variable response among individuals, it can provide a sense of peacefulness and comfort, helping relieve organic pain more than psychogenic pain.

Hypnosis can be modified by operant training, biofeedback, and sensory deprivation.

Cognitive-behavioral therapy (CBT)

CBT is based on the premise that cognition influences both emotion and behavior. Several cognitive styles, or thinking patterns, have been identified as particularly maladaptive and related to poor outcomes, distress, and likelihood of injury.

CBT is a multimodal treatment aimed at replacing maladaptive thinking patterns with more adaptive patterns and replacing maladaptive behavior patterns with functional alternatives. The therapy has been shown to affect emotions, pain behavior, and health-care use outcomes.

Cognitive approaches affect expectations, attitudes, and beliefs about pain, helping patients gain better control over their pain. Since behavior and actions are affected by how individuals see the world, correction of faulty thought processes decreases suffering and disability; maladaptive beliefs are replaced with new, more adaptive ones.

Cognitive approaches can be action oriented, limited, or structured, and they can be administered in group or individual settings.

Operant approaches

Operant approaches are based on the principle that a person's behavior is governed by both the positive and negative consequences of it. Positive reinforcers increase the likelihood of a behavior recurring and negative reinforcers decrease that likelihood. The goal is to replace learned behaviors with more "healthy" behaviors, ones that are incompatible with and in contrast to the "sick role."

Family members and health-care providers are instructed to reinforce healthy behavior and discourage pain behaviors, narcotic use, and inactivity. Other forms of therapy can be incorporated, including marital counseling, family therapy, and vocational training. The desired end state is decreased medication use and increased activity.

Physical modalities for pain control

Therapeutic heat and cold

Heat reduces muscle spasms, and an increase in muscle temperature reduces spindle afferant sensitivity and firing. The addition of cold to sensory terminals also tends to decrease the muscle spindle response.

While heat increases local blood flow, cold decreases it. In cases of acute injury, cold is preferred to reduce swelling. Heat reduces joint stiffness by increasing the extensibility of collagen tissue.

Superficial-heating modalities (with no effect beyond a depth of 1 cm) include hot packs, paraffin baths, hydrotherapy, and radiant heat. Although heat may be applied locally, it may still cause a reflex effect on other parts of the body, e.g., reduction in smooth muscle activity of the visceral organs when heat is applied to the abdomen. Available modalities use the principles of conduction, convection, and radiation.

Deep-heating modalities (heating structures to a depth of 3–5 cm) include ultrasound techniques and short- and microwave diathermy. Ultrasound converts high-frequency acoustic vibrations into heat, selectively heating bone and tissue without risk of superficial thermal burn. Absorption is determined by the protein content of the tissues.

Since ultrasound does not travel through air, topical application of gel or water is required to transmit the heat. Ultrasound may also produce nonthermal effects, increasing the extensibility of collagen and muscle. Nonthermal effects of concern include pseudocavitation, which is production of gas bubbles that carry a risk of subsequent tissue destruction.

In short-wave diathermy, high-frequency current is used to heat subcutaneous and deep tissues. It should not be used in the presence of a metal implant as this may lead to burns in the surrounding tissues.

Microwave diathermy uses electromagnetic radiation, with heat production depending on interface reflection and absorption characteristics of underlying tissues. Its use is limited mostly to hepatic lesions and is contraindicated in fluid-filled areas such as eyes or joints.

The use of therapeutic heat is contraindicated over anesthetic or ischemic areas, in delirious patients, near gonads or developing fetuses (except ultrasound), and in the presence of cardiac pacemakers or metal implants (especially short-wave and microwave diathermy).

Therapeutic cold reduces metabolism, the inflammatory response, nerve conduction velocity, and muscle spindle activity. It is used to reduce pain, inflammation, and edema in cases of acute injury. Commonly used techniques include cold packs (10–20 minutes); ice massage (through the stages of coolness, burning, and numbness); cold baths (13–18°C); vapocoolant spray (ethyl chloride and fluorimethane); and the spray and stretch technique on trigger points.

Therapeutic cold is contraindicated in patients with Raynaud's phenomenon or hypersensitivity to cold.

Transcutaneous electrical nerve stimulation (TENS)

In TENS, electrical energy is transmitted across the skin surface to the nervous system, stimulating large, myelinated A fibers and closing the gate for pain coming from C fibers.

Traditional TENS methodology is of low intensity and high frequency (pulse width of 50–80 microseconds and frequency of 80–100 Hz) with an immediate effect, mediated by serotonin but not reversible with naloxone. High-intensity and low-frequency ("acupuncture-like," pulse width > 200 microseconds, frequency < 10 Hz) methodologies may be reversed by naloxone, with a delayed effect (20–30 minutes).

Clinical indications include acute pain (such as that from sprains, lacerations, and fractures), postoperative pain, labor pain, and chronic pain (such as lower back pain, arthritis, phantom limb pain, neuropathies, and cancer pain).

Acupuncture

Acupuncture is the practice of inserting one or more needles into specific sites on the body surface for therapeutic purposes. In addition to needle insertion, acupuncture points can also be "stimulated" with heat, electrical currents, pressure, laser light, or shock waves.

Acupuncture works by stimulating A-delta fibers in the skin and muscles, conducting impulses to the spinal gray matter, and inhibiting painful stimuli from the periphery, thereby reducing pain perception. The activation of encephalin-containing interneurons in the substantia gelatinosa of the spinal gray matter inhibits conduction of pain signals to the brain.

Subsequent neuromodulatory effects include release of beta-endorphin and met-encephalin in the brain, activation of two descending pain control systems in the midbrain, and modulatory effects on the central pain network in the hypothalamus and the limbic system.

Acupuncture also induces relaxation by affecting a person's emotional state, evoking a pleasant sensation through theorized action on the reward system of dopamine and serotonin.

It may reduce gastric acid secretion and correct gastric arrhythmia, thereby reducing nausea and vomiting, and may also reduce bladder urgency and incontinence caused by an overactive or unstable bladder.

Evidenced-based studies of acupuncture benefits are limited. In a 2006 review article by Derry et al.[99] analyzing 35 systematic reviews of acupuncture that were published between 1996 and 2005, 17 of the reviews found no evidence of benefit, 12 found some benefit, and none could demonstrate evidence of benefit when strict criteria of quality, validity, and size were applied.

Nonserious adverse effects occur in 7–11% of all acupuncture patients, including severe tiredness and exhaustion, pain at the site of needling, and headache. Serious adverse effects include rare instances of pneumothorax or cardiac tamponade and infections such as hepatitis C or HIV.

Clinical pearls

- Physical modalities to reduce pain and muscle spasm should be considered in every patient.
- Explore cognitive behavioral therapies in all patients.
- Explore expressive supportive counseling in patients with psychosocial problems.
- Consider anesthetic and neurosurgical procedures where appropriate, e.g., celiac plexus block for pancreatic cancer pain.
- Counsel patients and explore spiritual issues complicating pain.
- A multidisciplinary approach is the key to successful pain management.

Risk evaluation and mitigation strategies (REMS) for opioid medications

With a concerning trend toward increasing opioid-related deaths and opioid misuse and addiction in the United States, the FDA has proposed extending Risk Evaluation and Mitigation Strategies (REMS) to opioid medications. The Food and Drug Administration Amendments Act of 2007 gave the FDA the authority to require REMs from manufacturers of certain prescription medications to "ensure that the benefits of a drug or biological product outweigh its risks."[100]

Initially targeting both long- and short-acting preparations, the application of REMS to opioids is now limited to long-acting preparations. The FDA hopes stricter controls on opioid prescribing will increase safety and minimize risks. From the prescriber's and patient's standpoint, decreased access to opioids as a result of stricter controls could potentially create a new barrier to effective pain control.

REMS for a particular opioid will require special certification and enrollment of pharmacists and health-care practitioners who dispense and prescribe a drug. The practitioner would only dispense the drug to patients with evidence of safe-use conditions (i.e., documentation of consent and understanding, as well as pregnancy and blood chemistry testing). Each patient using the drug will be enrolled in a registry and be subject to regular monitoring by a physician.

Ongoing discussions between the Industry Working Group (IWG), a committee composed of opioid manufacturers, and the FDA, are geared toward the collaborative development of new safety standards for opioid medications.[101] IWG recommendations to the FDA during a December 4, 2009, open hearing included developing a medication guide for patients and a detailed communication plan for prescribers to follow.

Recommendations also included the development of special certification or training for prescribers, unless already possessing specialty or subspecialty certification in such areas as hospice and palliative medicine.

A prescriber–patient agreement would provide information regarding opioid prescribing, storage, and use; a Patient Medication Information Sheet would make such information available to patients.

Recognizing the challenge of developing REMS for opioids, the FDA has been receptive to public contributions.

References

1. Foley KM (1979). Pain syndromes in patients with cancer. In Bonica JJ, Ventafridda V (Eds.), Advances in Pain Research and Therapy. New York: Raven Press, pp. 59–75.
2. Bonica JJ (1990). Cancer pain. In Bonica JJ (Ed.), The Management of Pain. Philadelphia: Lea & Febiger, p. 400.
3. Twycross RG, Fairfield S (1982). Pain in far-advanced cancer. Pain 14:303–310.
4. World Health Organization (1986). Cancer Pain Relief. Geneva: World Health Organization.
5. Levin D, Cleeland CS, Dar R (1985). Public attitudes toward cancer pain. Cancer 56:2337–2339.

6. Koshy RC, Rhodes D, Devi S, Grossman SA (1998). Cancer pain management in developing countries: a mosaic of complex issues resulting in inadequate analgesia. *Support Care Cancer* 6(5):430–437.

7. Rajagopal MR, Joranson DE, Gilson AM (2001). Medical use, misuse, and diversion of opioids in India. *Lancet* 358(9276):139–143.

8. Higginson IJ (1997). Innovations in assessment: epidemiology and assessment of pain in advanced cancer. In Jenson TS, Turner JA, Wiesenfeld-Hallin Z (Eds.), *Proceedings of the 8th World Congress on Pain, Progress in Pain Research and Management.* Vol. 8. Seattle, WA: IASP Press, pp. 707–716.

9. Portenoy RK, Hagen NA (1990). Breakthrough pain: definition, prevalence, and characteristics. *Pain* 41:273–281.

10. Bruera E, MacMillan K, Hanson J, et al. (1989). The Edmonton staging system for cancer pain: preliminary report. *Pain* 37:203–209.

11. Bruera E, Kuehn N, Miller MJ, Selmser P, MacMillan K (1991). The Edmonton Symptom Assessment System: a simple method for the assessment of palliative care patients. *J Palliat Care* 7:6–9.

12. Walker P. (2001). Impact of the Edmonton Labeled Visual Information System on the physician recall of metastatic cancer patient histories: a randomized controlled trial. *J Pain Symptom Manage* 21(1):4–11.

13. Derogatis LR, Marrow GR, Fetting J, et al. (1983). The prevalence of psychiatric disorders among cancer patients. *JAMA* 249:754.

14. Jacox A, Carr DB, Payne R, et al. (1994). *Management of Cancer Pain.* Clinical Practice Guidelines No. 9, AHCPR Publication 94–0592. Rockville, MD: US Department of Health and Human Services, Agency for Health Care Policy and Research.

15. World Health Organization (1990). Cancer pain relief and palliative care: report of a WHO Expert Committee. *World Health Organ Tech Ser* 804:11–12.

16. Sindrup SH, Andersen G, Madsen C, Smith T, Brosen K, Jensen TS (1999). Tramadol relieves pain and allodynia in polyneuropathy: a randomized, double-blind, controlled trial. *Pain* 83(1):85–90.

17. Afshari R, Maxwell S, Dawson A, Bateman DN (2005). ECG abnormalities in co-proxamol (paracetamol/dextropropoxyphene) poisoning. *Clin Toxicol (Phila)* 43(4):255–259.

18. Andersen G, Christrup L, Sjogren P (2003). .Relationships among morphine metabolism, and side effects during long-term treatment: an update. *J Pain Symptom Manage* 25(1):74–91.

19. Prommer, E (2006). Oxymorphone: a review. *Support Care Cancer* 14(2):109–115.

20. Bruera E, Sloan P, Scott J, Suarez-Almazor M (1996). A randomized, double dummy, crossover trial comparing slow release to immediate release hydromorphone for the treatment of cancer pain. *J Clin Oncol.* 14(5):1713–1717.

21. Portenoy RK, Taylor D, Messina J, Tremmel L (2006). A randomized, placebo-controlled study of fentanyl buccal tablet for breakthrough pain in opioid-treated patients with cancer. *Clin J Pain* 22(9):805–811.

22. Portenoy RK, Payne R, Coluzzi P, Raschko JW, Lyss A, Busch MA, Frigerio V, Ingham J, Loseth DB, Nordbrock E, Rhiner M (1999). Oral transmucosal fentanyl citrate (OTFC) for the treatment of breakthrough pain in cancer patients: a controlled dose titration study. *Pain* 79(2-3):303–312.

23. Tennant F, Hermann L (2002). Self-treatment with oral transmucosal fentanyl citrate to prevent emergency room visits for pain crises: patient self-reports of efficacy and utility. *J Palliat Care Pharmacother.* 16(3):37–44.

24. Skaer TL. (2006). Transdermal opioids for cancer pain. *Health Qual Life Outcomes* 4:24.

25. Gordon DB (2006). Oral transmucosal fentanyl citrate for cancer breakthrough pain: a review. *Oncol Nurs Forum* 33(2):257–264.

26. Portenoy RK, Messina J, Xie F, Peppin J (2007). Fentanyl buccal tablet (FBT) for relief of breakthrough pain in opioid-treated patients with chronic low back pain: a randomized, placebo-controlled study. *Curr Med Res Opin* 23(1):223–233.

27. Paix A, Coleman A, Lees J, et al. (1995). Subcutaneous fentanyl and sufentanil infusion substitution for morphine intolerance in cancer pain management. *Pain* 63:263–269.

28. Kunz K, Thiesen J, Schroder M (1993). Severe episodic pain management with sublingual sufentanil [letter]. *J Pain Symptom Manage* 8:189–190.

29. Belluck P (2003). Methadone, once the way out, suddenly grows as a killer drug. *New York Times*, February 9.

30. Mercadente S, Casuccio A, Fulfaro F, et al. (2001). Switching from morphine to methadone to improve analgesia and tolerability in cancer patients: a prospective study. *J Clin Oncol* 19(11):2898–2904.

31. Bruera EB, Pereira J, Watanabe S, et al. (1996). Systemic opioid therapy for chronic cancer pain: practical guidelines for converting drugs and routes. *Cancer* 78:852–857.

32. Shaiova L, Berger A, Blinderman CD, et al., (2008). Consensus guideline on parenteral methadone use in pain and palliative care. *Palliat Support Care* 6(2):165–176.

33. Weschules DJ, Bain KT (2008). A systematic review of opioid conversion rations used with methadone for the treatment of pain. *Pain Med* 9(5):595–612.

34. Nicholson AB (2007). Methadone for cancer pain. *Cochrane Database Syst Rev* 17;(4): CD003971.

35. Krants M, Martin J, Stimmel B, Mehta D, Haigney MC (2009). QTc interval screening in methadone treatment. *Ann Intern Med* 150(6):387–395.

36. Reddy S, Hui D, El Osta B, et al. (2010). The effect of oral methadone on the QTc interval in advanced cancer patients: a prospective pilot study. *J Palliat Med* 13:33–38.

37. Prommer, E (2007). Levorphanol: the forgotten opioid. *Support Care Cancer* 15(3):259–264.

38. Galer BS, Coyle N, Pasternak GW, Portenoy RK (1992). Individual variation in the response to different opioids—report of five cases. *Pain* 49:87–91.

39. Hanks G, Forbes K (1997). Opioid responsiveness. *Acta Anesthesiol Scand* 41:154–158.

40. Mystakidou K, Katsouda E, Parpa E, Vlahos L, Tsiatas ML (2006). Oral transmucosal fentanyl citrate: overview of pharmacological and clinical characteristics: *Drug Deliv* 13(4):269–276.

41. Bruera E, Chadwick S, Brenneis C, Hanson J, MacDonald RN (1987). Methylphenidate associated with narcotics for the treatment of cancer pain. *Cancer Treat Rep* 71(1):67–70.

42. Starreveld JS, Pols MA, Van Wijk HJ,Bogaard JW, Poen H, Smout AJ. The plain abdominal radiograph in the assessment of constipation. Z Gastroenterol 1990; 28:335–338.

43. Bruera E, Suarez-Almazor M, Velasco A, Bertolino M, MacDonald SM, Hanson J (1994). The assessment of constipation in terminal cancer patients admitted to a palliative care unit: a retrospective review. *J Pain Symptom Manage* 9(8):515–519.

44. Sykes NP (1996). An investigation of the ability of oral naloxone to correct opioid-related constipation in patients with advanced cancer. *Palliat Med* 10:135–144.

45. Thomas J, Karver S, Cooney GA, Chamberlain BH, Watt CK, Slatkin NE, Stambler N, Kremer AB, Israel RJ (2008). Methylnaltrexone for opioid-induced constipation in advanced illness. *N Engl J Med* 358(22):2332–2343.

46. Merimsky O, Reider-Grosswaser I, Wiggle N, Chaitchik S (1992). Encephalopathy in ifosfamide-treated patients. *Acta Neurol Scand* 86(5):521–525.

47. Crossen JR, Garrod D, Glatsein E, Neuwelt EA (1994). Neurobehavioral sequelae of cranial irradiation in adults; a review of radiation-induced encephalopathy. *J Clin Oncol* 12(3):627–642.

48. Reich A, Szepietowski JC (2009). Opioid-induced pruritis: an update. *Clin Exp Dermatol* 35(1):2–6.

49. Cherny NJ, Chang V, Frager G, et al. (1995). Opioid pharmacotherapy in the management of cancer pain: a survey of strategies used by pain physicians for the selection of analgesic drugs and routes of administration. *Cancer* 76:1288–1293.

49a. Indelicato RA, Portenoy RK (2002). Opioid rotation in the management of refractory cancer pain. *J Clin Oncol* 20(1):348–352.

50. Pickering G, Loriot MA, Libert F, Eschalier A, Beaune P, Dubray C (2006). Analgesic effect of acetaminophen in humans: first evidence of a central serotonergic mechanism. *Clin Phamacol Ther* 79:371–378.

51. Saito O, Aoe T, Yamamoto T (2005). Analgesic effects of nonsteroidal anti-inflammatory drugs, acetaminophen, and morphine in a mouse model of bone cancer pain. *J Anesth* 19(3):218–224.

52. Stockler M, Vardy J, Pillai A, Warr D (2004). Acetaminophen (paracetamol) improves pain and well-being in people with advanced cancer already receiving a strong opioid regimen: a randomized, double-blind, placebo-controlled cross-over trial. *J Clin Oncol* 22(16):3389–3394.

53. Watkins PB, Kaplowitz N, Slattery JT, Colonese CR, Colucci SV, Stewart PW, Harris SC (2006). Aminotransferase elevations in healthy adults receiving 4 grams of acetaminophen daily: a randomized controlled trial. *JAMA* 296(1):87–93.

54. Lane NE (1997). Pain management in osteoarthritis: the role of COX-2 inhibitors. *J Rheumatol* 24:20–24.

55. Fine PG, et al. (2002). The role of rofecoxib, a cyclooxygenase-2-specific inhibitor, for the treatment of non-cancer pain: a review. *J Pain* 3(4):272–283.

56. Bresalier RS, Sandler RS, Quan H, Bolognese JA, Oxenius B, Horgan K, Lines C, Riddell R, Morton D, Lanas A, Konstam MA, Baron JA (2005). Adenomatous Polyp Prevention on Vioxx (APPROVe) Trial Investigators. Cardiovascular events associated with rofecoxib in a colorectal adenoma chemoprevention trial. *N Engl J Med* 352(11):1092–1102.

57. Magni G (1991). The use of antidepressants in the treatment of chronic pain: a review of current evidence. *Drugs* 42:730–748.

58. Kolke M, Hoffken K, Olbrich H, Schmidt CG (1999). Antidepressants and anticonvulsants for the treatment of neuropathic pain syndromes in cancer patients. *Onkologie* 14:40–43.

59. Rowbotham M, Harden N, Stacey B, Bernstein P, Magnus-Miller L (1998). Gabapentin for the treatment of postherpetic neuralgia: a randomized controlled trial. *JAMA* 280:1837–1842.

60. Backonja M, Beydoun A, Edwards KR, et al. (1998). Gabapentin for the symptomatic treatment of painful neuropathy in patients with diabetes mellitus: a randomized controlled trial. *JAMA* 280:1831–1836.

61. Lyrica Study Group (2006). Pregabalin for peripheral neuropathic pain: results of a multicenter, non-comparative, open-label study in Indian patients. *Int J Clin Pract* 60(9):1060–1067.

62. Brietbart W (1998). Psychotropic adjuvant analgesics for pain in cancer and AIDS. *Psychooncology* 7:333–345.

63. Patt R, Propper G, Reddy S (1994). The neuroleptics as adjuvants analgesics. *J Pain Symptom Manage* 9:446–453.

64. Reddy S, Patt RB (1994). The benzodiazepines as adjuvant analgesics. *J Pain Symptom Manage*. 9:510–514.

65. Thiebaud D, Leyvarz S, von Fliedner V, et al. (1991). Treatment of bone metastases from breast cancer and myeloma with pamidronate. *Eur J Cancer* 27:37–41.

66. NagaroT, Shimizu C, Inoue H, et al. (1995). The efficacy of intravenous lidocaine on various types of neuropathic pain. *Masui* 44(6):862–867.

67. Brose W, Cousins M (1991). Subcutaneous lidocaine for the treatment of neuropathic cancer pain. *Pain* 45(2):145–148.

68. Clark JL, Kalan GE (1995). Effective treatment of severe cancer pain of the head using low-dose ketamine. *J Pain Symptom Manage* 10(4):310–314.

69. Mercadante S, Lodi F, Sapio M, et al. (1995). Long-term ketamine subcutaneous infusion in neuropathic cancer pain. *J Pain Symptom Manage* 10(7):564–568.

70. Ellison N, Loprinzi CL, Kugler J, et al. (1997). Phase 3 placebo-controlled trial of capsaicin cream in the management of surgical neuropathic pain in cancer patients. *J Clin Oncol* 15(8):2974–2980.

71. Kedlaya D, Reynolds L, Waldman S (2002). Epidural and intrathecal analgesia for cancer pain. *Best Pract Res Clin Anaesthesiol* 16:651–665.

72. Aldrete JA (1995). Epidural fibrosis after permanent catheter insertion and infusion. *J Pain Symptom Manage* 10:624–631.

73. Applegren L, Nordberg C, Sjoberg M, et al. (1997). Spinal epidural metastasis: implications for spinal analgesia to treat refractory cancer pain. *J Pain Symptom Manage* 13:25–42.

74. Yennurajalingam S, Dev R, Walker PW, Reddy SK, Bruera E (2010). Challenges associated with spinal opioid therapy for pain in patients with advanced cancer: a report of three cases. *J Pain Symptom Manage*. 39(5):930–935.

75. Hopwood P, Stephens RJ (2000). Depression in patients with lung cancer: prevalence and risk factors derived from quality-of-life data. *J Clin Oncol* 18:893–903.

76. Klepstad P, Hilton P, Moen J, et al. (2002). Self-reports are not related to objective assessments of cognitive function and sedation in patients with cancer pain admitted to a palliative care unit. *Palliat Med* 16:513–519.

77. Bruera E, Fainsinger RL, Miller MJ, Kuehn N (1992). The assessment of pain intensity in patients with cognitive failure: a preliminary report. *J Pain Symptom Manage* 7:267–270.

78. Parsons HA, Delgado-Guay MO, El Osta B, et al. (2008). Alcoholism screening in patients with advanced cancer: impact on symptom burden and opioid use. *J Palliat Med* 11:964–968.

79. Fainsinger RL, Nekolaichuk L, Lawlor PG, et al. (2005). A multicenter study of the revised Edmonton Staging System for classifying cancer pain in advanced cancer patients. *J Pain Symptom Manage* 29:224–237.

80. Krames ES (2002). Implantable devices for pain control:spinal stimulation and intrathecal therapies. *Best Pract Res Clin Anaesthesiol* 16:619–649.

81. Mayerson BA (1983). Electrostimulation procedures: effects, presumed rationale, and possible mechanisms. In Bounce JJ, et al. (Eds.), *Advances in Pain Research and Therapy*. New York: Raven Press, pp. 495–534.

82. Duncan GH, Bushnell MC, Marchand S (1991). Deep brain stimulation: a review of basic research and clinical studies. *Pain* 45:49–60.

83. Arner S (1982). The role of nerve blocks in the treatment of cancer pain. *Acta Anaesthesio. Scand* 74:104–108.

84. Cousins MJ, Bridenbaug PO (Eds.) (1988). *Neural Blockade*, 2nd ed. Philadelphia: JB Lippincott.

85. Brown DL, Bulley CK, Quiel EL (1987). Neurolytic celiac plexus block for pancreatic cancer pain. *Anesth Analg* 66:869–873.

86. Neurolytic Celiac Plexus Block for Pancreatic Cancer Pain? JWatch Gastroenterology. 2004;2004(414):6.

87. Lillemoe KD, Cameron JL, Kaufman HS, Yeo CJ, Pitt HA, Sauter PK (1993). Chemical splanch-nicectomy in patients with unresectable pancreatic cancer. A prospective randomized trial. *Ann Surg* 217(5):447–455; discussion 456–457.

88. Gilbert Y. Wong MD, Darrell R, et al. (2004). Effect of neurolytic celiac plexus block on pain relief, quality of life, and survival in patients with unresectable pancreatic cancer. A randomized controlled trial. *JAMA* 291:1092–1099.

89. Patt RB, Payne R, Farhat GA, Reddy SK (1995). Subarachnoid neurolytic block under general anesthesia in a 3-year-old with neuroblastoma. *Clin J Pain* 11(2):143–146.

90. Smith TJ, Staats PS, Deer T, et al. (2002). Randomized clinical trial of an implantable drug delivery system compared with comprehensive medical management for refractory cancer pain: impact on pain, drug-related toxicity, and survival. *J Clin Oncol* 20(19):4040–4049.

91. Davis MP, Walsh D, Lagman R, LeGrand SB (2003). Randomized clinical trial of an implantable drug delivery system. *J Clin Oncol* 21(14):2800–2801.

92. Ripamonti C, Brunelli C (2003). Randomized clinical trial of an implantable drug delivery system compared with comprehensive medical management for refractory cancer pain: impact on pain, drug-related toxicity, and survival. *J Clin Oncol* 21(14):2801–2802.

93. Meyerson BA (1982). The role of neurosurgery in the treatment of cancer pain. *Acta Anaesthesiol Scand* 74:109–113.

94. Weill A, Chiras J, Simon JM, Rose M, Soal-Martinez T, Enkaoua E (1996). Spinal metastases: indications for and results of percutaneous injection of acrylic surgical cement. *Radiology* 199:241–247.

95. Cotton A, Boutry N, Cortet B, et al. (1998). Percutaneous vertebroplasty: state of the art. *Radiographic* 18:311–322.

96. Macalusco C, Foley KM, Arbit E (1988). Cordotomy for lumbosacral, pelvic and lower extremity pain of malignant origin: safety and efficacy. *Neurology* 38:110.

97. Goetz MP, Callstrom MR, Charboneau JW, et al. (2004). Percutaneous image-guided radiofrequency ablation of painful metastases involving bone: a multicenter study. *J Clin Oncol* 15:22(2):300–306.

98. Mayerson BA (1983). Electrostimulation procedures: effects, presumed rationale, and possible mechanisms, In Bounce JJ, et al. (Eds), *Advances in Pain Research and Therapy*, New York: Raven Press, pp. 495–534.

99. Derry CJ, Derry S, McQuay HJ, Moore RA (2006). Systematic review of systematic reviews of acupuncture published 1996–2005. *Clin Med* 6(4):381–386.

100. U.S. Food and Drug Administration (2010). Approved risk evaluation and mitigation strategies (REMS). Available at http://www.fda.gov/Drugs/DrugSafety/PostmarketDrugSafetyInformation forPatientsandProviders/ucm111350.htm

101. Muir, JC (2010). Opioid REMS—tension between two competing public health crises: under-treatment of pain versus increased opioid-related deaths in the United States. *AAHPM Bull* Spring, pp. 6–7.

Fatigue

Sriram Yennurajalingam, MD

Definition and prevalence

The National Comprehensive Cancer Network defines cancer-related fatigue as "a distressing, persistent, subjective sense of <u>physical</u>, <u>emotional</u>, and/or <u>cognitive</u> tiredness or exhaustion related to cancer or cancer treatment that is not proportional to recent activity and interferes with usual functioning. " From 48% to 85% of cancer patients report or experience fatigue, and fatigue is most severe near the end of patients' lives.[1,2]

Although fatigue is the most common and severe symptom that patients experience while receiving palliative care,[3] it is also the most underdiagnosed and undertreated.[4] Fatigue has substantial adverse physical, psychosocial, and economic consequences for patients and caregivers and is an important predictor of patients' quality of life.[3,4]

However, because of its subjective nature and multifactorial causes, assessing and treating fatigue in the palliative setting can be complex. In this chapter we review the definition and prevalence of fatigue, its causes, clinical evaluation, and treatment in palliative care settings.

Most of the evidence presented in this chapter relates to studies in cancer patients. However, similar principles can be applied to fatigue in patients with other disease.

Causes

Fatigue is a multidimensional syndrome, often with multiple contributing causes (Fig. 5.1). Studies have shown that fatigue is correlated with the severity of psychological symptoms (e.g., anxiety and depression), pain, sleep disturbances, dyspnea, anorexia, anemia, and opioid dose (if used).[2]

Pro-inflammatory cytokines

Pro-inflammatory cytokines can induce fatigue by affecting mood, muscle mass, cognition, and metabolic status.[5,6] These cytokines can be induced by disease process or its treatment and can trigger alterations of immune homeostasis by 1) changing proportions or activating certain subsets and/or 2) altering the expression and signaling of Toll-like receptors, thereby activating latent virus reactivation.

Inflammatory cytokines (specifically interleukin-6, interleukin-1β, and tumor necrosis factor-α) also induce disturbances in the hypothalamic–pituitary axis that affect corticotrophin-stimulating and adrenocorticotropic hormone levels, which in turn influence adrenocorticoid secretion.[6]

Anemia

Anemia causes fatigue in patients receiving cancer therapy, and treating anemia in these patients has been shown to reduce their fatigue and improve their quality of life.

However, as the severity of other contributing factors—anxiety and depression, pain, cachexia, drug side effects, inactivity, infections and hypogonadism–tends to increase progressively at the end of a patient's life, anemia's relative contribution to fatigue diminishes.[7]

Symptoms caused by cancer and its treatment

Various correlative studies have established fatigue's association with pain, dyspnea, anorexia, sleep disturbances, and psychological symptoms such as anxiety and depression.

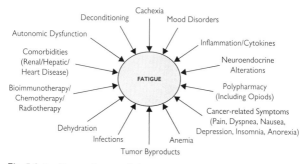

Fig. 5.1 Possible contributors to fatigue.

However, the intensity of an individual symptom in a given patient may determine its ultimate contribution to the cause of the patient's fatigue.[2]

Drug interactions

The combination of opioids and other medications (such as anticholinergics, antihistamines, anticonvulsants, neuroleptics, central α-adrenergic antagonists, beta-blockers, diuretics, selective serotonin reuptake inhibitors [SSRIs], tricyclic antidepressants [TCAs], muscle relaxants, and benzodiazepines) or the interaction between these medications may contribute to drowsiness and fatigue.

Clinical assessment

The clinical assessment of fatigue relies on complete evaluation in three areas: patient history, physical examination, and lab evaluation.[2,8]

Patient history

Characterizing the fatigue

A variety of clinical assessment tools, including 0–10 on visual analog scales, can be used to assess the intensity of a patient's fatigue, its onset and duration, and its effect on a patient's function and overall quality of life (Table 5.1).

However, one patient who presents with a fatigue score of 9 on a 0–10 scale may have fatigue caused mainly by anemia and cachexia, while another patient who presents with the same intensity may have fatigue caused primarily by depression.

Hence, using a simple Edmonton Symptom Assessment Scale or other multidimensional tool may help provide a more comprehensive assessment of a patient's fatigue.

Identifying possible causes and contributing factors

Patients should be evaluated for the following major reversible factors in fatigue: mood disorders (specifically depression and anxiety), cognitive disorders (dementia and delirium), pain, anemia, malnutrition, and deconditioning.

Other contributing factors may include sleep patterns, weight changes, infections, trauma, self-medication with over-the-counter drugs, prescription drugs, tobacco, alcohol, or illicit drugs, diet, and social changes (such as retirement).

Environmental assessment should be considered if necessary.

Physical examination

Physical examination should include an evaluation for orthostatic changes, an inspection of mucous membranes for pallor or icterus, and examination for lymphadenopathy, hepatosplenomegaly, murmurs, or bruits. A detailed neurological examination including an assessment of cognition should be performed.

Laboratory investigations

Laboratory investigations should include any blood tests and diagnostic imaging as suggested by the physical examination or history.[2]

Table 5.1 Fatigue assessment tools for patients with cancer or other conditions*

Measure/scale	Reliability (Cronbach coefficient)	Population base	Number of items	Comments
Multi-dimensional Fatigue Inventory	0.80 Validity (r ≤0.78)	Cancer patients receiving radiotherapy, patients with chronic fatigue syndrome, psychology students, medical students, army recruits, and junior physicians	20-item self-report instrument	Multidimensional scale including: general fatigue, physical fatigue, mental fatigue, reduced motivation and reduced activity
Multi-dimensional Assessment of Fatigue	0.93	Adults with rheumatoid arthritis, HIV, multiple sclerosis, coronary heart disease, or cancer	16 items, self-administered, 5 minutes	Subjective aspects of fatigue, including quantity, degree, distress, impact, and timing, are assessed
Multidimensional Fatigue Symptom Inventory (short form)	0.87–0.96	Patients with different types of cancer	30-item instrument	Global, somatic, affective, cognitive, and behavioral symptoms of fatigue
Revised Piper Fatigue Scale	0.85–0.97	Patients with cancer-related fatigue; or chronic hepatitis C infections	22-item measure	Multidimensional; assesses global fatigue severity to evaluate the efficacy of intervention strategies
Brief Fatigue Inventory	0.82–0.97	Cancer and cancer treatment	9 items, self-administered, 5 minutes	Severity and impact of fatigue on daily functioning in the past 24 hours

Fatigue Symptom Inventory	0.90	13 items, self-administered	Fatigue intensity and duration and interference with QOL in the past week
Functional Assessment of Chronic Illness Therapy – Fatigue (FACIT-F)	0.93–0.95 Test–retest reliability r = 0.87 over 3–7 days	Cancer and cancer treatment	41 items, self-administered or interview, 10 minutes	Multidimensional fatigue subscales of Functional Assessment of Cancer Therapy (FACT); assesses global fatigue severity and QOL
Edmonton Symptom Assessment Scale (ESAS) (Fig. 5.1)	0.79 Test–retest reliability 0.65	Elderly palliative care patients	Patients rate the severity of 9 symptoms, including fatigue (visual analogue scales); self-administered or interview, 5 minutes	Global fatigue severity
Profile of Mood States (vigor and fatigue)	0.89 Test–retest reliability r = 0.65	Cancer patients; patients with many other chronic conditions	8 items (vigor), 7 items (fatigue)	Global fatigue severity
Short Form-36-Version 1 Vitality (Energy/ Fatigue) Subscale	0.87	Adults with cancer and other populations	1–2 minutes for 4-item subscale	Vitality (energy level and fatigue)

*Reprinted with permission from Yennurajalingam S, Bruera E (2007). Palliative management of fatigue at the close of life: "It feels like my body is just worn out." *JAMA* 297:295–304. Copyright © (2009) American Medical Association. All rights reserved.

Management

Optimal fatigue management involves comprehensive symptom assessment and aggressive treatment of reversible causes, if possible (Fig. 5.2).[2] If the cause is not reversible or apparent, the fatigue should be treated symptomatically (Fig. 5.2).

Ideally, fatigue treatment should involve an interdisciplinary team with active participation by the physician, nurse, psychiatric counselor, social worker, chaplain, physical therapist, and occupational therapist, as appropriate.

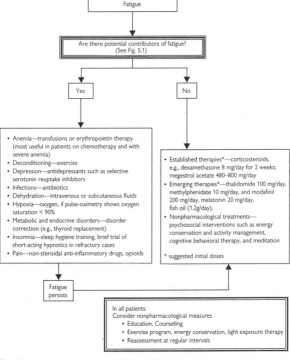

Fig. 5.2 Treatments for fatigue and its underlying causes.

Treatment of causes

Anemia

Anemia in palliative care patients is best managed by treating its underlying cause or (if the cause is not known) treating it symptomatically with transfusions of packed red blood cells.

Patients who receive repeated transfusions risk blood-borne infection, acute transfusion reaction, transfusion-associated graft-versus-host disease, subtle immune modulation that occurs with transfusion, and iron overload.

If repeated blood transfusions are not an option, recombinant human erythropoietin (rhEPO) therapy can help relieve fatigue and thus improve the quality of life in chronically anemic patients who have AIDS or end-stage renal disease or who are undergoing chemotherapy.

However, rhEPO therapy is expensive, and although treating anemia with rhEPO has been shown to decrease fatigue in patients receiving chemotherapy, concerns about the safety of rhEPO arose after several phase III studies showed increased mortality and thromboembolic complications in rhEPO-treated patients compared to controls.

Pain and opioid-induced neurotoxicity

Treating pain and opioid-induced neurotoxicity may benefit patients with chronic disorders and patients at the end of life. Successful management requires either reducing the opioid dose or administering a different opioid, as well as addressing other reversible precipitants such as dehydration. If opioid-induced sedation is persistent, a trial of methylphenidate may be helpful.

Because the combination of opioids and medications from different drug classes and the interaction of these medications may contribute to drowsiness and fatigue, it is appropriate to cease these medications or adjust their doses to reduce fatigue.

Depression

Antidepressants, counseling, and exercise can reduce the vegetative symptoms caused by depression. Clinical observations suggest that antidepressant therapy can increase energy levels without altering a patient's mood to the same degree.

Methylphenidate has been shown to reduce fatigue in cancer patients with depression. Counseling, and exercise are the other modalities of treatment that are found to be effective in the treatment of fatigue and depression in patients with cancer.[2]

Delirium and cognitive dysfunction

To successfully manage delirium and cognitive dysfunction, the physician must identify and correct the underlying reversible causes and the symptoms. Thus, the practitioner should evaluate the patient for opioid toxicity, dehydration, infection, medication interactions or adverse effects, metabolic disturbances, thyroid dysfunction, and anemia.

In an end-of-life setting, the intensity of the diagnostic workup and the treatment strategies for cognitive dysfunction and delirium must be individualized.

Weight loss

Fatigue and cachexia coexist in the great majority of patients with advanced cancer, and it is likely that malnutrition is a major contributor to fatigue. The inflammation in response to progressive cancer and loss of muscle mass resulting from progressive cachexia provide a reason for profound weakness and fatigue.

Treatment of fatigue as a symptom

Because of the complex nature of fatigue and limited number of randomized controlled studies that have been performed in the palliative care setting, there are few pharmacological options for effective fatigue treatment (Table 5.2). In this section, we review established drug therapies, investigational agents, and nonpharmacological treatment options.

Established pharmacological agents

Corticosteroids

Preliminary studies have shown that corticosteroids can reduce symptoms such as fatigue, pain, poor appetite, and nausea and improve the overall quality of life in patients with advanced cancer. It is unclear if there are any differences between types of corticosteroids, because dexamethasone appears to be the most intensively investigated.[2]

The overall adverse reaction profile of dexamethasone is well understood. It appears that the severity of most of its toxic effects is dose dependent. Side effects may include infection, oral thrush, insomnia, mood swings, myalgia, and elevation of blood glucose.

Prolonged use of dexamethasone (for more than 1 month) in some patients will cause gastritis (particularly if the patient is concurrently using nonsteroidal anti-inflammatory drugs [NSAIDs]), hiccups, edema, muscle weakness, easy bruising, dizziness, unusual hair growth, and slow wound healing.

Megestrol acetate

In randomized controlled trials, megestrol acetate (160–480 mg/day) increased appetite, activity levels, and overall well-being compared to placebo in anorexia patients with advanced cancer.

Megestrol is dosed orally, once daily. The response increases as the dose rises from 160 to 800 mg/day.

Investigational drugs

Psychostimulants

In patients receiving palliative care, fatigue and depression can be treated with psychostimulants such as dextroamphetamine and methylphenidate.

Psychostimulants act rapidly, are well tolerated, and are generally safe. However, they should be used with caution in patients with heart disease or cognitive disturbances (e.g., delirium).

The role of psychostimulants in management of fatigue in terminally ill patients needs to be defined further in randomized controlled trials.

Methylphenidate

In patients with cancer, methylphenidate has been effective against opioid-induced sedation, cognitive failure associated with brain tumors, and

Table 5.2 Medications for symptomatic treatment of fatigue at the end of life

Drug and indication	Initial dose	Side effects
Corticosteroids Disease-related fatigue (off-label use)	Dexamethasone: 8 mg/day for 2 weeks	Severity of most toxic effects is dose dependent. Adverse effects include infection, oral thrush, insomnia, mood swings, myalgia, and elevation of blood glucose. Prolonged use (>1 month): gastritis (especially with concurrent use of NSAIDs), hiccups, edema, muscle weakness, easy bruising, dizziness, hirsutism, and slow wound healing.
Methylphenidate Cancer-related fatigue (off-label use)	5 mg/day	Common adverse effects include loss of appetite, slurred speech, abnormal behavior, and restlessness. Serious adverse effects include hypertension, tachyarrhythmia, thrombocytopenia, and hallucinations.
Megestrol acetate FDA-approved treatment for cachexia in patients with AIDS and as a treatment for breast and endometrial cancer; also used for treating cancer-associated cachexia and anorexia (off-label use)	480–800 mg/day	Common adverse effects include hypertension, sweating, hot flashes, weight gain, dyspepsia, nausea, vomiting, insomnia, mood swings, and impotence. Serious adverse effects include thrombophlebitis, adrenal insufficiency, and pulmonary embolism.
Modafinil Fatigue related to cancer and multiple sclerosis (off-label use)	200 mg/day	Common adverse effects include diarrhea, nausea, dizziness, headache, insomnia, agitation, anxiety, nervousness, and rhinitis. Serious adverse effects include cardiac dysrhythmia, hypertension, and infectious disease.

depression. It stimulates the CNS by blocking presynaptic norepinephrine and dopamine reuptake.

Methylphenidate is usually administered orally twice a day, at breakfast and lunch, to minimize insomnia. Because of its rapid onset of action and short half-life, methylphenidate is effective at relieving fatigue. In an open-label study of 31 patients with advanced cancer who experienced fatigue, methylphenidate every 2 hours as needed significantly reduced fatigue.

In contrast, a randomized controlled trial of 112 patients with advanced cancer showed that although patients using methylphenidate plus nursing intervention and patients using placebo and the intervention both experienced a significant reduction in fatigue, there was no significant difference in improvements between the groups.

Modafinil

Modafinil, a psychostimulant, is an effective and well-tolerated agent used to treat excessive daytime sleepiness in patients with narcolepsy and other conditions such as Parkinson's disease and obstructive sleep apnea.

The exact mechanism of action is unclear; however, a recent preclinical house study implicated non-noradrenergic, dopamine-dependent adrenergic signaling in promoting wakefulness.

In a phase II study, patients with multiple sclerosis who received modafinil at 200 mg/day for 2 weeks experienced a significant reduction in their fatigue compared with patients who received placebo.

Nonpharmacological approaches

Exercise

Well-powered randomized controlled trials have demonstrated that exercise is the only effective nonpharmacological treatment for fatigue. Physical activity helps patients maintain their sense of well-being and enhance their quality of life.

Most palliative care patients experience multiple symptoms (e.g., fatigue, pain, dyspnea, and nausea) that may lead to diminished physical activity and thereby lead to deconditioning. Exercise rehabilitation during or after curative or palliative treatment is now considered an effective means of restoring patients' physical and psychological functioning.

For example, in a pilot study of 34 patients with incurable cancer a 50-minute, twice-a-week group exercise program improved patients' emotional functioning and reduced their physical fatigue.[2].

Psychosocial interventions

Psychosocial interventions have been found to be effective treatments for cancer-related fatigue. Randomized clinical trials have shown that both group and individual supportive interventions such as education and stress management groups, coping strategies training, and behavioral interventions can help cancer patients manage their fatigue.[9]

References

1. Lawrence DP, Kupelnick B, Miller K, et al. (2004). Evidence report on the occurrence, assessment, and treatment of fatigue in cancer patients. *J Natl Cancer Inst Monogr* 32:40–50.
2. Yennurajalingam S, Bruera E (2007). Palliative management of fatigue at the close of life: "It feels like my body is just worn out."*JAMA* 297:295–304.
3. Cella D, Davis K, Breitbart W, Curt G, for the Fatigue Coalition (2001). Cancer-related fatigue: prevalence of proposed diagnostic criteria in a United States sample of cancer survivors. *J Clin Oncol* 19:3385–3391.
4. Curt GA, Breitbart W, Cella D (2000). Impact of cancer-related fatigue on the lives of patients: new findings from the Fatigue Coalition. *Oncologist* 5:353–360.

5. Ahlberg K, Ekman T, Gaston-Johansson F, et al. (2003). Assessment and management of cancer-related fatigue in adults. *Lancet* 362:640–650.
6. Lee BN, Dantzer R, Langley K, et al. (2004). A cytokine-based neuroimmunologic mechanism of cancer-related symptom. *Neuroimmnomodulation* 11:279–292.
7. Munch TN, Zhang T, Willey J, Palmer JL, Bruera E (2005). The association between anemia and fatigue in patients with advanced cancer receiving palliative care. *J Palliat Med* 8:1144–1149.
8. Dittner AJ, Wessely SC, Brown RG (2004). The assessment of fatigue: a practical guide for clinicians and researchers. *J Psychosom Res* 56:157–170.
9. Wagner LI, Cella D (2004). Fatigue and cancer: causes, prevalence and treatment approaches. *Br J Cancer* 91:822–828.

Cachexia

Egidio Del Fabbro, MD

Definition

Cachexia is characterized by involuntary weight loss, regardless of caloric intake or appetite. Patients often experience a combination of muscle wasting, loss of body fat, and poor appetite, resulting in the cachexia–anorexia syndrome (CAS).

Cachexia should be distinguished from starvation and sarcopenia (see Table 6.1). However, all three conditions could be present to some degree in an individual

Cachexia may be found in many seemingly disparate conditions, including cancer, HIV, tuberculosis and malaria, rheumatoid arthritis, chronic obstructive pulmonary disease (COPD),[1] congestive heart failure,[2] chronic kidney disease, and liver failure.

Table 6.1 Distinguishing between cachexia, sarcopenia, and starvation*

	Starvation	Cachexia	Sarcopenia
Weight loss/BMI	↓↓	↓↓	↓/↔
Inflammatory markers (CRP and cytokines)	↔	↑↑	↑/↔/↓
Resting energy expenditure (REE)	↓↓	↑↑/↔/↓↑†	↑/↔/↓
Protein synthesis	↓↓	↓/↑↑‡	↓↓
Muscle/fat lossInsulin	↓/↓↓	↓↓/↓	↓/↔
Insulin	↓↓	↑↑	↔
Cortisol	↔	↑	↔
Effect of caloric intake on muscle mass	↑↑	↔	↔

*An individual patient may have components of all three conditions. Most patients with cancer cachexia are also sarcopenic, but most sarcopenic individuals are not considered cachetic.

†Cachexia patients may be hyper-, hypo-, or eumetabolic.

‡Increased acute-phase response proteins, decreased myosin (muscle)

↓ = decreased; ↔ = no change; ↑ = increased; / = and/or.

Mechanisms of cachexia–anorexia syndrome[3]

An aberrant inflammatory response is generated by the disease–host interaction. Cytokine-induced catabolism causes impaired synthesis and increased degradation of muscle and fat. Other disease-specific factors (e.g., lipid mobilizing factor in cancer) may also be involved (see Fig. 6.1).

There is also neurohormonal dysfunction. A loss of endocrine home-ostasis impairs anabolism and appetite. Abnormalities associated with the CAS include elevated cortisol levels, ghrelin and insulin resistance, low serum testosterone, and sympathetic activation.

Pro-inflammatory cytokines play a role in propagating these irregu-larities and alter hypothalamic sensitivity to orexigenic and anorexigenic peptides.

Exacerbating factors

Appetite loss experienced by many patients can be aggravated by symp-toms such as severe pain, nausea, early satiety, constipation, and depres-sion. Elderly or sedentary patients may have underlying sarcopenia and poor muscle reserves.

Deficiencies of particular substrates, such as amino acids and, L-carnitine, may also play a role.

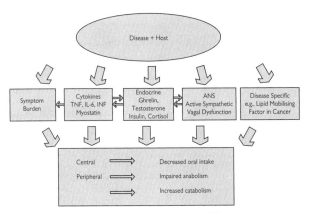

Fig. 6.1 Mechanisms of cachexia–anorexia syndrome. ANS, autonomic nervous system.

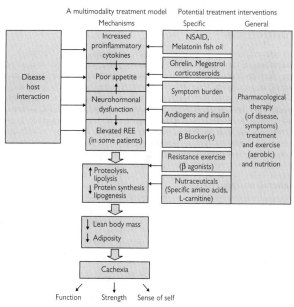

Fig. 6.2 Model of multimodality therapy directed at the mechanisms of cachexia.

Clinical assessment

Patient history

Patient history can be used to identify patients with involuntary weight loss of >5% within the past 6 months (if no prior weights are available). Ideally, these patients should be identified even earlier in the disease trajectory in order for interventions to produce the greatest impact.

Prior comorbid conditions such as endocrine abnormalities (hyper- or hypothyroidism, adrenal insufficiency, diabetes) and vitamin deficiencies (vitamin B_{12}, vitamin D) need to be determined.

Symptoms contributing to decreased oral intake are also important factors. A symptom assessment tool such as the Edmonton Symptom Assessment Scale (ESAS) can be used to identify symptoms such as pain, depression, and nausea. Additional factors may include early satiety, oral ulcers, dental problems, dry mouth, and dysphagia

Patient goals are crucial in determining the choice of therapy. For most patients, an improvement in strength and function is the goal. Others may want an improved appetite above all, to enjoy meals with family and friends. For some, body image and psychosocial issues may be more important, since cachexia is a very visible manifestation of illness.

Examination

Muscle wasting is often readily apparent but may be disguised in patients who were obese prior to their illness.

Body mass index (BMI = body weight divided by height in kg/m^2) is not useful in evaluating body composition or lean body mass.

Monitor the impact of therapy with relatively low-burden tests, such as arm muscle area[4]:

$$(\text{mid-arm circumference [MAC] in centimeters}) - \pi \times \text{tricipital skin fold thickness [in millimeters]})^2 / (4 \times \pi)^{5,6}$$

minus a correction factor of 10 for men and 6.5 for women.

Electrical bioimpedance analysis (BIA) can conveniently measure fat-free mass (FFM). The fat-free mass index (FFMI = FFM divided by height in kg/m^2) is especially useful in patients with COPD. Edema affects the accuracy of BIA.

Dual energy X-ray absorptiometry (DEXA) and computerized tomographic (CT) scanning for measuring muscle mass are possible in the research setting

Physical strength and function

- These should be assessed for longitudinal follow-up.
- Choose tests that are least burdensome to the patient.
- Use a 6-minute walk or 50-meter walk for assessing an intervention's impact on endurance.
- Use a hand-grip dynamometer and sit-to-stand for assessing strength.

Investigations

These depend on the history and exam, but could include all of the following.

Laboratory
- Complete blood count (CBC) to monitor polycythemia/anemia (androgen replacement, anti-inflammatory use)
- Electrolytes, creatinine, BUN, and glucose
- Calcium—hypercalcemia produces poor appetite and fatigue
- Liver function tests
- C-reactive protein (CRP)—consider immune modulation therapy if >5 mg/L
- Vitamin B_{12}, folate, vitamin D
- Thyroid-stimulating hormone (TSH) for hypothyroidism (especially in the elderly and after radiation for head and neck cancer), monitor replacement therapy
- Testosterone—early morning, preferably bioavailable (free and weakly bound). Decreased levels common in COPD, HIV, and cancer cachexia (75%)
- Cortisol—early morning (<3 mcg/dL is diagnostic, >18 mcg/dL is normal, mid-range requires additional tests of dynamic adrenal function)
- Albumin has prognostic value particularly in renal-failure cachexia.

Radiology
- Abdominal X-ray to evaluate for mechanical obstruction (cancer) or severe constipation

Metabolism
- Indirect calorimetry, if possible
  - Resting energy expenditure (REE) and caloric needs are more accurately measured, and hypermetabolic patients are identified. (hypermetabolic >110% of predicted REE as per Harris–Benedict Equation)

Treatment

Nutrition

The ideal goal of 34 kcal/kg/day or 1.5x REE may not be realistic[7] depending on the patients' condition. Usually, frequent small meals that are calorie dense are advised.

Counseling by a dietician can help with increasing caloric intake but does not necessarily improve clinical outcomes.

Specific amino acids given in patients with HIV and cancer cachexia (arginine-, glutamine-, and leucine-related products) increased lean body mass in two small placebo-controlled trials.[8,9]

Antioxidants and polyphenols have been used in open-label combination therapy for cancer cachexia.

Omega-3 oils used in short placebo-controlled trials to treat cancer cachexia had no benefit. Physical activity may increase, and high doses improve appetite, but GI side effects are problematic.

Symptoms and conditions contributing to poor appetite

- Oral—poor dentition, infection, mucositis, xerostomia
- Dysgeusia—trial of zinc for 2 weeks
- Nausea—5HT3 antagonists, metoclopramide
- Early satiety—metoclopramide
- Pain—opioid, NSAIDs
- Depression—tricyclic antidepressants, mirtazapine
- Constipation—laxatives
- Dysphagia—endoscopic intervention, enteral and parenteral nutrition if starvation is a large component of the weight loss
- Treat conditions contributing to CAS (see lab investigations)

Drugs for cachexia

No single pharmacological intervention is consistently effective for treating CAS. Multiple medications have demonstrated benefit in small trials.

Most cachexia treatments probably have some activity against the disease as well as independent anti-cachexia actions.

Some disease-specific drugs, e.g., beta-blockers for congestive heart failure (CHF), could modulate the mechanisms of cachexia in other conditions such as hypermetabolic cancer cachexia.

Conventional drugs

Corticosteroids are effective for multiple symptoms (poor appetite, fatigue, nausea) in the short term. Prolonged use increases the risk of infections and myopathy. They may be best for the last 2 months of life.

With megestrol acetate treatment, appetite increased in 50% and weight gain (predominantly fat /fluid) in 30%. Benefit was shown in patients with cancer, HIV, or COPD. The risk of thromboembolism is dose dependent and increases with chemotherapy. Hypogonadism and hypoadrenalism may require replacement therapy.[10]

Investigational drugs
- Cannabinoids are no better than placebo for cancer cachexia[11] but improve appetite in HIV patients. They may be more effective at higher doses but are limited by side effects.
- NSAIDs are given alone or combined[5] with appetite stimulants for cancer cachexia. Ibuprofen in combination with megestrol increased lean mass in patients with solid tumors. Celecoxib as part of multimodality therapy was also effective in small open label trials.
- Melatonin was effective in preventing and treating cancer cachexia in open-label trials. No double-blind, placebo–controlled trials have been conducted.
- Beta-blockers, angiotensin-converting enzyme (ACE) inhibitors, and angiotensin II receptor blockers (ARBs) are the standard of care for CHF and may be useful in other conditions, e.g., cancer cachexia.
- Androgens (testosterone, oxandrolone, nandrolone) have shown benefit in small trials of HIV, COPD, and possibly cancer cachexia.
- Muscle anabolism—beta agonists, myostatin inhibitors in the future
- Thalidomide is useful in HIV, tuberculosis, and preliminary cancer cachexia trials.[3]
- Ghrelin and ghrelin mimetics may be of benefit in treating cachexia in cancer, COPD, and CHF. Their safety needs to be established in cancer patients.
- Growth hormone is used for HIV cachexia. Patient tolerance may be a problem.
- Parenteral nutrition is used when starvation is a major component, the tumor is slow growing, and there is >6 weeks' survival.

Exercise

There is preliminary evidence of greater muscle strength with resistance training in patients with sarcopenia, chronic renal insufficiency, rheumatoid arthritis, HIV, or COPD.

Outcomes

Effective therapies should (ideally) achieve all of the following:
- Increased lean body mass
- Improved function (activities of daily living [ADL], see functional tests)
- Increased appetite
- Weight gain

Prognosis
- Weight loss >5% (CHF, HIV)
- BMI <20
- CRP >10 mg/L
- Hypoalbuminemia(renal cachexia)
- Combination in cancer cachexia may be more accurate[6]: weight loss ≥10%, CRP ≥10 mg/L, food intake ≤1500 kcal/day

What families and patients need to know

Many patients and families believe poor appetite and weight loss are the most burdensome issues they face. Unfortunately, their concerns are seldom addressed by health-care providers.

Opening a dialogue with patients and their families may resolve family conflict, increase confidence in health-care providers, and avoid unnecessary interventions. Explaining the mechanisms of cachexia without medical jargon may help families appreciate that increased caloric intake will not necessarily result in muscle gains or functional improvement.

An understanding of this counterintuitive concept could help avoid unnecessary enteral or parenteral supplementation and relieve pressure on patients perceived as not trying "hard enough" to eat.

Clinical pearls

- A pro-inflammatory state is likely the dominant mechanism causing muscle wasting.
- Frequently used medications such as corticosteroids and megestrol are associated with dose-dependent side effects.
- C-reactive protein levels are useful for diagnosis and prognosis
- Multimodality therapy (including pharmacological, nutritional, and exercise interventions) should be considered.
- Nutritional issues are important to patients and their families and need to be addressed (even when therapeutic options are not available or indicated).

References

1. Schols AM, Broekhuizen R, Weling-Scheepers CA, Wouters EF (2005). Body composition and mortality in chronic obstructive pulmonary disease. Am J Clin Nutr 82(1):53–59.
2. von Haehling S, Lainscak M, Springer J, Anker SD (2009). Cardiac cachexia: a systemic overview. Pharmacol Ther 121(3):227–252.
3. Baracos VE. Cancer-associated cachexia and underlying biological mechanisms. Annu Rev Nutr. 2006;26:435–461.
4. Gordon JN, Trebble TM, Ellis RD, Duncan HD, Johns T, Goggin PM (2005). Thalidomide in the treatment of cancer cachexia: a randomized placebo controlled trial. Gut 54(4):540–545.
5. Mantovani G, Madeddu C, Gramignano G, Serpe R, Massa E, Deiana L, Macciò A (2007). An innovative treatment approach for cancer-related anorexia/cachexia and oxidative stress: background and design of an ongoing, phase III, randomized clinical trial. Support Cancer Ther 4(3):163–167.
6. Fearon KC, Voss AC, Hustead DS (2006). Definition of cancer cachexia: effect of weight loss, reduced food intake, and systemic inflammation on functional status and prognosis. Am J Clin Nutr 83(6):1345–1350.
7. Hutton JL, Martin L, Field CJ, Wismer WV, Bruera ED, Watanabe SM, Baracos VE (2006). Dietary patterns in patients with advanced cancer implications for anorexia–cachexia therapy. Am J Clin Nutr 84(5):1163–1170.
8. Clark RH, Feleke G, Din M, Yasmin T, Singh G, Khan FA, Rathmacher JA (2000). Nutritional treatment for acquired immunodeficiency virus-associated wasting using beta-hydroxy beta-methylbutyrate, glutamine, and arginine: a randomized, double-blind, placebo-controlled study. JPEN J Parenter Enteral Nutr 24(3):133–139.
9. May PE, Barber A, D'Olimpio JT, Hourihane A, Abumrad NN (2002). Reversal of cancer-related wasting using oral supplementation with a combination of beta-hydroxy-beta-methyl-butyrate, arginine, and glutamine. Am J Surg Apr 183(4):471–479.
10. Dev R, Del Fabbro E, Bruera E. (2007). Association between megestrol acetate treatment and symptomatic adrenal insufficiency with hypogonadism in male patients with cancer. Cancer 110(6):1173–1177.
11. Strasser F, Luftner D, Possinger K, Ernst G, Ruhstaller T, Meissner W, Ko YD, Schnelle M, Reif M, Cerny T (2006). Comparison for orally administered cannabis extract and delta-9-tetrahydrocannabinol in treating patients with cancer-related anorexia-cachexia syndrome: a multi-center, phase III, randomized, double-blind, placebo-controlled clinical trial. J Clin Oncol 24(21):3394–3400.

Dehydration

Shalini Dalal, MD

Introduction

The vast majority of patients in the terminal phase of their illness experience severely reduced oral intake before death, which may arise due to a variety of causes related to their diagnosis or its treatment.

Commonly experienced symptoms such as decreased appetite, nausea and vomiting, bowel obstruction, dysphagia, cognitive impairment, and depression predispose to deficits in fluid status, which in turn can lead to distressful symptoms (such as confusion, fatigue) and/or death. See Figure 7.1.

In this chapter, we offer recommendations for an individualized approach in the management of fluid deficits in terminally ill patients that is based on symptom burden, patient and family preferences, and goals of care.

Fluid homeostasis

Fluid homeostasis is dependent on the maintenance of a relatively constant and stable composition of body fluids. It is achieved in normal individuals by matching daily water intake to fluid losses from the body.

In normal, healthy adults, water constitutes approximately 60% of total body weight (TBW) in men and 55% in women. This amount declines with aging, with shifts in body composition resulting in a 10%–15% of total body water.

Water in the body is in a constant state of motion, shifting between the various fluid compartments of the body. Two-thirds of the total body water is present in tissue cells. The remaining third is present as extracellular fluid and is divided between the plasma (intravascular compartment) and interstitial compartment.

The amount of these fluids is highly variable, and these compartments are generally ignored when considering body fluids.

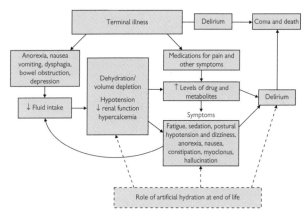

Fig. 7.1 Theoretical model of the effects of fluid deficits in terminally ill patients and the role of parenteral hydration on symptom distress and delirium.[2]

Dehydration

Classically, the medical literature has distinguished two forms of total body water fluid loss: 1) dehydration, which refers to a loss of body water mainly from the intracellular compartments, and 2) volume depletion, referring to a loss of extracellular fluid clinically affecting the vascular tree and interstitial compartment.

Dehydration can be defined as a complex condition resulting in a reduction in total body water. This can be due primarily to a water deficit (water loss dehydration) or both a salt and water deficit (salt loss dehydration).

In most cases, dehydration is due to disease and/or the effects of medication and not primarily due to lack of access to water. Clinically, it cannot be defined by a single symptom, sign, or laboratory value.[1]

The fluid requirement in terminal patients may be less; however, they are at an increased risk of fluid deficit, often precipitated by minor variations in fluid intake, infections, and other conditions.

Many patients are elderly, with renal and neurohormonal functions deteriorated by age and thereby not as effective as in younger individuals. The thirst mechanism diminishes with age, significantly impairing the ability of the elderly to maintain homeostasis and increasing the risk for dehydration. An age-related decrease in maximal urinary concentrating ability further increases the risk for dehydration.

Symptoms

Fluid deficits may cause cognitive impairment, altered behavior, decreased energy level, confusion, delirium, fainting, or syncope. A confused patient may be a danger to self or at risk for falls, or have aberrant behavior with paranoid delusions or hallucinations. They can also appear significantly distressed to their caregivers.

Studies noting a high prevalence of thirst and dry mouth in patients with advanced cancer have failed to show an association between these symptoms and biochemical markers of fluid deficit or dehydration.

Dry mouth can be alleviated by simple measures such as oral care, small sips of water, and lubrication.

Persistent subclinical dehydration is associated with anxiety, panic attacks, and agitation. Fluctuation in tissue hydration results in inattention, hallucinations, and delusions. Severe dehydration leads to somnolence, psychosis, and unconsciousness.[1]

Mechanisms include increased local cytokine production, glutamate toxicity, mitochondrial dysfunction, altered pharmacokinetics of drugs, and increased anticholinergic burden.[3]

Assessment of hydration status

Initial assessment
Determine the presence of fluid deficits.

History
- Urine output, third spacing, hemorrhage
- Cognitive impairment
- Altered behavior
- Constipation

Physical examination
- Dry mucous membranes,
- Reduced skin turgor
- Sunken eyes
- Dry axillae
- Postural hypotension, tachycardia, increased capillary refill time
- Cyanosis, mottling, reticulation

Laboratory
Clarification of the goals of treatment is important prior to ordering laboratory tests, as some may not be useful in determination of treatment.
- Increased plasma protein
- Increased hematocrit
- Increased sodium
- Increased blood urea nitrogen and serum creatinine

Symptom effects
Determine the symptom burden (with use of multidimensional assessment tools). Determine the impact of symptoms on quality of life, patient and family distress, and function.
- Thirst and dry mouth are distressing symptoms for both the patient and family.
- Not exclusive to dehydration
- May be a consequence of medication, radiation, mouth breathing, or thrush

Determine benefits vs. burden of artificial hydration
- Hydration may be beneficial if cognitive changes, delirium
- May not be beneficial for symptoms of thirst or dry mouth
- Determine disadvantages (hospitalization, mobility, discomfort)

Determine patient and family preferences and goals
- Discuss both the benefits and burdens of hydration.
- Disclose uncertainties.
- Discuss a trial of hydration to assess benefit.
- Provide alternatives if hydration is not considered.
- Provide emotional support.
- Inform the patient and family that hydration can be ethically withheld and withdrawn.

If hydration is considered

• Consider hypodermoclysis.
• Administer appropriate volumes (<1000 mL/day).
• Consider discontinuation if there are no perceived benefits.

Intravenous

The traditional route for hydration has been intravenous (IV) and usually via a peripheral line. In some patients with terminal illness, central venous access devices (CVADs) are placed. These CVADs are associated with an increased risk of complications during placement as well as ongoing use.

Patients have an increased frequency of local infections and catheter associated bacteremia.[4] Management of these catheters can be a difficult option in the home care setting.

The IV route should be limited to situations where subcutaneous (SC) administration of fluids is contraindicated, such as in patients with generalized edema or major coagulation disorders or who already have an IV line or CVAD in place for other purposes.

Enteral

This route is indicated for any malnourished patient with a functional GI tract who is unable to orally ingest sufficient nutrients as long as access can be achieved safely. This route is simpler, safer, more physiologic, and less costly than parenteral.

Common indications include dysphagia due to head and neck cancer, esophageal obstruction, gastric outlet obstruction, or critical illness requiring prolonged mechanical ventilation.

The choice of access device is dependent on anticipated duration of use, the underlying pathophysiology and anatomy, patient preference, and local expertise. Nasogastric (NG) tubes are best for patients who require enteral support for less than 30 days.

Placement of a percutaneous feeding tube is indicated in patients who will require long-term support.

Hypodermoclysis

Hypodermoclysis is the infusion of fluids into the SC space and can be used in reference to medication infusion. Several recent studies in patients with terminal illness and for infusion of analgesics have demonstrated its safety, efficacy, and practical advantages over IV routes.[5]

Hypodermoclysis involves insertion of a butterfly needle subcutaneously and attaching a line for fluids to be administered via an infusion pump or gravity in the home setting. In ambulatory patients, the abdomen, upper chest, and area above the breast may be used as the SC infusion site. In bedridden patients, preferred sites are the thighs, abdomen, and outer aspects of the upper arm. These sites can be used for 5–7 days.[6]

Approximately 1 L of fluid is sufficient for a 24-hour period and allows for normal urine output and adequate hydration in most patients. In home settings these fluids can be administered via gravity at a rate of 1–2 mL per minute at one site, allowing up to 1.5 L in a 24-hour period. Patients can receive overnight infusions or several 1-hour boluses, which will allow for mobility and freedom from tubing for most of the day.[4]

Commonly administered electrolyte fluid solutions such as normal (0.9%) and half-normal (0.45%) saline, saline-dextrose combinations such as one-third saline with two-thirds glucose (5%), have been used in studies involving hypodermoclysis and can be safely administered.[7]

The use of nonelectrolyte solutions is not recommended for hypodermoclysis as they can cause sloughing of tissue, mostly in pediatric patients.

Rapid or large-volume SC infusion of electrolyte-free solutions can cause circulatory collapse. Side effects can include local skin irritation and occasional itching, site bleeding, and infection. Colloidal and hyperosmolar solutions should not be given.

Hypodermoclysis is contraindicated in patients with generalized edema or clotting disorders. Patients at increased risk of pulmonary edema should be treated with caution and monitored to prevent respiratory distress due to fluid overload.

The risks of hypodermoclysis are minimal when it is administered within accepted indications and guidelines.

Proctolysis

Proctolysis is the rectal administration of fluids. This is an alternative for patients who require hydration but are unable to receive it by another route. The procedure is invasive, requiring insertion of a catheter about 40 cm into the rectum.

Disadvantages include enema effect with maximal rates of infusion, leakage of fluids, and pain during insertion of catheter and infusion of fluids.

Clinical pearls

- Hydration may benefit symptoms of delirium, fatigue, and opioid neurotoxicity.
- Hydration may not be beneficial for symptoms of thirst or dry mouth.
- Hypodermoclysis is an excellent alternative to intravenous hydration because of its simplicity, low cost, and feasibility.

References

1. Thomas DR, Cote TR, Lawhorne L, et al. (2008). Understanding clinical dehydration and its treatment. *J Am Med Dir Assoc* 9:287–288.
2. Dalal S, Del Fabbro E, Bruera E (2009). Is there a role for hydration at the end of life?. *Curr Opin Support Palliat Care* 3:72–78.
3. Wilson MM, Morley JE (2003). Impaired cognitive function and mental performance in mild dehydration. *Eur J Clin Nutr* 57:S24–S29.
4. Dalal S, Bruera E (2004). Dehydration in cancer patients: to treat or not to treat. *J Support Oncol* 2:467–479.
5. Bruera E, Legris MA, Kuehn N, et al (1990). Hypodermoclysis for the administration of fluids and narcotic analgesics in patients with advanced cancer. *J Pain Symptom Manage* 5:218–220.
6. Sasson M, Shvartzman P (2001). Hypodermoclysis: an alternative infusion technique. *Am Fam Physician* 64:1575–1578.
7. Slesak G, Schnurle JW, Kinzel E, et al (2003). Comparison of subcutaneous and intravenous rehydration in geriatric patients: a randomized trial. *J Am Geriatr Soc* 51:155–160.

Anxiety and depression

Paul W. Walker, MD

Management of psychological symptoms including anxiety and depression

Introduction

Changes in mood and coping are expected when a devastating illness is being treated. How to best manage these concerns, and when to medicate the patient for depression and anxiety, are important questions for the clinician to consider.

Understanding the differences between the more typical adjustment reactions and major depressive disorder is important. *Adjustment reactions* occur with an acute stressor such as a diagnosis of a serious illness or with other setbacks such as recurrences or relapses. They may also occur in the late stage of disease when treatment is no longer effective.

The patient often reacts with increased anxiety or depression that fluctuates and is usually limited to a period of weeks. This is generally an acute emotional reaction to the stressor and improves with time and psychotherapeutic support.

Depression is a more serious disorder that requires careful attention to diagnosis and management.

It is important to note that depression is underdiagnosed and undertreated. A survey of patients receiving palliative care for cancer revealed that 60% of patients with major depressive disorder were not being treated with antidepressants.

Depression

Prevalence

Variable rates of depression are reported for patients in the palliative setting, ranging from 1.5 to 50%. In the past, studies focused on cancer patients, but other diseases are now coming under the purview of hospice and palliative care.

Of these non-cancer diseases, patients with myocardial infarction show a prevalence of depression of 16–23%. Patients with Alzheimer's disease, diabetes type 1 or 2, or Huntington's disease may have prevalence for depression as high as 32%. Those with Parkinson's disease or multiple sclerosis have prevalence rates as high as 50%.

A family history of depression is the most widely recognized risk factor. An inherited depression may have an earlier age at onset and manifest recurrences.

Females are more at risk, which may be due to genetic influences. Other risk factors include impaired functional status, poor social support, uncontrolled pain, and external stressors.

Malignancies that have been linked to depression include retroperitoneal tumors (e.g., pancreatic cancer), primary brain tumors, and head and neck cancers.

Medications that increase the risk of depression include interferon, interleukin, intrathecal methotrexate, vincristine, and steroids. Drug withdrawal can also be a precipitating factor.

Diagnosis

Depressed mood is a complex and heterogeneous problem that has multiple manifestations and etiologies (see Table 8.1). The clinician should not fall under the illusion that all such patients will present alike.

In the DMS-III to DMS-IV-TR, the classification for the most severe patients has been the term *major depressive disorder*. An episode with evidence of psychotic features is a severe form termed *psychotic depression*. Bipolar disorder is differentiated by an episode of mania.[1,2]

Conditions that do not meet the full definition of the syndrome include dysthymia, recurrent brief depression, minor depressive disorder, normal bereavement, and adjustment disorder with depressed mood.

The full syndrome requires presentation with five of nine symptoms occurring for 2 consecutive weeks. There must be a change from the patient's previous level of functioning, and one of the symptoms must be depressed mood or anhedonia (loss of pleasure or interest). These symptoms must be present most of the day, nearly every day, during this period. The other symptoms include weight loss or gain or decrease or increase in appetite, insomnia or hypersomnia, psychomotor agitation or retardation, fatigue, feelings of worthlessness or inappropriate guilt, diminished concentration or indecisiveness, and thoughts of death or suicide.

However, many serious illnesses or their treatments can be the cause of some of these symptoms. An example of this would be cancer, which in many cases causes weight loss, fatigue, and anorexia.

One approach to the assessment of depression in cancer patients is to substitute the somatic symptoms that can be influenced by the cancer with other psychological symptoms (such as hopelessness, social withdrawal, brooding, pessimism, depressed appearance, tearfulness, and lack of reactivity).

A single screening question ("Are you depressed most of the time?") has been found to be a brief, reliable screen in terminally ill cancer patients. Asking about suicidal thoughts and plans for self-harm is important for any patient being screened for depression.

Table 8.1 Features of major depression

Depressed mood
Diminished interest of pleasure (anhedonia)
(one of the above must be present)
Weight loss or weight gain
Insomnia or hypersomnia
Psychomotor agitation or retardation
Fatigue or loss of energy
Feelings of worthlessness or excessive guilt
Diminished ability to think or concentrate, indecisiveness
Recurrent thoughts of death or suicide

These questions have not been found to increase the risk of suicide as some clinicians may fear, but rather greatly aid the detection of a patient at suicidal risk and enable interventions to minimize occurrences.

It is helpful to destigmatize the question posed to the patient. The question could be phrased as follows: "It would not be unusual for someone in your situation to have thoughts of harming themselves. Have you had thoughts like that?"

Depression is a problem associated with all serious illnesses. Short periods of sadness are expected when dealing with the troubles that accompany a medical illness. However, when a depressed mood persists and becomes pervasive, together with other symptoms of major depressive disorder, the diagnosis needs to be considered to direct effective management.

Treatment

As with any other condition that has multiple etiologies, diagnosing the underlying cause results in the most successful outcome. Delving into the various physical, drug and treatment, and psychosocial and spiritual issues involved can help direct management specific to the patient.

Two main interventions are psychotherapy and antidepressant medication. While these may be used separately, their combined use may prove most effective.[1,2] Also, altering other factors that may be adversely affecting the patient, such as discontinuing highly toxic therapies, can markedly improve depression.

The vicious circle of pain and depression is important to consider when caring for palliative patients. Recognizing that chronic pain can cause depression may aid effective treatment by focusing on analgesic strategies alone. Also, recognizing the converse, that depression causes an increase in pain expression, is important.

Depression has been closely associated with somatization or "total pain." An important finding of a survey of palliative care patients was that fully 82.9% of participants with both depression and anxiety reported a moderate to extreme degree of global suffering resembling "total pain."

Supportive psychotherapy that allows expression of the patient's worries, fears, and concerns, as well as validating and supporting the patient, is the basis of psychotherapy for the seriously ill. Often it is the social worker, chaplain, or psychologist that is available and inclined to provide this. However, interested and experienced nurses, physicians, or other professionals can also be effective.

Most critical to effective psychotherapy is the importance of a "therapeutic relationship." This supportive relationship between the two individuals is more important than which particular type of therapy is employed.

An important aspect of counseling the very ill is re-establishing their autonomy through attempts to empower the individual. This is necessary, as the illness has often robbed the patient of basic abilities and freedoms as well as privacy. Attempts to listen, provide information, and allow patients as much control as possible over their treatment and care options, as well as their day-to-day living, are often very significant to the individual.

Establishing what the patient's goals and priorities are and developing strategies to work toward achieving them often results in effective empowerment of the individual.

Other types of psychotherapy that have been recommended include individual and group, cognitive-behavioral, family, interpersonal, and mindfulness-based therapy.

Newer developments by experts in the field of psycho-oncology include the development of meaning-centered (developed by Breitbart) and dignity psychotherapy (developed by Chochinov).[3] These therapies are often directed to those who have expressed a desire for death or existential distress.

Meaning-centered group therapy is based on the principles of Viktor Frankl's logotherapy and deals with issues of sustaining meaning and hope in the context of illness and impending death.

Dignity psychotherapy focuses on bolstering the patient's sense of purpose, meaning, and worth. The concern that nothing in one's life will transcend death is approached through a life-review process that is intended to develop a sense of legacy.

Therapy with antidepressant medication is the mainstay of treatment for major depressive disorder (see Table 8.2). The selective serotonin reuptake inhibitors (SSRIs), serotonin-norepinephrine reuptake inhibitors (SNRIs), and psychostimulants are most frequently used because of their more tolerable side-effect profiles.

Since few psychiatric studies have focused on the palliative population, those in the general population have been used as a basis for treating

Table 8.2 Commonly used antidepressants

Generic (trade name)	Therapeutic daily dosage (mg)
Selective serotonin reuptake inhibitors (SSRIs)	
Citalopram (Celexa)	10–60
Escitalopram (Lexapro, Cipralex)	10–20
Fluvoxamine (Luvox)	50–300
Paroxetine (Paxil, Seroxat)	10–60
Sertraline (Zoloft, Lustral)	25–200
Combination agents (serontonin/noradrenergic)	
Mirtazapine (Remeron)	15–45
Venlafaxine (Effexor)	37.5–225
Duloxetine (Cymbalta)	40–60
Psychostimulants	
Methylphenidate (Ritalin)	5–30
Dextroamphetamine (Dexedrine)	5–30

depression in palliative care. Historically, clinical trials have shown that virtually all antidepressant strategies have similar efficacy in addressing major depression. Thus approaches to drug choice are based on either choosing agents with side effects that would benefit the patient or minimizing the risk of drug interaction.[3]

More recently, a large meta-analysis challenges this approach.[4] Although this study may not be generalizable to the palliative population, it reports that mirtazapine, escitalopram, venlafaxine, and sertraline were significantly more efficacious than duloxetine, fluoxetine, fluvoxamine, paroxetine, and reboxetine. Escitalopram and sertraline showed better acceptability, leading to fewer discontinuations than with duloxetine, fluvoxamine, paroxetine, reboxetine, and venlafaxine. The authors concluded that important differences exist among these antidepressants in terms of efficacy and acceptability, in favor of escitalopram and sertraline.

Also of note is that both of these drugs have fewer drug interactions via the cytochrome P450 system than most other agents.

Side effects of the SSRIs are commonly nausea, sleep disturbance, headache, and sexual dysfunction. The SNRI venlafaxine has been reported to cause more nausea and vomiting than that with the SSRIs. Mirtazapine has been linked to weight gain; trazodone to somnolence; sertraline to diarrhea; paroxetine and venlafaxine to discontinuation syndrome; and paroxetine to more sexual dysfunction and bupropion to less dysfunction.

Fluoxetine is not favored because of its long half-life. The onset of antidepressant effect with these medications is often after a minimum of 2–3 weeks, with 4–6 weeks being a typical trial period.

Psychostimulants such as methylphenidate and dextroamphetamine have the benefit of a more rapid effect, which may be particularly important for patients with a short life expectancy. These agents are usually taken in the morning and mid-day so as to not interfere with sleep.[5]

Combining psychostimulants with an SSRI or other antidepressants may be a useful strategy, especially in severely depressed or suicidal patients. With all medications, it is recommended that one start with a low dose and increase it gradually, especially considering the fragile nature of this population.[6]

For patients who are not improving despite treatment, there are other options. Increasing the dose of the initial antidepressant, switching to a different drug, augmenting it with agents that increase the effectiveness of the antidepressant, or combining antidepressants may be tried.

The assistance of a psychiatrist is helpful at this stage. Patients who present serious suicidal risk require increased clinician diligence. Verbally contracting with the patient to contact the clinician prior to any harmful actions is useful.

It is also judicious to ask family members to remove excess medications or weapons (e.g., a gun) that could be used for suicide. Again, expert psychiatric assistance is beneficial in these situations.

Bereavement and complicated grief

Family members and caregivers are at risk for bereavement throughout the illness but also especially following the patient's death. It is estimated that an average of 5 persons are left bereaved following each death.

Risk factors for a more difficult bereavement include a sudden or unexpected death, a perception of the patient suffering from pain or other symptoms, a stigmatized death (e.g., AIDS, suicide), substance abuse, psychiatric disorder, and dysfunction within the family. An important complication can be the development of bereavement-related major depressive disorder.

Another serious condition termed *complicated grief* occurs in approximately 10 to 20% of bereaved individuals. This condition shares similarities with and differences from major depression and posttraumatic stress disorder (PTSD).

It can be diagnosed 6 months after the death, by administering the Inventory of Complicated Grief. Important features include 1) a sense of disbelief regarding the death; 2) anger and bitterness over the death; 3) recurrent pangs of painful emotions, with intense yearning and longing for the deceased; and 4) preoccupation with thoughts of the loved one, often including distressing intrusive thoughts related to the death.

Avoidance behaviors are often part of this condition. This disabling condition leaves individuals in a protracted difficult mourning, unable to lead productive or enjoyable lives. The diagnosis of complicated grief can co-occur with major depression or PTSD, with rates as high as 50%.

Studies show that complicated grief does not respond to treatment for bereavement-related depression.

Innovative research by Katherine Shear[7] has produced a therapy that borrows from cognitive–behavioral therapy for trauma and PTSD. Similar to PTSD therapy, periods of re-experiencing the trauma of the loved one's death in a controlled way are an important part of the therapy. A randomized trial has shown that this complicated grief treatment produced higher response rates and faster times to response than the standard interpersonal psychotherapy.

Anxiety

Prevalence and diagnosis

Uncomfortable fear or apprehension is understandably common in terminally ill patients. *Anxiety* is a term that includes many different presentations and multiple causes. It is estimated that the prevalence of anxiety in the individual with cancer is in the range of 25%.

This problem often occurs as an "adjustment disorder with anxiety" or "adjustment disorder with mixed anxiety and depressed mood" commonly triggered by the breaking of bad news. Patients may have prior conditions such as generalized anxiety disorder, panic disorder, or phobias that increase their experience of anxiety during their illness. An example of this is claustrophobia, a common difficulty exacerbated by the requirements of MRI imaging.

Agitated depression can present with symptoms of anxiety. In cancer patients, a mix of anxiety and depressive symptoms is found to occur more frequently than anxiety alone.

Not surprisingly, anxiety often increases with progression of disease and worsening of physical health.

Medical complications such as sepsis, pulmonary embolism, and other acute problems do induce apprehension. Poor control of pain or dyspnea, and drug withdrawal states also incur anxiety. Adverse drug reactions also need to be considered.

A common side effect of metoclopromide is akathisia. This is an extrapyramidal syndrome that can occur with dopamine antagonists and causes patients to feel as if they cannot sit still. The ambulatory patient is often seen pacing; the bed-bound individual is more difficult to diagnosis. Both can have their presentation misinterpreted as being due to emotional distress. Patients with agitated delirium may be misdiagnosed as having anxiety or pain if a careful assessment for cognitive failure is not undertaken.

More commonly, lucid individuals have normal fears and worries related to death or existential issues. Issues around death usually relate to concern about separation from family and the future well-being of family members.

Financial and legal issues can also be important at this time. Also, fear about worsening pain or other symptoms may preoccupy the patient. Existential issues may focus on loss of autonomy and meaning.

Over the course of a prolonged illness, individuals suffer multiple losses of their normal health. This may result in difficulty coping with their new restrictions and loss of the life they used to enjoy. Important questions to ask may be "What is your biggest fear, or what things worry you now?"

Treatment

Determining the likely etiology of the patient's anxiety and addressing it is the most fruitful approach. Too often the reflex reaction of the clinician is to simply add an antianxiety medication without a careful evaluation of the underlying causes, resulting in needless side effects.

Excellent communication skills are needed to listen empathically to the patient's story and concerns. This is time well invested, as patients often feel that they have not had their concerns heard. Taking time to address issues and answer questions may be all that is required.

Commonly, questions related to the present status of the disease and to the benefits and complications of possible treatments remain troubling and undiscussed. A catharsis of emotion may be necessary for healing.

Do not be afraid of this happening; come prepared to supply tissues to catch the tears. Taking the time to open effective communication is the first and most important step.

If the physician is unable to do this, other team members, such as the chaplain or social worker, may serve in this role. Individuals skilled in relaxation techniques and guided imagery can aid the patient in new ways to handle anxious feelings.

Family meetings are an important intervention, as the patient does not live in isolation but is usually closely connected to family members. Addressing openly the worries, concerns, and fears of the patient and family members helps to break down the "conspiracy of silence" that so often accompanies a family's adaptation to serious illness. More functional communication may result. Addressing the family members' anxiety may also result in a less anxious patient.

Pharmacological treatment of anxiety needs to be considered carefully.[6] Benzodiazepines may be necessary for patients who have profound symptoms related to anxiety, including pervasive worry, insomnia, and autonomic hyperactivity.

However, the many concerns about these agents' use in the frail terminally ill need to be considered, including their predisposition to causing sedation, delirium, falls, and disturbance of normal sleep pattern, as well as inducing tolerance.

A careful assessment of the risks and benefits of such treatment is needed as well as consideration for discontinuing the drug after a course of initial management. Shorter-acting benzodiazepines, such as lorazepam or alprazolam, are less likely to cause toxicity.

Commonly, doses of lorazepam are 0.5–2.0 mg tid–qid po or IV. Doses of alprazolam are 0.25–2.0 mg tid–qid po. If frequent breakthrough anxiety occurs or concerns such as depersonalization or derealization are present, then a longer-acting benzodiazepine such as clonazepam may be useful; doses are typically 0.5–2.0 mg po bid–qid.

For patients with agitation related to delirium, management with a neuroleptic such as haloperidol, chlorpromazine, or olanzapine is preferable. These agents may also be preferred for individuals with anxiety who are deemed fragile and at risk for delirium secondary to administration of a benzodiazepine.

For patients with panic attacks that are frequent and severe, administering both a benzodiazepine and an SSRI provides immediate treatment with the sedative while waiting for the SSRI to become effective, which usually takes 2–3 weeks. Treatment of anxiety related to uncontrolled pain or dyspnea with a strong opioid is standard management.[6]

Clinical pearls

- Asking about suicidal thoughts is an important part of assessing depression.
- Psychotherapy is an important modality for treating depression and adjustment reaction.
- Pain and depression can function in a vicious cycle, one causing the other.
- Complicated grief occurs in 10–20% of bereaved individuals and requires specialized treatment.
- Excellent communication skills help in managing anxiety.

References

1. Skakum K, Chochinov HM (2005). Anxiety and depression. In MacDonald N, Oneschuk D, Hagen N, Doyle D (Eds), Palliative Medicine—A Case-Based Manual. New York: Oxford University Press, pp. 97–110.
2. McClement SE, Chochinov HM (2009). Depression. In Walsh D, Caraceni AT, Fainsinger R, Foley K, et al. (Eds). *Palliative Medicine*. Philadelphia: Saunders-Elsevier, pp. 865–870.
3. Breitbart W, Chochinov HM, Passik D (2004). Psychiatric symptoms in palliative medicine. In Doyle D, Hanks G, Cherny N, Calman K (Eds), *Oxford Textbook of Palliative Medicine*. New York: Oxford University Press, pp. 746–771.
4. Cipriani A, Furukawa TA, Salanti G, et al. (2009). Comparative efficacy and acceptability of 12 new-generation antidepressants: a multiple-treatments meta-analysis. *Lancet* 373:746–758.
5. Wilson KG, Chochinov HM, Skirko MG, et al. (2007). Depression and anxiety disorders in palliative cancer care. *J Pain Symptom Manage* 33(2):118–129.
6. Qaseem A, Snow V, Denberg TD, et al. (2008). Using second-generation antidepressants to treat depressive disorders: a clinical practice guideline from the American College of Physicians. *Ann Intern Med* 149:725–733.
7. Shear K, Frank E, Houck PR, et al. (2005). Treatment of complicated grief, a randomized controlled trial. *JAMA* 293(21):2601–2608.

Sleep disturbance

Marvin Omar Delgado Guay, MD
Sriram Yennurajalingam, MD

Introduction

Sleep is a fundamental physiological process that performs a restorative function for the brain and body. It improves energy and the sense of well-being, and for persons living with cancer, sleep provides respite from physical discomfort and psychological stressors.[1-3]

Disturbances in both sleep architecture and circadian factors account for the majority of sleep disturbances encountered in the context of cancer.[4]

Sleep disturbances constitute a significant source of distress for patients with cancer as they move through the course of treatment and advanced illness.[1-3] Sleep disturbance results in decline in cognitive function, inability to engage in work or recreational activities, and reduced quality of life.[1-4] It is extremely important to identify, recognize, and properly manage these sleep disturbances in order to reduce suffering and improve the quality of life of our patients (see Box 9.1).

This chapter focuses on the impact of sleep disturbances in patients with cancer and other advanced illness and on the appropriate assessment and management of these sleep disturbances.

Box 9.1 Assessment and management of sleep disturbances in patients with advanced cancer

Assess

a. Characterize the sleep complaint intensity using a scale from 0 to 10, and characterize the type and duration of the sleep disturbance with the use of sleep diaries and logs, e.g., difficulty initiating sleep, recurrent nocturnal awakenings.
b. Take a comprehensive history, perform an exam, and use objective measures such as actigraphy and polysomnography as indicated to rule out common causes:
   1. Cancer-related symptoms, including pain, delirium, anxiety, depression, nausea and vomiting, and dyspnea
   2. Side effects of medications, including corticosteroids; psychostimulants, such as modafinil methylphenidate (short and long acting), caffeine, and herbal remedies; antihypertensives, including diuretics and benzodiazepines; and medication withdrawal from alcohol, sedative hypnotics, or opioids
   3. Issues affecting the sleep–wake cycle, such as polyuria, nocturia, and disruption in normal schedule, e.g., multiple hospital admissions, poor sleep hygiene
   4. Conditions affecting sleep—brain metastasis, sleep apnea, restless leg syndrome, heart failure, severe COPD

Treat

Interdisciplinary approach

a. Treat the underlying symptom and/or cause.
b. Symptom management using a combination of pharmacological and nonpharmacological approaches should be explored if the primary cause cannot be treated.

Pharmacological treatments

- Consider use of hypnotics on an individual basis but only for short-term use.
- Consider issues such as drug interaction, drug pharmacokinetics and pharmacodynamics, drug side-effect profile, tolerance, addiction, and dependency.

Nonpharmacological treatments

- Sleep hygiene
- Cognitive-behavioral therapy
- Muscle relaxation training
- Biofeedback
- Supportive brief psychotherapy

Sleep disturbance and cancer patients

Patients living with cancer can experience significant disruptions of the normal behaviors and physiology that lead to restful sleep.[1,4] Behaviors of cancer patients that disrupt the sleep cycle include spending more time in bed, reduced daytime activity, and mental stimulation.[1,5]

Cancer patients also have a higher probability of being hospitalized or institutionalized, worsening the sleep disturbance.[6]

The prevalence of sleep disturbances in patients living with cancer ranges from 24% to 95%.[1,4,7] This wide range in percentages reflects the use of different definitions of *insomnia* in assessment tools.

According to the International Classification of Sleep Disorders[8] and the *Diagnostic and Statistical Manual of Mental Disorders*,[9] the diagnostic criteria for insomnia syndrome include difficulty initiating sleep (greater than 30 minutes to sleep onset) and/or difficulty maintaining sleep (greater than 30 minutes nocturnal waking time); the presence of sleep difficulty at least 3 nights per week, and sleep difficulty that causes significant impairment of daytime functioning.[4,7–9]

One of the major factors that affect sleep quality in patients living with cancer is the presence of poorly controlled symptoms, especially pain. Patients with pain can experience difficulty with sleep onset and sleep maintenance.[1,4,7]

Psychosocial distress, such as depression[10] and anxiety,[11] also plays an important role in the development of sleep disturbances in patients with cancer.[1,4]

The most commonly reported sleep disturbance is frequent waking.[12,13] Forty-four percent of patients surveyed reported trouble achieving sleep, and one-third of patients reported waking for extended periods of time (35%) or waking too early (33%).[14]

More than half of patients (52%) attributed their sleep disturbance to "intrusive thoughts" and 45% attributed their sleep disturbance to physical discomfort.[1,14]

Silberfarb et al.[15] reported that patients with lung cancer stayed in bed significantly longer than other groups. These patients reported poorer sleep efficiency and more difficulty falling asleep and staying asleep than either patients with breast cancer or normal sleepers.

Women with breast cancer who have completed chemotherapy have lighter sleep, less deep sleep, less REM sleep, and lower sleep efficiency compared to normal sleepers.[4,16] In addition, the presence of hot flashes in breast cancer patients is associated with a higher percentage of wake time, lower percentage of stage 2 sleep, and less efficient sleep compared to nights with no hot flashes.[17]

When the patients receiving hospice care were queried, 70% reported difficultly sleeping, and frequent waking was the most common problem.[18] Interestingly, these patients receiving hospice care reported more than 60% of uncontrolled symptoms.

In another study, Mercadante et al.[19] showed that 30% of patients in an inpatient palliative care unit had insomnia (reported as less than 5 hours of sleep per night). These patients had difficulty with early waking, and waking and falling asleep were associated with fewer hours of sleep. In that study, the presence of depression and anxiety as also associated with insomnia.[19]

Sleep disturbance has a negative impact on quality of life.[20] The presence of sleep deprivation heightens the physical, psychological, social, and existential suffering of cancer patients.[20]

It also contributes to diminished coping capacity and exacerbates symptoms, such as pain and discomfort, and increases the perception of illness severity.[20] Furthermore, the patient's family members also experience these symptoms of distress.[21]

Assessment of sleep disturbances

Insomnia is underreported; Engstrom et al.[22] showed that only 16% of cancer patients with sleep disturbances reported their problem to health-care providers. Thus, objective measures of sleep disturbance and enhanced questioning by caregivers is necessary.

Objective measurement of sleep disturbances

It is important to assess sleep disturbances and identify related factors and symptoms associated with them.

There are several tools used to evaluate sleep disturbances, one being the Edmonton Symptom Assessment System (ESAS),[23] which assesses multiple symptoms. The ESAS has been widely used in the clinical setting[23] and has been validated for use in patients with advanced cancer.[24] It consists of 10 questions, rated on a scale of 0 to 10, that evaluate a mix of psychological and physical symptoms, which may include sleep disturbance as an "other symptom."

In addition to the ESAS, it is also very important to evaluate for the presence of delirium, which can be related to insomnia in patients with advanced illnesses.[1]

One of the most frequently used tools to evaluate sleep disturbances is the Pittsburgh Sleep Quality Index (PSQI).[25] It is an effective instrument to measure the quality and patterns of sleep.

This instrument enables differentiation of "poor" from "good" sleep through measurement of seven areas: subjective sleep quality, sleep latency, sleep duration, habitual sleep efficiency, sleep disturbances, use of sleeping medication, and daytime dysfunction over the last month. The patient self-rates each of the seven areas of sleep.

The scoring of the answers is based on a 0 to 3 scale, and the seven component scores are added to obtain a global score ranging from 0 to 21. A global sum of 5 or greater indicates a "poor" sleeper.

The PSQI can be used for both an initial assessment and ongoing comparative measurements across all health-care settings. The PSQI has an internal consistency and a reliability coefficient (Cronbach's alpha) of 0.83 for its seven components.[25]

However, because of its length and its relatively complex scoring, it may be difficult to use the PSQI in the clinical setting, particularly in palliative care patients who also require frequent assessments of many other symptoms such as pain, delirium, dyspnea, and fatigue.

Another method for measuring sleep disturbances is an actigraph. It is a simple, noninvasive device approximately the size of a watch that is worn on the wrist. It is used to measure levels of daytime and nighttime activity that can be used to accurately estimate the duration of both daytime and nighttime sleep.

Activity data are stored to memory, typically in 30- to 60-second epochs for 24-hour intervals. These data provide diurnal activity counts, nocturnal activity counts, and the means by which to infer sleep continuity parameters, for example, time in bed (sleep period), time awake after sleep onset, total sleep time, and, potentially, sleep latency.

Once uncontrolled symptoms are identified it is important to treat them properly to reduce suffering in these distressed patients. We will address several methods for treating sleep disturbances in cancer patients in the next section.

Management of sleep disturbances

The management of sleep disturbances, as in the case of fatigue, requires a multimodal approach, including pharmacological (Table 9.1) and non-pharmacological interventions. However, research on the efficacy of any specific modality in patients at the end of life is limited.

Table 9.1 Pharmacological management of sleep disturbances in patients with advanced illnesses

Activity	Initial dose	Considerations
Ultra-short acting		
• Zaleplon	5–10 mg	Little to no anxiolytic effect; costly
Short-onset, brief duration		
• Triazolam	0.125 mg	Rapid sleep induction; limited effect on sleep maintenance
• Alprazolam	0.5–1 mg	
Short-onset, intermediate duration of action		
• Zolpidem	5–10 mg	No clear advantage over benzodiazepines; costly; minimal anxiolytic effect
• Zopiclone	5–7.5 mg	
• Eszopiclone	3 mg	
Intermediate onset, duration		
• Lorazepam	0.5–4 mg	Adequate effect on sleep induction and maintenance; risk of daytime drowsiness
• Temazepam	7.5–15mg	
Longer latency to onset, prolonged activity (half-life, metabolites)		
• Clonazepam	0.5–2 mg	Slow sleep induction with increased risk of accumulation of metabolites; high risk of daytime sedation
• Chlordiazepoxide	50–100mg	
• Diazepam	5–10 mg	
Longer latency to onset, prolonged activity (off-label treatment for insomnia)		
• Amitryptilene	25–100 mg	Increased risk of daytime sedation, confusion, constipation, and cardiac conduction abnormalities
• Imipramine	25–100 mg	
• Doxepin	25–100 mg	
• Trazodone	25–100 mg	
• Mirtazapine	15–30 mg	Start with 15 mg at bedtime.
Variable activity (off-label treatment for insomnia)		
• Haloperidol	0.5–5 mg	Used mainly in sleep disturbance related to delirium or psychosis
• Risperidone	0.5–1 mg	
• Olanzapine	5–10 mg	
• Quetiapine	25 mg	

Pharmacologic management

Benzodiazepines

Benzodiazepines are used because of their sedative properties to reduce the time to sleep onset and to improve sleep efficiency. Unfortunately, tolerance to these medications occurs rapidly and their prolonged use can cause sleep disturbances, such as fragmented sleep and dependence on medication for sleep onset.[26]

Despite their effect on sleep patterns and architecture, agents acting at on the gamma-amino-butyric acid/benzodiazepine receptor, such as zaleplon and zolpidem, do not have a clear clinical advantage for cancer patients with sleep disturbances.[27]

In addition, several side effects have been observed with benzodiazepines, such as daytime sedation, delirium, and fatigue, particularly in the elderly and in those with impaired processing of the medications.[26,27]

Furthermore, benzodiazepines have the potential to exacerbate respiratory suppression when combined with opioids, as has been described with methadone, even at a low dose.[28]

Antidepressants

Antidepressants are the first choice if the patient presents with major depression complicated by insomnia. It is important to mention, however, that data on the use of most of these antidepressant agents for primary insomnia is not compelling.[29]

Some antidepressants, especially tricyclics, have been used in persons with neuropathic pain or headache disorders with insomnia.[30] Antidepressant medications can produce desirable side effects, such as sedation, but can also produce undesirable side effects, such as orthostasis, constipation, and anticholinergic activity. In addition, tricyclic antidepressants are associated with the development of cardiac arrhythmias.[29]

Data on the use of antidepressants for sleep disorders is described below.

Selective serotonin reuptake inhibitors (SSRIs) do not have a role in the treatment of insomnia other than depression-related insomnia, because of their very low sedating effects.[1]

The serotonergic antidepressant, trazodone has been used for insomnia related to depression because of its sedative and hypnotic effects. However, there are no conclusive data evaluating the minimum effective dose for treating sleep disorder.[31]

Mirtazapine, another antidepressant, acts on different receptors, including serotonin and histamine receptors. It is sedating, can stimulate appetite, and is less toxic than other antidepressants.[32,33]

Antihistamines do not have a role in the treatment of insomnia associated with cancer because of their side-effect profile, which includes cognitive impairment, delirium, and constipation.[1]

There are limited data regarding the safety and efficacy of alternative or complementary agents, such as valerian root, kava, and melatonin. Melatonin has demonstrated some usefulness in primary insomnia in persons with sleep disturbances secondary to a "phase-shift" disruption of the sleep cycle,[1] although it has not been studied in advanced cancer patients with insomnia.[1]

Paltiel et al.[34] reported that cancer patients with sleep disturbances taking tranquilizers and sleeping pills had poorer quality of life and increased severity of physical symptoms when compared with cancer patients who were not taking those medications.

Antipsychotic medications have an important role in managing insomnia in patients with delirium,[35] a common and distressing disorder that affects the advanced-cancer population.[1]

Nonpharmacological management

Nonpharmacological interventions, such as *cognitive-behavioral therapies, sleep hygiene,* and *muscle relaxation* have been demonstrated to be effective in the treatment of primary insomnia.[35–37] The use of these techniques in cancer patients is sometimes limited because of the progressive and debilitative illness and the amount of energy required to learn new behaviors.[1,38]

Another promising method used in the treatment of sleep disturbances in advanced cancer patients is bright light therapy.[39] Patients with advanced illnesses not only have disruption in the architecture of sleep but also alterations in the circadian rhythm, causing sleep disturbances. Thus, a light, which is the main stimulus for coordinating the circadian system with the external environment, may improve sleep disturbances in these patients.

Ancoli-Israel et al.[39] presented a preliminary report about the effect of bright light on sleep in 11 breast cancer patients receiving chemotherapy, concluding that bright white light may increase the number of hours of sleep in women undergoing chemotherapy, as well as decrease sleep latency and improve sleep quality. No side effects were reported in that study.

Bright light therapy also has been effective in sleep disturbances among demented nursing home patients.

Light therapy has also been used for the treatment of seasonal affective disorder and has some effect in nonseasonal depression.[40]

Nonpharmacological therapies demonstrate some advantages over pharmacological interventions in patients with sleep disturbances, including persistent efficacy and no risk of drug interactions or severe adverse effects, although behavioral treatments may have limited application in patients with advanced disease because of the time and energy required to acquire new skills.

Bright light therapy may improve the quality of life of cancer patients with sleep disturbances with minimal side effects and no medication interactions.

Clinical pearls

- Sleep disturbance is underreported and undertreated. Sleep disturbance affects the quality of life of patients with advanced illnesses and their caregivers and family members.
- A comprehensive evaluation of all symptoms related to sleep disturbances is extremely important.
- In the setting of sleep disturbances in advanced illnesses, always evaluate for the presence of delirium.
- When treating patients with sleep disturbances, it is very important to use a multimodal approach that includes both pharmacological and nonpharmacological interventions.

References

1. Mystakidou K, Parpa E, Tsilika E, et al. (2007). Sleep quality in advanced cancer patients. *J Psychosom Res* 62:527–533.
2. Zisapel N (2007). Sleep and sleep disturbances: biological basis and clinical implications. *Cell Mol Life Sci* 64:1174–1186.
3. Maquet P (2001). The role of sleep in learning and memory. *Science* 294:1048–1052.
4. Graci G (2005). Pathogenesis and management of cancer-related insomnia. *J Support Oncol* 3:349–359.
5. Morgan K (2003). Daytime activity and risk factors for late-life insomnia. *J Sleep Res* 12:231–238.
6. Sheely L (1996). Sleep disturbances in hospitalized patients with cancer. *Oncol Nurs Forum* 23,:109–111.
7. Fiorentino L., Ancoli-Israel S (2006). Insomnia and its treatment in women with breast cancer. *Sleep Med Rev* 10:419–429.
8. The International Classification of Sleep Disorders. Rochester, MN: American Sleep Disorders Association, 1997.
9. American Psychiatric Association (1994). *Diagnostic and Statistical Manual of Mental Disorders*, 4th ed. Washington DC: American Psychiatric Association.
10. Shuster JL Jr, Breitbart W, Chochinov HM (1999). Psychiatric aspects of excellent end-of-life care. Ad hoc committee of end-of-life care. The Academy of Psychosomatic Medicine. *Psychosomatics* 40:1–4.
11. Stark D, Kiely A, Smith A, Velikova G, House A, Selby P (2002). Anxiety disorders in cancer patients: their nature, associations, and relation to quality of life. *J Clin Oncol* 20:3137–3148.
12. Koopman C, Nouriani B, Erickson V, et al. (2002). Sleep disturbances in women with metastatic breast cancer. *Breast J* 8:362–370.
13. Savard J, Simard S, Blanchet J, Ivers H, Morin CM (2001). Prevalence, clinical characteristics, and risk factors for insomnia in the context of breast cancer. *Sleep* 24:583–590.
14. Davidson J, MacLean A, Brundage M, Schulze K (2002). Sleep disturbance in cancer patients. *Soc Sci Med* 54:1309–1321.
15. Silberfarb P, Hauri P, Oxman T, Schnurr P (1993). Assessment of sleep in patients with lung cancer and breast cancer. *J Clin Oncol* 11:997–1004.
16. Fiorentino L, Mason W, Parker B, Johnson S, Amador X, Ancoli-Israel S (2005). Sleep disruption in breast cancer patients post-chemotherapy. *Sleep* 28:A294.
17. Savard J, Davidson J, Ivers H, et al. (2004). The association between nocturnal hot flashes and sleep in breast cancer survivors. *J Pain Symptom Manage* 27:513–522.
18. Hugel H, Ellershaw J, Cook L, Skinner J, Irvine C (2004). The prevalence, key causes, and management of insomnia in palliative care patients. *J Pain Symptom Manage* 27:316–321.
19. Mercadante S, Girelli D. Casuccio A (2004). Sleep disorders in advanced cancer patients: prevalence and factors associated. *Support Care Cancer* 12:355–359.

20. Fortner B, Stepanski E, Wang S, et al. (2002). Sleep and quality of life in breast cancer patients. *J Pain Symptom Manage* 24:471–480.

21. Katz D, McHorney C (2002). The relationship between insomnia and health-related quality of life in patients with chronic illness. *J Fam Pract* 51:229–235.

22. Engstrom C, Strohl R, Rose L, Lewandowski L, Stefanek M (1999). Sleep alterations in cancer patients. *Cancer Nurs* 22:143–148.

23. Bruera E, Kuehn N, Miller MJ, Selmser P, Macmillan K (1991). The Edmonton Symptom Assessment System (ESAS): a simple method for the assessment of palliative care patients. *J Palliat Care* 7:6–9.

24. Chang VT, Hwang SS, Feuerman M (2000). Validation of the Edmonton Symptom Assessment Scale. *Cancer* 88:2164–2171.

25. Buysee DJ, Reynolds CF, Monk TH, Berman SR, Kupfer DJ (1989). The Pittsburgh Sleep Quality Index: a new instrument for psychiatric practice and research. *Psychiatry Res* 28:193–213.

26. Ohayon M, Lader M (2002). Use of psychotropic medication in the general population of France, Germany, Italy, and the United Kingdom. *J Clin Psychiatry* 63:817–825.

27. Drover D (2004). Comparative pharmacokinetics and pharmacodynamics of short-acting hypnosedadives: zaleplon, zolpidem, and zopiclone. *Clin Pharmacokinet* 43:227–238.

28. Corkery J, Schifano F, Ghodse A, Oyefeso A (2004). The effects of methadone and its role in fatalities. *Hum Psychopharmacol* 19:565–576.

29. Fava M, Hoog S, Judge R, Kopp J, Nilson M, Gonzalez J (2002). Acute efficacy of fluoxetine versus sertraline and paroxetine in major depressive disorder including effects of baseline insomnia. *J Clin Psychopharmacol* 22:137–147.

30. Sindrup S, Jensen T (1999). Efficacy of pharmacological treatments of neuropathic pain: an update and effect related to mechanism of drug action. *Pain* 83:389–400.

31. Saletu-Zyhlarz G, Abu-Bakr M, Anderer P, et al. (2002). Insomnia in depression: differences in objective and subjective sleep and awakening quality to normal controls and acute effects of trazodone. *Prog Neuropsychopharmacol Biol Psychiatry* 26:249–260.

32. Theobald D, Kirsh K, Holtsclaw E, Donaghy K, Passik S (2002). An open-label, crossover trial of mirtazapine (15 to 30 mg) in cancer patients with pain and other distressing symptoms. *J Pain Symptom Manage* 23:442–447.

33. Davis M, Khawan E, Pozuelo L, Lagman R (2002). Management of symptoms associated with advanced cancer: olanzapine and mirtazapine. A World Health Organization project. *Expert Rev Anticancer Ther* 25:288–291.

34. Paltiel O, Marzec-Boguslawska A, Soskolne V, et al (2004). Use of tranquilizers and sleeping pills among cancer patients is associated with a poorer quality of life. *Qual Life Res* 13:1699–1706.

35. Morin C, Colecci C, Stone J, Sood R, Brink D (1999). Behavioral and pharmacological therapies for late-life insomnia. *JAMA* 281:991–999.

36. Quesnel C, Savard J, Simard S, Ivers H, Morin CM (2003). Efficacy of cognitive-behavioral therapy for insomnia in women treated for nonmetastatic breast cancer. *J Consult Clin Psychol* 71:189–200.

37. Chesson A, Anderson W, Littner M (1999). Practice parameter for the non-pharmacologic treatment of chronic insomnia. *Sleep* 22:1128–1133.

38. Edinger J, Wohlgemuth W, Radtke R, Marsh G, Quillian R (2001). Cognitive behavioral therapy for treatment of chronic primary insomnia. *JAMA* 285:1856–164.

39. Ancoli-Israel S, Rissling M, Trofimenko V, Parker A (2007). Preliminary effects of bright light on sleep in women with breast cancer. *J Clin Oncol ASCO Annual Meeting Proc Suppl*, p. 9094.

40. Eagles J (2006). Light therapy and seasonal affective disorder. *Psychiatry* 5:199–203.

Chronic nausea and vomiting

Shalini Dalal, MD

Definition and prevalence

Chronic nausea and vomiting are common symptoms in patients with advanced-stage disease and significantly impact quality of life.[1] In advanced cancers, the reported prevalence is between 40% and 70%, depending on patient characteristics and assessment methods used.

There is no standardized definition for chronic nausea. For research purposes it is often defined as nausea lasting more than 4 weeks. In the terminally ill, however, the presence of nausea for more than 1 week, in the absence of a well-identified, self-limiting cause (e.g., chemotherapy or radiotherapy), is used.

Pathophysiology

The pathophysiology of chronic nausea and vomiting is complex. In the palliative care population, multiple mechanisms may be simultaneously involved in the generation of symptoms. Figure 10.1 illustrates the various pathways and centers known to be involved in the emetic pathway. These are briefly described below.

Two areas in the brainstem (medulla) are critical for the control of emesis: the vomiting center (VC) and the chemoreceptor trigger zone (CTZ). The VC, located in the lateral reticular formation of the medulla, is the physiological control center. It is not a discrete anatomic site, but represents interrelated neuronal networks, including the nucleus tractus solitarius (NTS) and the dorsal motor nucleus of the vagus (DMV).[2]

The NTS receives various afferent neuronal pathways, which include (1) cortical pathways from higher cortical centers, which respond to increased intracranial pressures, sensory (pain, sight, smell) and psychogenic (memory, conditioning, fear) stimuli; (2) vestibular pathways, which respond to vertigo and visuospatial disorientation; (3) peripheral pathways (via the vagus and splanchnic nerves) from the gastrointestinal (GI) tract, visceral capsules, and the parietal serosal surfaces; and (4) neuronal connections from the CTZ.

The CTZ, located in the area postrema of the medulla, also receives afferent input from the GI tract via the vagus and splanchnic nerves. Unlike the VC, the CTZ is functionally located outside the blood–brain barrier and is therefore able to sample emetogenic toxins, metabolic abnormalities, such as uremia or hypercalcemia, or drugs in the blood and spinal fluid. It cannot, however, initiate emesis independently and does so only via stimulation of the NTS.

Once the vomiting center (NTS) receives signals from the various afferent sources mentioned above, the information is processed and the DMV puts out an appropriate vasomotor efferent response (respiratory, salivatory, gut, diaphragm, and abdominal muscles) inducing nausea, retching, or vomiting, depending on the intensity and duration of received signals.

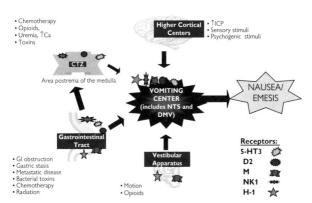

Fig. 10.1 Pathophysiology of nausea and vomiting. CTZ, chemoreceptor trigger zone; ICP, intracranial pressure; 5-HT3 serotonin; D2, dopamine; M, muscarinic/cholinergic; NK-1, neurokinin-1; H-1, histamine.

Etiology

Chronic nausea has many etiologies. Some of the more common ones are illustrated in Figure 10.2. In many patients, the underlying cause(s) may be difficult to determine.

Opioids are one of the most common causes of chronic nausea in terminally ill patients. Although opioid-induced nausea is usually transient and responds well to antiemetics, some patients, particularly those receiving high doses of opioids may continue to experience chronic and severe nausea. Other medications causing nausea include nonsteroidal anti-inflammatory drugs (NSAIDs) and antibiotics.

Delayed chemotherapy-induced nausea and vomiting (CINV) refers to symptoms that occur 24 hours after chemotherapy administration and that may last for as many as 6 to 7 days.

Patients with HIV may have nausea, which is a side effect of all the drugs of the antiretroviral therapy (ART) regimen.

Constipation is a common complication in terminally ill patients and may cause or aggravate nausea. Factors that predispose to the development of constipation include opioid analgesics, immobility, poor oral intake and dehydration, autonomic failure, and other medications.

The etiology of nausea may be related to the underlying disease. For instance, in cancer patients, nausea is often present in association with intra-abdominal disease, such as liver metastasis, bowel obstruction from mechanical compression by tumor, or peritoneal carcinomatosis.

The stomach and duodenum can be compressed, causing the "squashed-stomach syndrome." Nausea may be present secondary to primary or metastatic brain involvement by tumor or leptomeningeal disease. Radiation therapy to the spine or abdomen may be followed by nausea and vomiting.

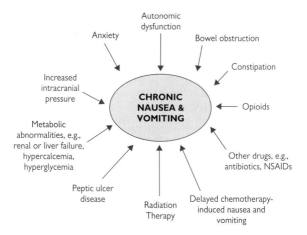

Fig. 10.2 Etiology of chronic nausea and vomiting.

Assessment

As nausea is a subjective symptom, its expression varies from patient to patient. From a practical point of view, this occasionally leads to a lack of correlation between the observed expression of nausea and the presumed pathophysiology of the underlying condition.

It is also important to note that the term *nausea* may mean different things to different people and be used by some patients to describe other symptoms, including abdominal discomfort, pain, distention, or early satiety.

There are a number of ways to assess nausea intensity, such as visual analog scales, numerical scales, and verbal descriptors, but there is no gold standard for nausea assessment. Because the causes of chronic nausea and vomiting are often multifactorial, the assessment needs to be multidimensional, with awareness that these symptoms are dynamic processes and may frequently change in intensity.

Further, it is important to assess the symptom of nausea in the context of other commonly experienced symptoms, such as pain, appetite, fatigue, depression, and anxiety. This multidimensional assessment allows formulation of an overall therapeutic strategy. An example of a validated multidimensional assessment tool is the Edmonton Symptom Assessment System (ESAS).[3]

A detailed history and physical examination is essential and may provide clues to the underlying etiology of symptoms (see Table 10.1). Intensity, frequency, exacerbating and relieving factors, onset, and duration of nausea should be documented. If there is coexistent vomiting, the nature and volume of vomiting can give a clue to the etiology.

Large-volume emesis may indicate gastric outflow obstruction, whereas small-volume emesis may indicate gastric stasis. The extent to which emesis interferes with oral intake should be noted, as large and frequent volume vomiting puts the patient at risk of dehydration. A history of syncopal episodes or early satiety should alert the physician of the possibility of autonomic insufficiency.

Investigations to exclude renal impairment, hepatic failure, and other metabolic abnormalities such as hypercalcemia, hypokalemia, and hyponatremia should be undertaken.

A computed tomography scan of the brain may be indicated when brain metastases are suspected. Abdominal X-rays may be useful in assessing nausea.

A supine X-ray may indicate the presence of stool and fecal impaction. Erect or decubitus views may show air and fluid levels in the bowel, which is typical of bowel obstruction.

Table 10.1 Clues from history and physical examination to the etiology of chronic nausea and vomiting

Findings on history and physical examination	Possible etiology
Pattern of infrequent large-volume vomitus that relieves nausea	Bowel obstruction—partial or complete Gastric outlet obstruction
Symptoms of nausea or vomiting related to movements	Vestibular dysfunction; mesenteric traction
History of polyuria and polydipsia	Hyperglycemia Hypercalcemia
Associated changes in mental status	Brain metastasis, metabolic abnormalities (examples: hyperglycemia, hypercalcemia, hyponatremia, renal failure, liver failure [elevated ammonia levels])
Papilledema	Raised intracranial pressure as with brain metastasis
Orthostatic blood pressures, absence of heart rate variability with valsalva, syncopal episodes	Autonomic insufficiency
Decreased frequency of bowel movements	Constipation
History of a mood disorder or anxiety	Anxiety
Medication/treatment history Chemotherapy or radiation Antibiotics; HIV medications	Treatment-specific syndromes (delayed chemotherapy-induced nausea and vomiting [CINV])
Epigastric pain, anemia; melena Use of NSAIDs	Peptic ulcer disease (use of NSAIDs or corticosteroids)
Distended abdomen, shifting dullness, fluid wave	Ascites
Distended abdomen, absent bowel sounds	Bowel obstruction

Management

Appropriate management of chronic nausea and vomiting depends on a detailed assessment. General supportive measures should be instituted in all patients. These include maintenance of good oral hygiene (poor oral hygiene can contribute to nausea), the creation of a comfortable environment for the patient, regular baths to prevent unpleasant body odors, and attention to diet.

Small volumes of food at regular intervals should be considered for patients with early satiety associated with nausea.

Specific interventions

When an underlying cause or causes of nausea and vomiting have been identified, there should be an attempt to correct these (Table 10.2). Metabolic abnormalities should be corrected if this is possible and appropriate for the clinic setting.

In situations where opioid toxicity is suspected, a change of opioids using equianalgesic doses can be expected to improve symptoms of nausea while maintaining pain control. Unnecessary medications should be discontinued.

Aggressive bowel care, including cleansing enemas and regular laxatives, should be instituted when constipation or stool impaction is suspected.

In some cases, such as in patients with brain metastases, symptom control may be attempted with radiation therapy or corticosteroids. If peptic ulcer disease is suspected, appropriate treatment should be instituted.

Pharmacological interventions

Given the lack of well-designed relevant studies, there are no convincing data for the best pharmacological strategy for treatment of nausea and vomiting. Current management is based on expert opinion rather than on

Table 10.2 Examples of specific interventions when the etiology of nausea and vomiting is known or suspected

Etiology	Intervention
Hypercalcemia	Hydration, bisphosphonates
Opioid toxicity	Opioid rotation or decrease dose
Constipation	Aggressive bowel regimen. Consider X-rays
Gastric ulceration	Proton pump inhibitors (PPIs), H2-antagonists
Infection	Antibiotics
Tense ascites	Paracentesis, consider intraperitoneal (IP) catheter
Anxiety	Counseling, anxiolytics
Brain metastases	Radiation therapy, steroids
Bowel obstruction	Conservative vs. surgical procedures (e.g., resection, bypassing, or stenting, venting gastrostomy)

evidence. Both mechanistic-based and empiric regimens have been used with no head-to-head comparisons of these approaches.

The various classes of antiemetics and their site of receptor action, if known, are presented in Table 10.3 and briefly discussed further. Important considerations in choosing an antemetic should be likely etiology and severity of symptoms, the drug's potential adverse effect, available routes of administration, and cost.

Dopamine antagonists

Agents from this group exert their antiemetic effects centrally (predominantly CTZ) by antagonizing dopamine (D2) receptors. These agents do not increase GI motility and so are useful in patients presenting with bowel obstruction. Drugs in this group differ on the basis of their additional activities.

Haloperidol is a narrow-spectrum agent, with mainly D2 antagonistic activity with negligible anticholinergic or antihistaminic effects. Its oral bioavailability is approximately 65%. It is highly protein bound and is not cleared by the kidney, making it safe in the presence of renal failure.

Initial doses range from 0.5 to 2 mg/mL, which can be given orally or parenterally at 4-hour intervals. When used subcutaneously, it is recommended that the concentration of haloperidol be kept below 1.5 mg/mL to avoid precipitation of haloperidol crystals.[4]

The broader-spectrum agents include chlorpromazine, prochlorperazine, and promethazine and have dopaminergic, cholinergic, and histamine receptor antagonism. Side effects may include extrapyramidal reactions, hypotension, urinary retention, constipation, dry mouth, and sedation.

Prochlorperazine has a low oral absorption (14%) and is usually administered via the rectal or parenteral routes. Promethazine has a slightly better oral bioavailability (25%) than that of prochlorperazine.

Table 10.3 Antiemetic agents

Class	Examples
Dopamine antagonists	MetoclopramideHaloperidol, prochlorperazine, chlorpromazine
Prokinetic agent	Metoclopramide
Antihistaminics	Diphenhydramine, meclizine, hydroxyzine, promethazine
Anticholinergics	Scopolamine (transdermal), hyoscyamine, glycopyrrolate
Serotonin antagonists	Ondansetron, granisetron, dolasetron
Cannabinoids	Dronabinol, nabilone
Corticosteroids	Dexamethasone, methylprednisolone
Other useful agents	Lorazepam, octreotide

Prokinetic agents

Metoclopramide hydrochloride, a substituted benzamide, has a dual mechanism of action. It is predominantly a dopaminergic antagonist but also has prokinetic effects via the cholinergic system in the myenteric plexus. Local acetylcholine release, mediated by the 5-HT4 receptor, appears to play an important role in reversing gastroparesis and bringing about normal peristalsis in the upper GI tract.

Because of its short half-life (3 hours), metoclopramide requires frequent administration via oral or parenteral routes. Continuous infusion of metoclopramide can be given when intermittent doses fails to control nausea.

Side effects include akathisia and extrapyramidal reactions (more likely in younger patients), which may not be dose dependent. Anticholinergic medications, including tricyclic antidepressants (TCAs), antagonize the prokinetic effect so should not be coadministered.

Antihistaminics

Antihistaminics, such as cyclizine, promethazine, and dimenhydrinate, are useful antiemetics, particularly if a vestibular component to the nausea is identified. Drowsiness is a major side effect.

Antimuscarinic/anticholinergic agents

This group includes tertiary and quaternary ammonium derivatives. Tertiary compounds such as atropine and scopolamine are lipophilic, cross the blood–brain barrier, and frequently cause sedation and confusion.

Glycopyrrolate, a quaternary compound, has little CNS penetration and is therefore preferred. Anticholinergics have been used to reduce symptoms of nausea and abdominal colic when they are associated with mechanical bowel obstruction.

Serotonin antagonists

These agents are widely used and effective in the management of chemotherapy- and radiotherapy-induced nausea and vomiting. In addition, they may also have a role in other situations, such as for refractory nausea in the palliative care setting, although more research is needed.

Trials comparing serotonin antagonists and metoclopramide have either had methodological problems or used inadequate doses of metoclopramide (e.g., 10 mg three times per day). There have been some reports of its effectiveness in treating patients' refractory nausea.

Neurokinin-1-receptor antagonists

In clinical studies, neurokinin-1 (NK-1) receptor antagonists have shown efficacy in reducing both acute and delayed CINV when added to other antiemetics.[5] The potential role of NK-1-receptor antagonists in the treatment of chronic nausea and vomiting in advanced cancer or other palliative care population is currently unknown.

Cannabinoids

The proposed mechanism of action of dronabinol is through brainstem cannabinoid receptors. Several studies have demonstrated its efficacy as an antiemetic agent for the treatment of CINV.

In a study of patients with AIDS-related cachexia, dronabinol showed significant improvement in nausea, appetite, and mood, without weight gain.[6] Side effects, such as somnolence, confusion, and perceptual disturbance, are common, particularly in the elderly. Euphoria is more common than dysphoria in younger patients.

Larger studies are needed to assess the value of cannabinoids as antiemetics in patients with advanced disease.

Corticosteroids

Corticosteroids have powerful nonspecific antiemetic effects that are not well understood. They may act by modulation of prostaglandin release. They can decrease peritumoral edema, thus reducing intracranial pressure, a known cause of nausea.

Corticosteroids are beneficial in combination with other antiemetic agents such as 5-HT3 antagonists or metoclopramide in the prevention and management of acute and delayed chemotherapy-induced emesis.[7] Corticosteroids are also useful in the management of other symptoms that may coexist with nausea in the palliative care population, such as pain, anorexia, and asthenia.

Nonpharmacologic interventions

Behavioral and complementary therapies

Much of the research on psychological and nonpharmacological interventions has been conducted in chemotherapy or postoperative patients.

Acupuncture and acupressure have been shown to augment the effect of antiemetics during chemotherapy and to reduce postoperative nausea and vomiting.

Transcutaneous electrical nerve stimulation (TENS) has also been shown to enhance the effect of antiemetic drugs. Its effects may be mediated by endogenous opioid peptides.

A meta-analysis of 19 randomized trials found equivalent benefit of nonpharmacological treatment of nausea in postsurgical patients compared to traditional therapy.[8] This benefit was not found in children. The modalities studied were acupuncture, electroacupuncture, TENS, acupoint stimulation, and acupressure.

Similar analysis has not been performed in patients with advanced disease. Other studies have included progressive muscle relaxation and guided mental imagery during periods of chemotherapy and have shown beneficial effects.

Cognitive therapy has been found to be effective in providing relief of psychological morbidity associated with physical symptoms in advanced cancer.[9] Adaptation of these techniques to palliative care patients with nausea warrants research.

Surgical interventions

In patients with nausea or emesis caused by mechanical obstruction, surgical procedures such as percutaneous gastrostomy for gastric outlet obstruction, colostomy, intestinal bypass, or laparotomy for obstruction (such as secondary to tumors or adhesions) may be considered for symptom control and to improve life expectancy and quality of life. This is provided the patient's general physical condition suggest a life expectancy long enough to result in benefit from surgery.

Based on current evidence, there is no consensus on the indications for conservative vs. surgical treatment of patients with advanced cancer. Thus, consideration for surgical interventions should be individualized, weighing risks and benefits of the procedure.

Even when patients appear to be candidates for surgical procedures, these procedures are associated with complications and may not be successful in relieving symptoms.[10] Published data show operative mortality ranging from 9% to 40% and complication rates from 9% to 90%.

Newer endoscopically placed stents for gastric outlet obstruction offer the advantage of lower cost, the possibility of an outpatient procedure, and low risk of complications.

Abdominal paracentesis or a permanent intraperitoneal catheter may be helpful in the patient with nausea and ascites that does not respond to conventional therapy.

Conclusion

Chronic nausea and vomiting are common and distressing symptoms in patients with terminal cancer. These symptoms are likely to be due to several factors, including autonomic failure, opioid analgesics, metabolic abnormalities, constipation, and cachexia.

Promotility agents (sometimes in combination with corticosteroids) are in most cases the drug of choice for management of chronic nausea and vomiting. Pharmacological agents, such as progestational drugs and thalidomide, need further evaluation of their potential beneficial effects in patients with chronic nausea.

Despite significant ongoing research of acute chemotherapy-induced and postoperative emesis, research is lacking for treatment of chronic nausea. Drugs that have been found to be effective in acute vomiting, such as serotonin and neurokinin-1-receptor antagonists, require further evaluation in advanced-cancer patients with chronic nausea.

References

1. Portenoy RK, Thaler HT, Kornblith AB, et al (1994). Symptom prevalence, characteristics and distress in a cancer population. *Qual Life Res* 3:183–189.
2. Carpenter DO (1990). Neural mechanisms of emesis. *Can J Physiol Pharmacol* 68:230–236.
3. Bruera E, Kuehn N, Miller MJ, et al (1991). The Edmonton Symptom Assessment System (ESAS): a simple method for the assessment of palliative care patients. *J Palliat Care* 7:6–9.
4. Storey P, Hill HH, St Louis RH, et al (1990). Subcutaneous infusions for control of cancer symptoms. *J Pain Symptom Manage* 5:33–41.
5. Hesketh PJ, Grunberg SM, Gralla RJ, ,et al. (2003). The oral neurokinin-1 antagonist aprepitant for the prevention of chemotherapy-induced nausea and vomiting: a multinational, randomized, double-blind, placebo-controlled trial in patients receiving high-dose cisplatin—the Aprepitant Protocol 052 Study Group. *J Clin Oncol* 2:4112–4119.
6. Beal JE, Olson R, Lefkowitz L, et al (1997). Long-term efficacy and safety of dronabinol for acquired immunodeficiency syndrome-associated anorexia. *J Pain Symptom Manage* 14:7–14.
7. Ioannidis, JPA, Hesketh, PJ, Lau J (2000). Contribution of dexamethasone to control of chemotherapy-induced nausea and vomiting: a meta-analysis of randomized evidence. *J Clin Oncol* 18:3409–3422.
8. Lee A, Done ML (1999). The use of nonpharmacologic techniques to prevent postoperative nausea and vomiting: a meta-analysis. *Anesth Analg* 88:1362–1369.
9. Greer S, Moorey S, Baruch JD et al (1992). Adjuvant psychological therapy for patients with cancer in a prospective randomized trial. *BMJ* 304:675–680.
10. Ripamonti C, Conno FD, Ventafridda V, et al. (1993). Management of bowel obstruction in advanced and terminal cancer patients. *Ann Oncol* 4:15–21.

Chapter 11

Constipation and bowel obstruction

Nada Fadul, MD
Zohra Nooruddin, MD

Bowel obstruction

Definition and prevalence

Bowel obstruction is a common and distressing complication of intra-abdominal cancer.[1] Impairment to the aboral passage of intestinal contents may result from either mechanical obstruction or failure of normal intestinal motility in the absence of an obstructing lesion (ileus).

Intestinal obstruction may be categorized according to the degree of obstruction to the flow of intestinal contents (partial or complete), the absence or presence of intestinal ischemia (simple or strangulated), and the site of obstruction (small intestinal or colonic).

The three most common causes of small bowel obstruction (SBO) are postoperative intra-abdominal adhesions, hernias, and neoplasms. In the palliative care setting, cancer is usually the underlying cause. Bowel obstruction is particularly common in patients with intra-abdominal malignancies.[1]

Malignant bowel obstruction (MBO) can lead to multiple distressing symptoms that require urgent palliative interventions. In a consecutive series of 163 patients referred with malignant ovarian tumors, 24 (14.7%) patients developed major bowel complications. In terminal patients with recurrent ovarian cancer, the incidence is estimated to be around 42%.

Once an MBO occurs, median survival is approximately 3 months.[2]

Causes

Malignant bowel obstruction is an odious complication of numerous malignancies, most notably ovarian and colorectal cancers. The two most common primary malignancies causing SBO in a series of 32 patients were colorectal (41%) and ovarian adenocarcinoma (28%).

Hematogenous metastases from breast adenocarcinoma, melanoma, or Kaposi sarcoma also may involve the intestine and can cause MBO.

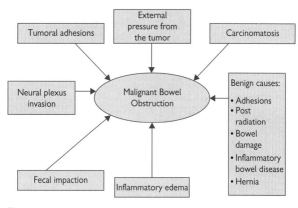

Fig. 11.1 Common causes of malignant bowel obstruction.

Primary neoplasms of the small bowel are the cause of SBO in less than 3% of cases. Both carcinoid tumors and adenocarcinoma have been reported as the most common malignancies of the small intestine to cause symptoms of obstruction.

Mechanisms of bowel obstruction in malignancy are illustrated in Figure 11.1.

Pathophysiology

Bowel obstruction results in an accumulation of gastric, pancreatic, and biliary secretions that are a potent stimulus for further intestinal secretions; reduced absorption of water and sodium from the intestinal lumen; and an increase in water and sodium secretion because of increased gastric distension. Depletion of water and salt in the lumen is considered the most important toxic factor in bowel obstruction.[3]

Intestinal obstruction causes the profound accumulation of fluid and swallowed air within the lumen proximal to the obstruction. Impaired water and electrolyte absorption and enhanced secretion cause the net movement of isotonic fluid from the intravascular space into the intestinal lumen. The accumulation of swallowed air and, to a lesser extent, hydrogen, carbon dioxide, and methane generated by bacterial overgrowth within the obstructed bowel contribute to intestinal dilatation.

The failure of normal intestinal motility with SBO allows the overgrowth of bacteria within the small intestine and loss of the normally increasing concentration gradient of bacteria from the jejunum to the ileum.

In one study using a porcine model of ileal obstruction, there was a 10,000-fold increase in the concentration of *Escherichia coli* in the ileum and a 40 million–fold increase in the jejunum over counts in normal controls. Data in humans and in animals suggest that the overgrowth of enteric bacterial flora occurs within a few hours of obstruction and is maximal by 24 hours.

Clinical presentation

The clinical picture of MBO can vary greatly from patient to patient, depending on the location of the obstruction, whether there are single or multiple points of obstruction, the mechanism of obstruction, exacerbating medications, and the extent and sites of tumor recurrence.[4]

The symptoms, which are almost always present, include nausea and vomiting, intestinal colic, and continuous abdominal pain.

Vomiting generally develops early in high intestinal-tract occlusion (gastric or duodenal and small bowel), whereas it occurs later in patients with large-bowel obstruction. Its frequency can be related to gastrointestinal (GI) involvement.

Abdominal colic is present in 72–76% of cases with advanced ovarian cancer and bowel involvement, and it this is usually due to bowel distension. Continuous abdominal pain is experienced by more than 90% of these patients.[2]

The absence of stool and flatus passage is a common symptom reported by patients, especially those with complete bowel obstruction. Patients with bowel obstruction can also suffer from diarrhea, which is caused by bacterial liquefaction. In palliative care patients, management of these symptoms can be challenging.

Diagnosis and clinical assessment

History and physical exam

The diagnosis of SBO requires a thorough assessment. It is usually established on clinical grounds and supported or confirmed by radiographic testing.

History of previous episodes and intra-abdominal surgery is highly suggestive of obstruction. The abdomen should be inspected for any surgical scars and the degree of distention.

Auscultation may reveal high-pitched or hypoactive bowel sounds and is therefore not very helpful in making a diagnosis.

Laboratory and imaging data

Laboratory investigations have a limited role in the diagnosis of SBO but can be help in the determination and management of metabolic and electrolyte abnormalities. Radiological examinations include an upright chest film to rule out the presence of free air, as well as supine and upright abdominal films.

Contrast X-rays may help in defining the site and the extent of the obstruction, including the accompanying dismotility. Barium provides excellent radiological definition, but it is not absorbed and may interfere with subsequent endoscopic procedures or cause severe impaction.

Gastrografin is preferable because it offers similar radiological definition. In some circumstances, it is useful in restoring the intestinal transit in reversible obstruction.

An abdominal CT scan is useful in evaluating the global extent of malignancy and aids in making therapeutic decisions regarding further treatment. CT findings of obstruction are similar to traditional radiographic findings: disparate dilation of proximal bowel loops compared with more distal ones.

Comparative studies have shown that CT is superior to plain-film radiography in detecting intestinal obstruction and in determining the cause of obstruction. Studies have shown CT sensitivities ranging from 90% to 95% in detecting obstruction, with no false-positive examinations.

Differential diagnoses

The differential diagnoses include the possibility of other causes of nausea and vomiting, constipation, and abdominal pain of other causes, including progressive intra-abdominal malignancy.

It is important to assess the possibility of metabolic abnormalities such as hypercalcemia or hypokalemia, the type and dosage of different medications that could have effects on intestinal motility, and nutritional and hydration status.[3]

Management

Symptom relief is the first aim of palliative care for these patients, although management of this situation is not well defined.

Surgical approach

Surgical palliation is a complex issue in patients with advanced cancer. The decision to proceed with a surgical approach should be individualized to the disease stage, patient's condition, and possibility of future antineoplastic therapy. Patients with a life expectancy of >2 months are more likely to benefit from surgery.

There are few possibilities for relieving a second episode of occlusion when a diagnosis of persistent or recurrent cancer is made. Therefore, the decision to proceed with a surgical approach should be individualized.

Surgery should not be routinely undertaken in patients with advanced and end-stage cancer who do not have a benign cause of occlusion. It will only benefit select patients with mechanical obstruction and/or limited tumor or a single site of obstruction and those with a reasonable chance of further response to antineoplastic therapy.

Nonsurgical approach

In inoperable patients, the usual treatment consists of drainage with a nasogastric tube associated with parenteral hydration. This treatment can cause great discomfort to the patient and a number of complications. Therefore, it should be considered a temporary measure to reduce the gastric distension while pharmacological treatment is initiated to control the amount of secretion and vomiting.

If continued drainage is required, a gastrostomy is much more tolerable for medium- and long-term decompression of the GI tract.

In patients with single-site colonic obstruction, the use of endoscopically inserted, self-expanding metallic stents is a rapid and effective nonsurgical means of relieving left-sided colonic obstruction.

Pharmacological measures

Several drugs have proved useful in controlling symptoms and avoiding use of a nasogastric tube, which leads to several complications, such as nasal cartilage erosion, aspiration pneumonia, otitis, esophagitis, and bleeding.

The main drugs used are analgesics, antiemetics, and drugs to decrease bowel secretions. Other agents commonly used include anticholinergic drugs, steroids, and smooth muscle relaxants such as atropine, scopolamine, and its analogs.[4]

Most patients with MBO cannot tolerate the oral route, so alternative routes should be considered for drug administration.

Opioids

Opioids are the most effective drugs for management of abdominal pain associated with bowel obstruction. These drugs can be administered subcutaneously, transdermally, or intravenously.

Anticholinergic drugs

Anticholinergic drugs such as scopolamine butylbromide or scopolamine hydrobromide can be added to opioids for colicky pain if the opioids alone are not effective.

Butylbromide and scopolamine have less penetration to the blood–brain barrier and thus have much fewer CNS side effects than those with other anticholinergic agents. Scopolamine and butylbromide can be given intravenously or subcutaneously.

Corticosteroids

Corticosteroids are used commonly in the medical management of MBO. They exert their effect through reducing intestinal and tumor-associated edema.

A recent systematic review of the role of corticosteroids in management of MBO in patients with ovarian and colorectal cancer showed evidence that corticosteroids in the dose range of 6–16 mg dexamethasone given intravenously may resolve bowel obstruction.[5]

Metoclopramide

Metoclopramide is the first-line antiemetic for patients with partial bowel obstruction in the absence of colicky pain. It is contraindicated in patients with complete obstruction because it might produce vomiting and pain due to its prokinetic activities.

Other pharmacological agents and antiemetics

Other pharmacological agents and antiemetics include neuroleptics such as haloperidol or prochlorprazine, or antihistamines such as dimenidrante or cyclizine. Haloperidol is considered the first-line antiemetic because it can be added to morphine and to scopolamine butylbromide or octreotide in the same subcutaneous (SC) infusion.

Somatostatin and its analogs (octreotide and vapreotide)

Somatostatin and its analogs have been used either alone or in combination to alleviate symptoms from an MBO in ovarian cancer and other malignancies. Somatostatin inhibits hormones such as glucagon and insulin, reduces acid secretion, slows intestinal mobility, decreases bile flow, and reduces splanchnic blood flow.

Among the antisecretory drugs, octreotide has been shown to reduce nausea and vomiting in bowel-obstructed patients through a reduction of GI secretions, thus allowing removal of the nasogastric tube and alleviation of associated distress in most patients.

Octreotide exerts actions similar to those of somatostatin, but it has a longer half-life and more potently inhibits growth hormone, glucagon, and insulin. Octreotide suppresses luteinizing hormone (LH) response to gonadotropin-releasing hormone (GnRH) and inhibits release of gastrin, secretin, vasoactive intestinal peptide (VIP), motilin, and pancreatic polypeptide. Its duration of action is 8–12 hours and it has been used successfully for management of MBO.

Octreotide can be administered by SC or IV infusion, or by bolus parenteral injection with duration of approximately 12 hours.

In a recent study of octreotide (300 mcg/day) used for bowel obstruction in 43 evaluable terminally ill cancer patients, the symptom score as evaluated by the M.D. Anderson Symptom Inventory improved in 59–72% of patients and overall quality of life improved in 56% of patients.[4]

Summary

Bowel obstruction is a distressing condition in patients in palliative care. Malignant bowel obstruction is the most common type. Symptom relief should be the fundamental focus of management in these patients. Surgical approaches have limited benefit in patients with MBO.

Pharmacological decompression is the mainstay of management. Some patients may require a temporary nasogastric tube or a long-term gastrostomy tube for decompression.

Constipation

Definition and prevalence

Constipation is a clinical syndrome, rather than a symptom. It is defined as infrequent or difficult defecation with reduced number of bowel movements, which may or may not be abnormally hard with increased difficulty or discomfort.[6]

Constipation is one of the most common complaints in the general population, the prevalence ranging from 1.9% to 27.2% (an average of 15% has been described in most studies). Constipation affects more than 50% of patients in a palliative care unit or hospice. This might actually underestimate the problem, since many of these patients are already on stool softeners and/or laxatives.

In clinical practice, constipation is defined using the Rome criteria: the presence of two or more of the following symptoms for at least 3 months:
- Straining at least 25% of the time
- Hard stools at least 25% of the time
- Incomplete evacuation at least 25% of the time
- Two or fewer bowel movements per week

Practically, these criteria might be difficult to apply in palliative care patients. In addition, there is a wide interindividual variability in normal bowel patterns. Therefore, constipation in an individual patient should be defined according to that patient's experience.

Causes of constipation in palliative care patients

In the palliative care population, the etiology of constipation can be related to the primary illness or secondary associated factors such as autonomic failure; drugs, especially opioids; dehydration; and electrolyte abnormalities.

Figure 11.2 illustrates the most common causes contributing to constipation in palliative care patients.

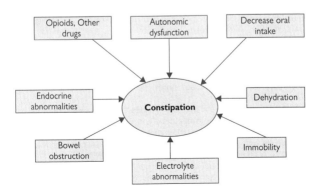

Fig. 11.2 Common causes of constipation in palliative care patients.

Primary causes
- Intestinal abnormality
- Tumor compression
- Neural plexus invasion
- Idiopathic constipation
- Slow-transition constipation
- Dyssynergic defecation

Secondary causes

Electrolyte imbalance
- Hypercalcemia
- Hyperkalemia

Endocrine abnormality
- Hypothyroidism
- Diabetes mellitus

Neurogenic disorders
- Multiple sclerosis
- Spinal cord injury

Drugs
- Analgesics (mainly opioids)
- Anticholinergic drugs (antidepressants, antispasmodics, antipsychotics)
- Chemotherapeutic agents

Other causes
- Dehydration
- Immobility
- Decreased oral intake

Pathophysiology

In palliative care patients, disturbance in normal bowel habits can be multifactorial, and pathologies at different levels can contribute to altered bowel function. These include dysmotility syndromes secondary to central and autonomic dyssenergy between neurohormonal and myogenic pathways, and fluid and electrolyte imbalance.

Normal bowel function requires the coordination of motility, mucosal transport, and defecation reflexes.

Motility of the small intestine, colon, and sphincteric regions is controlled by myogenic characteristics, central nervous system mechanisms, activity of the peripheral autonomic nervous system, and circulating GI hormones.

The autonomic nervous system regulates colonic movements through both of its divisions: the sympathetic and parasympathetic nervous systems. Constipation, as a sign of peripheral nerve damage, is seen in generalized as well as localized autonomic dysfunction. The most frequent observed condition is diabetic autonomic neuropathy.

Histopathological studies of the vagus nerve in patients with diabetes and GI manifestations have shown reductions in the number of unmyelinated fibers, indicating a role for autonomic dysfunction (AD) in these symptoms.

Clinical assessment

History and physical

Initial management includes a thorough history of the individual's previous normal bowel habits. Recent variation in bowel habits requires defining of the pattern of change in terms of frequency, consistency, straining, drug history, and associated symptoms. Since it is mainly patient's perception, in certain cases, obtaining a diary of bowel habits can be useful.

Subjective measures of constipation, such as questionnaires or visual analog (VAS) or adjectival scales, are easy to use and valid. One less time-consuming questionnaire, the Constipation Assessment Scale (CAS) designed by McMillan and Williams, determines constipation severity.

Physical examination includes abdominal auscultation for quality of bowel sounds, inspection, palpation, and percussion. Digital rectal exam is an important component of assessment to rule out fecal impaction and obstruction.

Diagnostic tests

Check for correctable causes such as electrolyte imbalance or endocrine disorders. Sometimes the history and physical examination may not be very reliable in palliative care patients and an objective study is required to assess constipation.

Although a static tool, Bruera et al. showed that radiographic studies provide good correlation with fecal load in the palliative care population.[7]

Management

Management of constipation can be divided into preventive measures and therapeutic measures. Figure 11.3 illustrates general guideline for the assessment and management of constipation.

Preventive measures

- Patient education
- Increase dietary and fluid intake
- Prophylaxis laxatives when initiating the patient on opioids
- Encourage patients to increase mobility
- Providing a comfortable environment for defecation

Therapeutic measures

Therapeutic modalities to treat existing constipation can also be divided into general interventions and pharmacological treatment.

Pharmacological approaches

Oral laxatives include emollients, bulk-forming agents, osmotic (saline) agents, hyperosmolar agents, contact cathartics, prokinetic drugs, and opioid antagonists (Table 11.1).

Rectal preparations include suppositories and enemas (Table 11.1). The rectal route may be very unpleasant for sick patients, but the quick satisfactory results in most cases makes them an acute short-term choice of treatment for intractable constipation.

Apart from their specific mechanisms of action, rectal agents act by stimulating the anocolonic reflex to induce defecation. They are contraindicated in patients with thrombocytopenia and neutropenia.

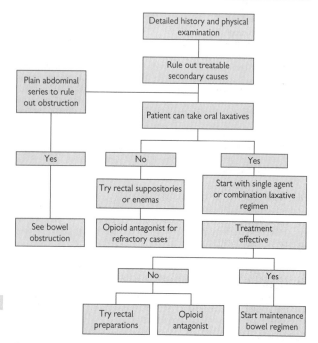

Fig. 11.3 General guidelines for assessment and management of constipation. Opioid antagonists are approved only for treatment of opioid-induced constipation.

Several forms of lubricant, osmotic, surfactant, and polyphenolics laxatives are available as rectal preparations, including suppository and enemas, but the latter form is reserved for constipation unrelieved by suppository.

Investigational and new approaches

In recent years, new pharmacological agents have been studied that have shown promising results. These include opiate antagonist, chloride channel activators, neurotrophins, and serotonergic enterokinetic agents.

Opioid antagonist

Opioid-induced constipation (OIC) is mediated by mu receptors in the GI system. Methylnaltrexone, a quaternary derivative of naltrexone, has restricted ability to cross the blood–brain barrier and does not affect opioid analgesic effects or induce opioid withdrawal symptoms. It has been recently approved for OIC in patients with advance illness.[8]

Chloride channel activator
Chloride channel activators enhance chloride-rich intestinal fluid secretion and increase intestinal motility.

Lubiprostone has been approved on the basis of two placebo-controlled trials in which it achieved significant results to relieve constipation and abdominal symptoms in patients with chronic idiopathic constipation. The most common adverse effect observed was nausea, which was dose related. The approved dose is 24 mcg twice a day with food.

Neurotrophins
The neurotrophic factor involved in the development of the nervous system has been studied in a phase II, randomized, double-blind trial. Subcutaneous neurotrophin-3, three times per week, significantly increased the frequency of bowel movements and improved other measures of constipation.

Serotonergic enterokinetic agents
Serotonin is involved in regulating gut motility, visceral sensitivity, and intestinal secretion through serotonin 5-HT4 receptors, which are expressed mainly by enteric nervous system interneurons.

Serotonergic enterokinetic agents stimulate 5-HT4 receptors on these enteric nervous system interneurons to enhance the peristaltic reflex and have shown efficacy for the treatment of chronic constipation.

Nonpharmacological approaches
The nonpharmacological measures used in prevention can also be incorporated into treatment of constipation

Biofeedback has proved to be beneficial in patients with dyssynergic defecation but has not shown any significant improvement in patients with slow-transit constipation.

In a Cochrane database review, aromatherapy and massage were not found to be effective for the treatment of constipation in cancer patients.

Summary
Constipation is a common symptom in patients with advanced illnesses that is underestimated even by palliative care physicians. The focus of treatment should start with proactive interventions. Disease processes should be taken into account for individualized management to effectively treat this debilitating complaint.

A lack of evidence-based clinical research leaves us with little guidance as to which laxative regimen to choose over another. Convenience of use, cost, tolerance, and effectiveness of the particular agent should be taken into consideration when managing constipation in palliative care patients.

Table 11.1 Commonly used laxatives for treatment of constipation

Laxatives	Mechanism	Recommended doses	Onset of action	Comments
Emollients				
Docusate	Act as detergents and help lower surface tension	Start 300 mg/day. Maximum 800 mg/day	1–3 days	Ensure adequate fluid intake
Mineral oil		15–45 mL/day	Oral: 6–8 hours Rectal: 2–15 minutes	Lipid pneumonitis with aspiration
Bulk forming				
Psyllium	Natural or synthetic; act by absorbing water in the intestine, increasing stool bulk, thereby promoting peristalsis and reducing transit time	Start 5–7 g/day	12–72 hours	Requires at least 300–500 mL of water ingestion, otherwise impaction may occur
Methylcellulose		Start 4–7 g/day	12–72 hours	
Hypersomolar agents				
Lactulose	These laxatives are undigestible, unabsorbable compounds that remain within the colon and retain the water that already is in the colon. The result is softening of the stool.	Start: 15–30 mL/day Max: 60 mL/day in 1–2 divided doses	24–48 hours	Abdominal bloating, colic, and flatulence
Polyethylene glycol		17–34 g/day	48–96 hours	Urticaria
Sorbitol		30–150 mL (as 70% solution)	24–48 hours	Pulmonary edema and hyperglycemia
Stimulants				
Bisacodyl	Stimulate peristalsis by directly irritating smooth muscle of the intestine, possibly the colonic intramural plexus; after water and electrolyte secretion, producing net intestinal fluid accumulation and laxation	Start: 5 mg/day Max: 30 Mg/day	6–10 hours	Electrolyte and fluid imbalance
Senna		Start 15 mg/day Max 70–100 mg/day	6–12 hours	Nausea, vomiting, melanosis coli

Prokinetic agents Metochlopromide	Promote colonic transit by increasing colonic motor activity	40–120 mg/day 30–80 mg/day	Variable Variable	Extraprymidal symptoms. Results are not impressive. Consider for refractory constipation. Avoid in cardiac patients.
Opioid antagonists Methylnaltrexone	Mu-receptor antagonist	38–<62 kg: 8 mg 62–114 kg: 12 mg >114 kg: 0.15 mg/kg (round dose up to nearest 0.1 mL of volume)	30–60 minutes	Only approved for opioid-induced constipation
Rectal preparation Sorbitol/Lactulos enemas	Hyperosmolar agent	120 mL of sorbitol 25–30% solution 200–300 mL of lactulose solution should be mixed with 700 mL of water or saline and retained for 30 to 60 minutes.	0.5–3 hours	Also used for hepatic encephalopathy
Saline enemas	Saline enemas cause water to be drawn into the colon.	Dose varies by the type of saline laxative	0.5–6 hours	Repeated enemas may result in electrolyte disturbances
Glycerine suppository	Glycerin suppositories act by irritating the rectum	Single dose 2-3 g/day	0.5–3 hours	May cause local irritation
Bisacodyl suppository	Bisacodyl act as a stimulant laxative	10 mg daily	Less than 1 hour	

Clinical pearls

Bowel obstruction
- Once MBO is diagnosed, median survival is 3 months.
- Surgery has little or no role in the management of MBO.
- Metoclopramide and prokinetics are contraindicated in patients with complete MBO.
- Octreotide can be beneficial in reducing intestinal secretions and motility.

Constipation
- Constipation can present as pseudo-diarrhea.
- Always perform a thorough medication history and discontinue constipating drugs when possible.
- Fiber supplements should be discouraged in palliative care patients.
- When in doubt, a plain abdominal X-ray can confirm the diagnosis of constipation.
- Opioid antagonists can be beneficial in patients with opioid-induced constipation.

References
1. Mangili, G, Aletti G, Frigerio L, et al. (2005). Palliative care for intestinal obstruction in recurrent ovarian cancer: a multivariate analysis. *Int J Gynecol Cancer* 15(5):830–835.
2. Baines M, Oliver DJ, Carter RL (1985). Medical management of intestinal obstruction in patients with advanced malignant disease. A clinical and pathological study. *Lancet* 2(8462):990–993.
3. Ripamonti, C, Bruera E (2002). Palliative management of malignant bowel obstruction. *Int J Gynecol Cancer* 12(2):135–143.
4. Hisanaga T, Shinjo T, Morita T, Nakajima N, et al. (2010). Multicenter prospective study on efficacy and safety of octreotide for inoperable malignant bowel obstruction. *Jpn J Clin Oncol* 40(8):739–745.
5. Feuer DJ, Broadley KE (2000). Corticosteroids for the resolution of malignant bowel obstruction in advanced gynaecological and gastrointestinal cancer. *Cochrane Database Syst Rev* 2000(2):CD001219.
6. Bruera E, Fadul N (2004). Constipation and diarrhea. In *Oxford Textbook of Palliative Medicine*. Oxford, UK: Oxford University Press.
7. Bruera E, Suarez-Almazor M, Velasco A, et al. The assessment of constipation in terminal cancer patients admitted to a palliative care unit: a retrospective review. *J Pain Symptom Manage* 9(8):515–519.
8. Thomas J, Karver S, Cooney GA, et al. (2008). Methylnaltrexone for opioid-induced constipation in advanced illness. *N Engl J Med* 358(22):2332–2343.

Delirium

Shirley H. Bush, MBBS, MRCGP, FAChPM
Ahmed Elsayem, MD

Definition and prevalence

Delirium is a multifactorial syndrome that results from global organic cerebral dysfunction. It is a severe neuropsychiatric syndrome that is frequently overlooked or misdiagnosed by health care professionals. Its early symptoms, such as anxiety, insomnia and mood changes, may be treated with anxiolytics and antidepressants, which may actually worsen the delirium.

Delirium is present in 26–44% of advanced-cancer patients at the time of admission to an acute care hospital or palliative care unit, and over 80% of patients with advanced cancer will develop delirium in the last hours and days before death.[1]

Delirium causes significant distress to patients, their families, and caregivers, with up to 75% of advanced cancer patients recalling their delirium episode.[2] It impairs patient communication and makes the assessment of pain and other symptoms difficult.

Agitated delirium and accompanying disinhibition may be misinterpreted as increased pain intensity, with the resulting increased opioid administration exacerbating the delirium severity. Delirium also causes significant morbidity and prognosticates an increased likelihood of death.

Pathophysiology

Many neurotransmitters are thought to be involved in the pathogenesis of delirium. The most important hypothesized mediators are an excess of dopamine and a deficiency of acetylcholine. Circulating cytokines and other neurotransmitters have also been implicated.[3]

Causes

The etiology of delirium is usually multifactorial (Fig. 12.1), with a median of 3 (range 1–6) precipitants per delirium episode. Causes of delirium can be categorized into predisposing and precipitating factors, but often a specific cause remains unidentified.

Predisposing factors increase a patient's baseline susceptibility for developing delirium—for example, pre-existing cognitive impairment and ↓ sensory input with poor vision or deafness.

Precipitating factors are the actual causative triggers for the delirium episode—for example, sepsis or electrolyte disturbance.

Urinary retention and constipation are factors capable of aggravating agitation, especially in the elderly.

Drug-induced delirium

Many drugs can cause a patient to become acutely confused. Commonly implicated medications are opioids, benzodiazepines, corticosteroids, and anticholinergics. Other causative drugs include antidepressants, neuroleptics, certain antiemetics and antivirals, antibiotics (quinolones), cimetidine and ranitidine, anticonvulsants, and chemotherapeutic agents.

Opioid-induced neurotoxicity (OIN) is a syndrome of neuropsychiatric side effects seen with opioid therapy. The components of OIN are severe sedation, hallucinations, cognitive impairment or delirium, myoclonus and seizures, and hyperalgesia/allodynia.

There is no specific order of development of these symptoms—they may occur as a single feature or in any combination.

The health care professional must remain vigilant as any patient prescribed opioids is at potential risk of OIN with the accumulation of toxic opioid metabolites. See Chapter 4 on pain management with opioids.

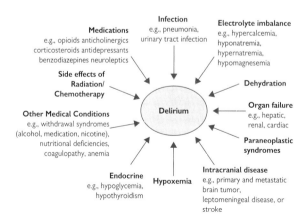

Fig 12.1 Factors contributing to delirium in cancer patients.

Presentation and diagnosis

Early identification is important and enables earlier treatment of delirium and education. An essential feature for the clinical diagnosis of delirium on the DSM-IV-TR criteria (Table 12.1) is a disturbance of consciousness.

Non-core clinical features of delirium include sleep–wake cycle disturbance, altered psychomotor activity, delusions, and emotional lability.

Three clinical subtypes of delirium have been described:

• *Hyperactive*: confusion + agitation ± hallucinations ± delusions ± myoclonus ± hyperalgesia (may be mistaken for anxiety or extrapyramidal side effects)
• *Hypoactive*: confusion + somnolence ± withdrawal (may simulate depression)
• *Mixed*: alternating symptoms of both hyperactive and hypoactive delirium.

Approximately two-thirds of delirium episodes are either of the hypoactive or mixed subtype. Hyperactive and mixed subtypes are highly associated with drug-induced delirium. Predominantly hypoactive delirium is associated with dehydration and encephalopathies.

Differential diagnosis
Dementia
• Little or no clouding of consciousness, insidious onset

Lewy body dementia
• Fluctuating symptom severity: cognitive impairment, visual hallucinations, delusions, and parkinsonism

Depression
• Hypoactive delirium in particular may be misdiagnosed as depression.

Screening and diagnostic tools
There are multiple validated delirium-specific assessment tools available, but only a few will be detailed in this chapter. The Mini-Mental State

---

Table 12.1 DSM-IV-TR (2000)* core diagnostic criteria for delirium

A. Disturbance of consciousness (i.e., reduced clarity of awareness of the environment) **with** reduced ability to focus, sustain, or shift attention

B. A change in cognition (such as memory deficit, disorientation, language disturbance) **or** the development of a perceptual disturbance that is not better accounted for by a pre-existing, established, or evolving dementia

C. The disturbance develops over a short period of time (usually hours to days) and tends to fluctuate during the course of the day.

D. There is evidence from the history, physical examination, or laboratory findings that the disturbance is caused by the direct physiological consequences of a general medical condition.

* Reprinted from the *Diagnostic and Statistical Manual of Mental Disorders*, Text Revision, Fourth Edition, (Copyright 2000). Washington, DC: American Psychiatric Association.

Examination (MMSE) for identifying cognitive impairment is not a delirium-specific instrument. Screening tools should be used in all patients, even with no overt signs of delirium, to make an early diagnosis.

The *Confusion Assessment Method* (CAM)[4] is a brief, easy-to-use, four-item diagnostic algorithm based on the DSM-III-R criteria. It does not measure delirium severity. It has recently been validated in the palliative care setting.

The *Memorial Delirium Assessment Scale* (MDAS)[5] is a 10-item, 4-point, clinician-rated instrument (possible range 0–30). It was originally designed to measure severity, but can be used as a diagnostic tool. A cutoff of total MDAS score of ≥7/30 may be used for delirium diagnosis.

The *Nursing Delirium Screening Scale* (Nu-DESC)[6] is an observational five-item scale (possible range 0–10) that includes the four items of the Confusion Rating Scale (CRS) and an additional assessment of psychomotor retardation. It is a low-burden tool that takes less than 2 minutes to complete. It can be used for screening and monitoring delirium severity.

Clinical assessment and investigations

▶ 50% of delirium episodes in advanced-cancer patients are reversible, so it is important to identify reversible causes and treat as appropriate.

Clinical history

In addition to a comprehensive medical history, including a history of alcohol or substance abuse, and multidimensional symptom assessment, ask the patient specifically about hallucinations (they are more often tactile than visual) and delusional thoughts, as patients frequently do not volunteer these symptoms. Medication history (new and continuing drugs) should also be reviewed.

It may be necessary to obtain a surrogate history from a family member or caregiver, and to ascertain the patient's baseline mental status.

Physical examination

Look for clinical signs of sepsis, OIN, other medication side effects, dehydration, metabolic abnormalities, and other potential causes of delirium (see Fig. 12.1, p. 155).

Investigations

Order investigations as appropriate to the patient's condition, such as CBC, electrolytes, calcium (with albumin), renal and liver function, urinalysis, chest X-ray, and O_2 saturation. Other tests may be indicated, such as radiological imaging of the brain with CT or MRI scan (see Fig. 12.2).

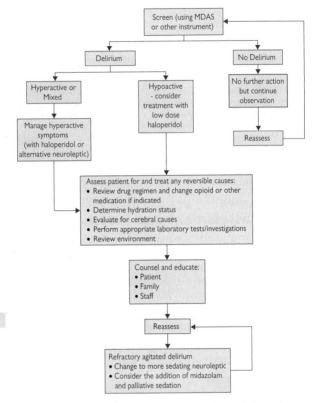

Fig. 12.2 Delirium assessment and treatment algorithm. MDAS, Memorial Delirium Assessment Scale.

Management

Comprehensive management should involve the multidisciplinary team.

Treatment of underlying causes

For patients who are at the end of life, these treatment strategies should be individualized.

- *Opioid toxicity*: Rotate or switch opioids. The equianalgesic dose of the new opioid should be reduced by 30–50%. See Chapter 4 on pain management and opioid rotation.
- *Sepsis*: Start appropriate antibiotics after discussing treatment options with the patient and the patient's family.
- *Other drugs*: Discontinue all implicated medications when possible.
- *Dehydration*: Start hypodermoclysis with normal saline at 60–100 mL/hour, or alternatively give subcutaneous (SC) boluses of 250 cc administered over 1 hour, three or four times daily. If an IV line is already established, hydration can easily be administered through it.
- *Hypercalcemia*: Treat with hydration, using saline, and bisphosphonates.
- *Hypoxia*: Treat the underlying cause and administer oxygen.
- *Brain tumor or metastasis*: Consider high-dose corticosteroids, e.g. dexamethasone 8–16 mg daily, in divided doses.

Pharmacological treatment of delirium symptoms

Neuroleptics are considered to be first-line agents. Haloperidol is most commonly used (see Table 12.2). Titrate the dose of neuroleptic to delirium severity, as long as there are no rate-limiting side effects. Once symptoms are under control, start reducing the neuroleptic dose to the minimal effective dose as soon as possible.

Regular low-dose haloperidol has also been used by some specialists for the management of hypoactive delirium.

More sedating neuroleptics, such as chlorpromazine and methotrime-prazine (levomepromazine) (not available in the United States), may be helpful for patients with severe agitation.

▶ Dose reduction of neuroleptics and slower titration are often needed for the elderly.

▶ Exercise caution when using benzodiazepines, as they can worsen the delirium. They should not be used as single agents. For acutely disturbed patients, lorazepam has been used in conjunction with haloperidol.

▶ Neuroleptics can reduce the seizure threshold, thereby potentially increasing the risk of seizures in susceptible patients.

▶ QTc interval prolongation can occur with many neuroleptics, including atypical antipsychotics (also see Table 12.3, p. 162).

Although extrapyramidal side effects are less likely with atypical antipsychotics, they can occur at higher doses, especially risperidone >6 mg/day.

⚠ Risperidone is reported to significantly increase risk of cerebrovascular events in elderly dementia patients. A U.S. Food and Drug Administration (FDA) warning also now extends to olanzapine and aripiprazole.

Table 12.2 Guide to commonly used neuroleptics for symptomatic treatment of delirium in palliative care

Drug (generic) name	Route	Commonly used starting doses (reduced in elderly)	Other comments
Conventional neuroleptics			
Haloperidol	PO (tablet and oral solution), SC, IV, IM	0.5–2 mg every 6 hours and 0.5–2 mg every 2–4 hours as needed	Average oral bioavailability of haloperidol is 60%
		For severe agitation:	∴ parenteral doses are
		↑ to 1–2 mg SC/IV every 30 minutes as needed during first hour, then every hour as needed	~ twice as potent as oral
Chlorpromazine	PO, IV, IM	12.5–25 mg every 4–12 hours	More sedating than haloperidol
			Adverse effect of orthostatic hypotension
Methotrimeprazine (levomepromazine Not available in U.S.	PO, SC, IV, IM	12.5–25 mg every 4–12 hours	More sedating than haloperidol
			Adverse effect of orthostatic hypotension
Atypical antipsychotics			
Risperidone	PO (tablet & oral solution), ODT	0.5–1 mg every 12–24 hours	
Olanzapine	PO, ODT, IM	2.5–5 mg every 12–24 hours	Sedating
			Metabolic syndrome can occur, but ? significance as usually only short-term use in delirium
Quetiapine	PO	12.5–25 mg every 12–24 hours	Less likely to cause EPS

EPS, extrapyramidal effects; ODT orally disintegrating tablet.

⚠ The use of typical and atypical antipsychotics in the treatment of dementia-related psychosis in the elderly has been associated with an increased risk of mortality.

Dementia-related agitation should be managed with a comprehensive biopsychosocial model. Alternative medications that have been suggested include cholinesterase inhibitors and SSRIs, and possibly anticonvulsants, lithium and anxiolytics.[7]

Psychostimulants, such as methylphenidate, have been used in the management of hypoactive delirium symptoms. However, caution is needed with their use. They may exacerbate or cause agitation and cause hallucinations, restlessness, insomnia, and cardiovascular effects.

In 2005, the FDA released a Public Health Advisory relating to atypical antipsychotics. The advisory is available at www.fda.gov.

More recently in 2008, the FDA announced a follow-up alert to health care professionals to also include conventional neuroleptics. This alert is available at www.fda.gov.

Nonpharmacological approaches

Simple environmental measures are often underutilized.
- Ensure a physically safe environment and minimize noise and excessive light.
- Ensure presence of familiar objects, and a visible clock and calendar.
- Enlist family members to assist with reorientation.
- Use clear and simple communication (do not forget the importance of glasses, hearing aids, dentures).

Psychosocial support and education

Confusion and agitation are expressions of brain malfunction and not necessarily of discomfort or suffering. Disinhibition is one of the main components of delirium that must be appropriately explained to families and, at times, to other health care professionals.

Counseling

Counsel the patient's family with expressive supportive therapy, as well as the patient when possible, to minimize distress. Hypoactive delirium is just as distressing for patients as hyperactive delirium.

Refractory agitated delirium

This will often necessitate the use of more sedative medications for patient symptomatic relief and comfort when other interventions have failed (see Chapter 13 regarding palliative sedation).

Table 12.3 Adverse effects of haloperidol*

Extrapyramidal side effects (EPS)	Comments	Management
• Acute dystonias (typically within days) • Acute akathisia (typically within weeks) • Neuroleptic-induced parkinsonism (usually after several weeks) • Triad: bradykinesia, tremor, rigidity • Tardive dyskinesia (usually after months of treatment)	→ with parenteral administration → with coadministration of anticholinergic ↑ with CYP2D6 substrateslow metabolizers	Acute dystonias/akathisia: • If possible, reduce or cease causative drug. • Prescribe an antimuscarinic antiparkinsonian drug, such as orphenadrine, benztropine. • Prescribe an antihistaminic antimuscarinic drug, such as diphenhydramine. • Consider switching to an atypical antipsychotic. • Neuroleptic induced parkinsonism: • If possible, reduce or cease causative drug. • Prescribe an antimuscarinic antiparkinsonian drug. • Consider switching to an atypical antipsychotic. Tardive dyskinesia: • Often poor response to drug treatment • Withdrawal of causative drug may lead to slow improvement, but sometimes irreversible • May be worsened by antimuscarinic antiparkinsonian drugs

MANAGEMENT 163

	Risk factors	

QTc interval prolongation

With any prolongation of QTc interval, especially >500 msec, patient is at risk of developing torsades de pointes (polymorphic ventricular tachycardia), with the threat of sudden cardiac death in the absence of medical intervention.

FDA alert (9/2007)
Recommends ECG monitoring if haloperidol given by IV route

Risk factors
- High-dose haloperidol (any route)
- IV haloperidol
- Congenital long QT syndrome
- Electrolyte abnormalities ($\downarrow$ K, $\downarrow$ Mg, $\downarrow$ Ca)
- $\uparrow$ Age (>65 years)
- Female
- Cardiac disease
- Bradycardia
- Concomitant administration of other drugs associated with QTc interval prolongation

1. Review and correct electrolyte levels if low ($\downarrow$ K, $\downarrow$ Mg, $\downarrow$ Ca)
2. Review other administered drugs that also have the potential to $\uparrow$ QTc interval
3. May require dose reduction or discontinuation of haloperidol (and other contributory medications) if QTc >450 msec, or increases >25% from baseline APA guidelines (1999)[†]
4. Consider cardiology consultation.

Sedation

Neuroleptic malignant syndrome
- Severe muscle rigidity
- Hyperthermia
- Altered mental status
- Autonomic dysfunction

Rare
- Infrequent and idiosyncratic Potentially fatal

- Cease causative drug
- General supportive care
- Benzodiazepines may help muscle rigidity.
- In severe cases, consider bromocriptine (IV dantrolene has been used in acute medical settings).

[*] Note: There is often marked variation in patient sensitivity.

[†] In: Practice guideline for the treatment of patients with delirium. Am J Psychiatry 1999; 156 (5 Suppl):1–20).

Clinical pearls

- To avoid missing the diagnosis of delirium, screen regularly using a validated delirium-specific assessment tool.
- Approximately 50% of delirium episodes in patients with advanced cancer are reversible.
- Routinely review for contributing factors, especially opioids and psychoactive medications, as well as other potentially reversible causes.
- Agitated delirium and accompanying disinhibition with grimacing and moaning may be incorrectly interpreted as pain, with the resulting inappropriate increased opioid administration worsening the agitated delirium and thus creating a vicious cycle.
- Providing psychosocial support and education may help to reduce the distress of patients, families, and professional caregivers.

References

1. Centeno C, Sanz A, Bruera E (2004). Delirium in advanced cancer patients. *Palliat Med* 18:184–194.
2. Bruera E, Bush SH, Willey J, et al. (2009). The impact of delirium and recall on the level of distress in patients with advanced cancer and their family caregivers. *Cancer* 115:2004–2012.
3. Agar M, Lawlor P (2008). Delirium in cancer patients: a focus on treatment-induced psychopathology. *Curr Opin Oncol* 20:360–366.
4. Inouye SK, van Dyck CH, Alessi CA, et al. (1990). Clarifying confusion: the Confusion Assessment Method. A new method for detection of delirium. *Ann Intern Med* 113:941–948.
5. Breitbart W, Rosenfeld B, Roth A, et al. (1997). The Memorial Delirium Assessment Scale. *J Pain Symptom Manage* 13:128–137.
6. Gaudreau JD, Gagnon P, Harel F, et al. (2005). Fast, systematic, and continuous delirium assessment in hospitalized patients: the Nursing Delirium Screening Scale. *J Pain Symptom Manage* 29:368–375.
7. Passmore MJ, Gardner DM, Polak Y, et al. (2008). Alternatives to atypical antipsychotics for the management of dementia-related agitation. *Drugs Aging* 25:381–398.

Clinical issues related to palliative sedation

Shirley H. Bush, MBBS, MRCGP, FAChPM
Ahmed Elsayem, MD

Definition[1–3]

Palliative sedation (PS) is the monitored use of proportionate sedative medication to reduce patients' awareness of intractable and refractory symptoms near the end of life when other interventions have failed to control them.

Consultation with a palliative care specialist is strongly recommended before initiating PS. See Table 13.1.

Appropriately titrated PS to relieve intractable distress in the dying is an ethically and legally accepted intervention. See Chapter 24 on ethics of palliative sedation.

PS is distinct from euthanasia, as the aim of PS is to relieve suffering by controlling distressing symptoms, not to shorten life. During PS, consciousness should be maintained, if possible.

Refractory agitated delirium is the most common indication for PS. Other indications include severe dyspnea or respiratory distress, pain, hemorrhage, severe seizures, and uncontrolled myoclonus.

The American Academy of Hospice and Palliative Medicine (AAHPM) position statement on PS (2006) is available at www.aahpm.org/positions/sedation.html. See Chapter 24 for more discussion of the AAHPM position statement.

Table 13.1 Checklist for palliative sedation

⚠ Consultation with a palliative care specialist is advisable before initiating PS.

1. Establish symptom(s) as severe, intractable, and refractory to treatment.

2. A symptom is *refractory* when all possible interventions known to control that symptom (including consultation with other providers) have been exhausted and failed, "or it is estimated that no methods are available for palliation within the time frame and the risk–benefit ratio that the patient can tolerate".[3]

3. Confirm that the patient is in the terminal phase of illness or close to death.

4. Discuss reasons and goals of palliative sedation with the patient (if possible) and/or family, and other members of the interdisciplinary health care team (including primary team if applicable). Reinforce that the goal is to relieve refractory symptoms and not to shorten life.

5. Document these discussions in the medical record.

6. Select the appropriate sedative medication and use the smallest effective dose to achieve symptom relief.

7. Only increase the dose (in appropriate increments) if lower doses have been ineffective, and document the indication for the dose increase.

8. Continue other ongoing symptom control management, e.g., opioid for pain and dyspnea, and other comfort measures.

9. Continue to provide emotional support to the family and health care team.

10. Regularly re-evaluate the need to continue PS. It may be possible to reduce or discontinue sedative medications if the indication for PS has improved.

Medications used

Midazolam is the drug of first choice for PS. It has a rapid onset of action, short half-life, and dose-dependent sedative effect. Use the lowest dose possible to provide comfort, e.g., commence a continuous SC or IV infusion of midazolam at 1 mg/hour and titrate according to clinical response.

Other medications that have been used for refractory delirium and PS include lorazepam, phenobarbital (phenobarbitone), propofol, and methotrimeprazine (levomepromazine; not available in the U.S.).

- Phenobarbital usual dosing: 50–100 mg SC bolus stat, then 200–800 mg/24 hours by continuous SC infusion. Occasionally, higher doses are needed. Phenobarbital needs to be administered as a separate infusion, as it is not compatible with most other drugs.
- Propofol is an ultrafast-acting IV anesthetic agent. Use requires specialist input.

Clinical pearls

- Consultation with a palliative care specialist is advisable before initiating PS.
- Establish symptom(s) as severe, intractable, and refractory to treatment.
- Confirm that the patient is in the terminal phase of illness or close to death.
- Discuss, and document, the indications and goals for initiation of PS with the patient (if possible), family, and health care team.
- Midazolam is the drug of first choice for PS. Commence with the lowest effective dose and then appropriately titrate according to clinical response.

References

1. Elsayem A, Curry Iii E, Boohene J, et al. (2009). Use of palliative sedation for intractable symptoms in the palliative care unit of a comprehensive cancer center. *Support Care Cancer* 17:53–59.
2. Lo B, Rubenfeld G (2005). Palliative sedation in dying patients: "we turn to it when everything else hasn't worked". *JAMA* 294:1810–1816.
3. de Graeff A, Dean M (2007). Palliative sedation therapy in the last weeks of life: a literature review and recommendations for standards. *J Palliat Med* 10:67–85.

Dyspnea

Jeff Myers, MD
Deborah Dudgeon, MD

Definition and epidemiology

Breathlessness is a distressing symptom experienced commonly by patients with advanced disease. Universal agreement on a definition does not exist; however, the most widely cited description is from the American Thoracic Society consensus statement outlining breathlessness as "a subjective experience of breathing discomfort that consists of qualitatively distinct sensations that vary in intensity. The experience derives from interaction among multiple physiologic, psychological, social, and environmental factors, and may induce secondary physiologic and behavioral responses."[1]

Reported prevalence varies and is dependent on the underlying diagnosis and the extent and stage of disease as well as choice of both assessment tool and the words or phrases used by investigators. At least 60% and 90% of patients with advanced heart disease and advanced COPD, respectively, will report feeling breathless.[2]

In the cancer population, breathlessness prevalence is dependent on the primary tumor site (46%, advanced lung cancer; 7%, advanced gastric cancer) and stage of disease.[2] In the final 6 weeks of life, 70% of all patients with cancer will experience breathlessness.

The distress associated with the perception of breathlessness can be severe, significantly impact quality of life, and is one of the most common reasons for an emergency room visit by all patients.

Pathophysiology

Although the neural pathways influencing the perception of breathlessness are not fully understood, Figure 14.1 outlines the current understanding of the contributing pathophysiological mechanisms.

A combination of central neural, chemical, mechanical, and emotional afferent impulses influence both the brainstem respiratory network (medulla and pons) and the higher brain centers located in the somatosensory and association cortices. Sensory input can be divided into four main categories.

Biochemical

- Both central and peripheral chemoreceptors (detect changes in pH, pCO_2, and pO_2) via vagus nerve

Vascular

- Baroreceptors (stretch sensitive mechanoreceptors) in the carotid and aortic bodies via vagus nerve

Mechanical

Sensory input is via receptors in the following:
- *Nasopharynx:* (cold, air flow) via trigeminal nerve
- *Airway:* rapidly adapting receptors within epithelium from trachea to bronchioles (lung irritants); slow-adapting receptors close to smooth

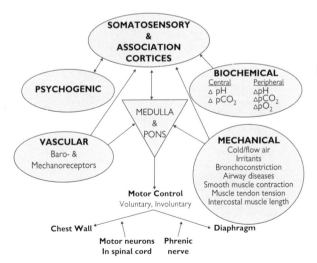

Fig. 14.1 Pathophysiology of Breathlessness

muscle of extra- and intrathoracic lower airway (airway wall tension); *bronchial C* fibers (irritants). All are via the vagus nerve.
- *Lung parenchyma:* pulmonary C-fibers within alveolar wall (pulmonary congestion, embolism, infection, chemicals) via vagus nerve
- *Muscles:* Golgi tendons (tension), intercostal muscles (length), diaphragm via spinal and supraspinal reflexes

Psychogenic

An affective state (i.e., anxiety and distress) can elicit changes in ventilation and sensation.

The control of respiratory motor activity resides in the brainstem (medulla and pons), and efferent impulses from here produce voluntary and involuntary contraction of the muscles in both the chest wall and the diaphragm.

In summary, respiratory motor drive is integrated with sensory input from several sites that, in connection with cognitive input, mediate the perception of breathlessness.

Etiology

In the setting of advanced disease, breathlessness may be multifactorial in etiology and categorized on the basis of both underlying disease and acuity of onset.

Malignant

Acute (within minutes)
- Pulmonary embolism
- Pneumothorax
- Aspiration
- Anxiety

Subacute (within hours to days)
- Pneumonia
- Pleural effusion (can also be chronic)
- Pericardial effusion
- Superior vena cava obstruction
- Anemia
- Radiation-induced pneumonitis (can also be chronic)
- Progressive metastatic disease (can also be chronic)

Chronic (within days to weeks)
- Radiation-induced pneumonitis/fibrosis
- Chemotherapy-induced (pulmonary fibrosis, cardiomyopathy)
- Contributing factors may include cachexia, ascites, and/or hepatomegaly.

Nonmalignant

Acute (within minutes)
Pulmonary
- Pneumothorax
- Pulmonary embolism
- Bronchospasm
- Acute bronchitis
- Asthma (with previous history)

Cardiac
- Acute myocardial ischemia or infarction
- Anxiety disorder

Subacute (within hours to days)
- Pneumonia
- CHF exacerbation
- Anemia

Chronic (within days to weeks)
Pulmonary
- Obstructive lung disease
- Restrictive lung disease
- Interstitial lung disease
- Pleural effusion

Cardiac
- CHF or ventricular dysfunction
- Neuromuscular disease
- Renal disease

Clinical evaluation

History: key questions

- Acuity? (onset and course)
- Severity? (use VAS or NRS; see below)
- Pattern?
- Triggering factors?
- Effect on activities of daily living?
- Mood and psychological state? (mental status, current or history of anxiety, current or history of depression)
- Meaning? (Is patient fearful of dying?)
- Current and previous medications?
- Underlying or concurrent diagnosis?
- Associated symptoms: cough (sputum production and color), fever and chills, sweats, chest pain, wheeze, chest tightness, hemoptysis, hoarseness, edema, weight loss or gain
- Advance directives and substitute decision maker?

Clinical pearls

- It is the patient's opinion of the severity of the symptoms that is the gold standard for symptom assessment.
- Often patients with advanced disease will have previously expressed or discussed their goals of care. This can provide clear guidance when formulating a plan for further assessment and management.

A visual analog scale (VAS) is a valid and reliable tool used to assess symptom intensity using a 100-mm vertical or horizontal line. Word anchors are attached to each end of the line to indicate the extremes of the sensation, with 0 representing no breathlessness and 100 representing worst possible breathlessness. The patient places a mark along the line to correspond with his or her symptom intensity, allowing the clinician to measure the distance from 0 to the patient's mark.

An example of a numerical rating scale (NRS) is the Edmonton Symptom Assessment System (ESAS), which is a valid and reliable assessment tool to assist in the assessment of nine common symptoms experienced by patients with advanced disease. The severity at the time of assessment of each symptom is rated from 0 to 10 on an NRS, 0 meaning that the symptom is absent and 10 that it is of the worst possible severity.[3]

Several scales have been developed specifically for dyspnea; however, as yet, there is no one scale that can accurately reflect breathlessness for all patients with advanced disease. For general clinical questions (e.g., effectiveness of medication), a VAS or the Modified Borg Scale (numerical scale with associated descriptors like "very, very slight" to "very, very severe") is most appropriate. Alternatively, if overall quality of life is the emphasis, then a multidimensional tool is preferable.

A unidimensional scale (e.g., VAS or NRS) should be combined with a disease-specific scale (if available) or a multidimensional scale in conjunction with other methods (such as qualitative techniques) to gauge psychosocial distress for assessment of breathlessness in advanced disease.

Physical exam

In the setting of advanced disease, the physical exam should be focused and guided by history and underlying illness.

Vital signs
- Heart (HR) and respiratory rate (RR), BP, O_2 sat., walking oximetry

Observe
- Overall level of distress
- Use of accessory muscles
- Elevated jugular venous pressure
- Pursed lips
- Cyanosis
- Ability to speak

Palpate
- Presence of dullness to percussion
- Decreased tactile fremitus

Auscultate
- Absent breath sounds?
- Adventitious breath sounds?
- Audible third heart sound (S3) or distant heart sounds?
- Wheeze?
- Pulses paradoxus?

Clinical pearls
- Tachypnea does not equate with breathlessness.
- Superior vena cava obstruction (SVCO) is a medical emergency and characterized by swelling and redness of face, distension of superficial and deep neck and upper arm vasculature, and cough.

Laboratory investigations and imaging

In patients with advanced disease, the appropriateness of an investigation will depend on the stage of disease and the goals of care. It is important to consider the burden of procedures and weigh this against the risk.

Investigations may contribute meaningful information in the assessment of breathlessness for patients with advanced disease; however, the results may not affect treatment. The choice of an appropriate test(s) will be guided by history, physical exam, and clinical scenario.

Investigations to be considered may include the following:
- CBC, serum K^+, PO_4, Mg
- Chest X-ray
- Blood gas
- Pulmonary function test
- CT
- Echocardiogram

Many clinicians make the mistake of equating breathlessness with hypoxemia, but very poor correlation has been reported between patient reports of breathlessness and oxygen levels or abnormalities in pulmonary function. In addition, patients may not show signs of hypoxia but report high levels of breathlessness. Oximetry (in particular, walking oximetry) may unmask the etiology for the breathlessness.

Management

The mainstay of management of breathlessness is to, if possible, identify a potentially reversible underlying cause, begin an appropriate and targeted treatment or intervention, evaluate the effectiveness of the treatment or intervention, and ensure that the symptom of breathlessness is well managed throughout.

An example of this is found in the setting of breathlessness and malignant pleural effusions. For appropriate patients, thoracentesis, pleurodesis, and/or ongoing drainage procedures should be offered.

Basic nonpharmacological and pharmacological interventions for breathlessness, based on severity, are summarized in Fig. 14.2.[3]

Nonpharmacological interventions

A recent Cochrane review examined efficacy for nonpharmacological and noninvasive interventions in advanced cancer and advanced non-cancer populations.[4] Both *neuroelectrical muscle stimulation* and *chest wall vibration* achieved a high level of evidence in their benefit in relieving breathlessness.

The use of *walking aids* and *breathing training* achieved a moderate level of benefit, and *acupuncture and acupressure* were found to have low evidence for efficacy in relieving breathlessness.

For patients with COPD-associated chronic dyspnea, given the resulting pattern of limbic system activation, effective management for this population includes structured cognitive-behavioral and self-management strategies to ensure that the affective dimension is adequately addressed.

Opioids

Although reports are limited for medications other than morphine, strong evidence from multiple studies and meta-analyses confirms the usefulness of oral and/or parenteral opioids in providing significant clinical benefit in the setting of acute, subacute, and chronic breathlessness.[5] This is true for both cancer and non-cancer populations.

In addition, incident breathlessness can be relieved rapidly with the use of breakthrough opioids.

With the exception of one study examining hydromorphone, nebulized opioids in general have not shown to be of any greater benefit than systemic opioids in reducing breathlessness.[5] It is suggested that when using opioids, only oral and systemic routes be considered.

Respiratory depression is a commonly feared side effect of opioids. Although some studies have shown a decrease in respiratory rate with the use of opioids, this has not been found to be clinically significant, as neither hypercapnia nor hypoxygenation result.

Another possible role of opioids in the setting of breathlessness may be to reduce the emotional reaction to the anxiety, fear, and panic that often occurs.

	Mild (VAS/ESAS 1-3)	Moderate (VAS/ESAS 4-6)	Severe (VAS/ESAS 7-10)
Clinical Features	• Usually can sit/lie quietly • Intermittent or persistent • Increase with exertion • No or mild anxiety • Patient does not appear uncomfortable	• Usually persistent • May be new or chronic • Settles partially with rest • Patient pauses while talking every 30 seconds • Breathing appears mildly labored	• Often acute on chronic • Has worsened over days to weeks • Anxiety present • Patient pauses while talking every 5-15 seconds • Patient appears uncomfortable
Management Strategies	• Consider oxygen (if hypoxemic or deemed helpful by patient) • If opioid naive, consider low dose routine or prn opioid (morphine 2.5-5.0mg or hydromorphone 0.5-1.0mg) • If on opioids, increase by 25% • Ensure breakthrough avail q2h • Titrate opioid short acting opioid by 25% every 3 to 5 hours until relief	• Start oxygen (if hypoxemic or deemed helpful by patient) • If opioid naive, consider low dose routine or prn opioid (morphine 2.5-5.0mg or hydromorphone 0.5-1.0mg) • If on opioids, increase by 25% • Ensure breakthrough avail q1h prn • Titrate opioid dose by 25% every 2-3 doses until relief	• Start oxygen (up to 6L/min by NP or higher with mask) • Use only short acting opioids to titrate • If opioid naive, begin either morphine PO 5-10mg q4h and 5mg q1h prn or hydromorphone 1-2mg q4h and 1mg q1h prn • Titrate opioid dose by 25% every 1-2 doses until relief • Consider adjuvant (midazolam, promethazine)

Clinical Pearl

When available, opioids can and should be administered subcutaneously, particularly if breathlessness is severe. ½ of the PO dose is equivalent to the SC dose and can be safely offered q30min prn

For all:
• Ensure access to fresh air or fan directing air on the face
• Open door, window(s), curtain(s)
• Encourage rest as needed
• When laying – elevate head of bed
• When sitting – use reclining chair and footrest
• When moving– use assistive devices (walker, wheelchair)

Fig. 14.2 General Features and Quick Reference Management of Breathlessness

Nonopioid medications

Nonopioid medications either play a role as an adjunct medication specifically for breathlessness management or are intended to treat or address the underlying disease or mechanism resulting in breathlessness.

Although it may seem counterintuitive, evidence does not support the use of benzodiazepines in the direct management of breathlessness.[5] Given the distinct psychogenic role in the severity of breathlessness, however, aggressively managing comorbid psychiatric conditions (anxiety and/or depression) warrants consideration.

Based on a recent systematic review of breathlessness management in patients with cancer, the following recommendations outline the evidence for use of nonopioid medications[5]:

- Oral promethazine may be used to manage dyspnea, as a second-line agent if systemic opioids cannot be used or in addition to systemic opioids. *(Promethazine must not be used parenterally.)*
- Prochlorperazine is not recommended as therapy for managing dyspnea.
- No comparative trials are available to support or refute the use of other phenothiazines, such as chlorpromazine and methotrimeprazine, for managing dyspnea.

No evidence exists for the use of corticosteroids in management of breathlessness in cancer patients.[6] Anecdotal reports suggest a role for corticosteroids when targeting specific cancer-related conditions:

- Obstruction (SVCO and/or airway)
- Lymphangitic carcinomatosis
- Radiation pneumonitis

In patients with cancer, nebulized furosemide has been found to relieve breathlessness when standard treatments (morphine and oxygen) are no longer effective. In this setting, no significant reduction in objective measures (i.e., arterial blood gases [ABGs], O_2 sat, HR, and RR) occurs.

In the setting of COPD, nebulized furosemide resulted in significant improvement in both the FEV_1 and the patient's perception of their dyspnea.

Other nonopioid medications in the appropriate setting may include

- Antibiotics
- Anticoagulants
- Bronchodilators
- Nebulized saline

Oxygen

In the setting of patients with COPD, ambulatory oxygen therapy increases exercise performance and improves exertional breathlessness. The mechanism is thought to be through the reduction in hyperinflation.

For patients with advanced cancer and advanced heart disease a consistent beneficial effect of oxygen has not been shown.[7] This result is limited by the small volume of research studies available for inclusion, small numbers of participants, and methods used in the studies.[7]

Summary

Breathlessness is a common and distressing symptom for patients with advanced disease. Assessment and management plans should be targeted to the individual patient. Reversible conditions contributing to breathlessness should be addressed and the symptom should be well managed using patient self-report in determining efficacy.

References

1. American Thoracic Society (2001). Dyspnea: mechanisms, assessment, and management: a consensus statement. *Am J Respir Crit Care Med* 163:951–957.
2. Solano JP, Gomes B, Higginson IJ (2006). A comparison of symptom prevalence in far advanced cancer, AIDS, heart disease, chronic obstructive pulmonary disease and renal disease. *J Pain Symptom Manage* 31(1):58–69.
3. Dyspnea management guidelines for palliative care. In *Kingston, Frontenac, Lennox and Addington (KFL and A) Palliative Care Integration Project: Symptom Management Guidelines.* 2003 (August); pp. 26–36.
4. Bruera E, Kuehn N, Miller MJ, Selmser P, Macmillan K. (1991). The Edmonton Symptom Assessment System (ESAS): a simple method for the assessment of palliative care patients. *J Palliat Care* 7(2):6–9.
5. Bausewein C, Booth S, Gysels M, Higginson IJ (2008). Non-pharmacological interventions for breathlessness in advanced stages of malignant and non-malignant diseases. *Cochrane Database Syst Rev* Issue 2:CD005623.
6. Viola R, Kiteley C, Lloyd NS, Mackay JA, Wilson J, Wong RKS (2008). The management of dyspnea in cancer patients: a systematic review. *Support Care Cancer* 16:329–337.
7. Cranston JM, Crockett A, Currow D. (2008). Oxygen therapy for dyspnea in adults. *Cochrane Database Syst Rev* Jul 16;(3):CD004769.

Emergencies in palliative care

Meiko Kuriya, MD
Rony Dev, DO

Hypercalcemia

Introduction

Approximately 10 to 30% of patients with cancer have complications of hypercalcemia at some time during the course of their illness.[1] Hypercalcemia is responsible for a significant number of hospitalizations and results in distressing symptoms in patients with cancer.

Hypercalcemia is also an indicator of poor prognosis; however, treatment with bisphosphonates may be decreasing the incidence and outcome for cancer patients.

Clinical presentation

Hypercalcemia results in nonspecific clinical symptoms: "bones, stones, abdominal groans, and psychic moans."

Symptoms include the following:
- Anorexia
- Nausea
- Abdominal pain
- Muscle weakness and fatigue
- Nephrolithiasis
- Dehydration
- Boney tenderness
- Complications of severe hypercalcemia
- Acute pancreatitis
- Acute renal failure
- Altered mental status and coma

Pathogenesis

Hypercalcemia associated with cancer can be classified into four types (Table 15.1).

Diagnosis

Formulas to correct total calcium level are often used; however, serum ionized calcium levels should be measured and are more reliable.

Corrected Calcium Formula (mg/dL) =
([4.0 − Albumin (g/dL)]] × 0.8) + Serum Total Calcium (mg/dL)

Hypercalcemia	Serum calcium level (mg/dL)	Serum calcium level (mmol/L)
Mild	10.5–11.9	2.6–2.9
Moderate	12.0–13.9	3.0–3.4
Severe	≥14.0	≥3.5

Table 15.1 Types of hypercalcemia associated with cancer

Type	Frequency (%)	Bone metastasis	Causal agent	Typical tumors
Local osteolytic hypercalcemia	20	Common, extensive	Cytokines, chemokines, PTHrP	Breast cancer, multiple myeloma, lymphoma
Humoral hypercalcemia of malignancy	80	Minimal or absent	PTHrP	Squamous cell cancer (e.g., of head and neck, esophagus, cervix, or lung), renal cancer, ovarian cancer, endometrial cancer, HTLV-associated lymphoma, breast cancer
1,25 (OH)2D-secreting lymphomas	<1	Variable	1,25(OH)2D	Lymphoma (all types)
Ectopic hyper-parathyroidism	<1	Variable	PTH	Variable

PTH, parathyroid hormone; PTHrP PTH-related protein; 1,25(OH)2D, 1,25-dihydroxyvitamin D; HTLV, human T-cell lymphotrophic virus

Management

Hydration with intravenous (IV) saline is essential to reverse decreased glomerular filtration rate (GFR) and impaired renal calcium excretion. Furosemide can also promote calcium excretion by inhibiting Na/K/Cl transporter in the loop of Henle; however, diuretics are not recommended in cancer patients, who are often volume depleted.

Bisphosphonates are first-line medical therapy and work by blocking osteoclastic bone resorption.[2] They include pamidronate and zolendronate. Bisphosphonates should be given intravenously since they are poorly absorbed when given orally. Common adverse effects include fever, nausea, vomiting, renal toxicity, and osteonecrosis of the jaw.

Second-line medications include glucocorticoids (useful in lymphoma patients with elevated 1,25(OH)2 vitamin D) and calcitonin, which results in rapid transient reduction in calcium levels.

Supportive care measures include removal of calcium in vitamin supplementations and from parenteral feeding solutions, discontinuation of medications that may lead to hypercalcemia (e.g., calcitriol, vitamin D, lithium, and thiazides), and replacement of phosphorous orally if serum phosphorous is <3 mg/dL.

IV phosphorous replacement should be avoided unless phosphorous is critically low (<1.5 mg/dL), since it can cause seizures, hypocalcemia, renal failure, and arrythmias.

Bleeding

Mild to severe bleeding is an emergent complication that occurs in approximately 6–10% of cancer patients and 1.5% of patients receiving palliative care.[3] Active bleeding can be very distressing for patients, families, and health-care providers.

For patients with a poor prognosis, advanced care planning is critical in order to anticipate possible catastrophic bleeding.

Etiology

Tumor invasion

Cancer infiltration of both small and large vessels and factors secreted by tumors that promote angiogenesis predispose patients to bleeding. Past radiation exposure can often weaken vessels, resulting in bleeding complications.

Head and neck tumors, lung, gastrointestinal, and gynecological malignancies are often associated with tumor destruction of small and large vessels.

Hepatocellular carcinoma may be complicated by bloody ascites and is a poor prognostic indicator. Vascular tumors, including renal cell carcinoma, choriocarcinoma, and melanoma, are also prone to bleeding.

Treatment side effects

Mucositis secondary to chemotherapy or radiation treatment and the complication of graft-versus-host disease can increase risk for bleeding.

Thrombocytopenia

Bone marrow suppression, bone marrow invasion of the cancer, disseminated intravascular coagulation (DIC), or splenomegaly secondary to portal hypertension from hepatocelluar carcinoma can result in thrombocytopenia.

Nutritional deficiencies

Vitamin K, zinc, folate, and vitamin B_{12} deficiencies can also promote bleeding.

Drugs

Coumadin, heparin products, and COX inhibitors can potentiate bleeding.

Coagulation abnormalities

DIC, primary fibrinolysis, and liver disease can result in coagulopathy contributing to increased bleeding risk.

Presentation

Bleeding can happen in several ways; oozing from the tumor, intracranial hemorrhage, epistaxis, hemoptysis, hematemesis, melena, hematochezia, hematuria, and vaginal bleeding.

Work up

In cases of noncatastrophic bleeding, it is important to detect and treat any reversible causes while initiating measures to control bleeding and anxiety in patients and families associated with visible blood loss.[3,4]

Labs should include complete blood count (CBC), platelet count, activated partial thromboplastin time (PTT), and international normalization ratio (INR). A liver function test could be included if liver dysfunction is suspected.

In cases of catastrophic bleeding, the priority is to control the bleeding and associated symptoms before reversing underlying factors.

Management

Interventions should be consistent with a patient's goals of care and are formulated on the basis of overall prognosis, performance status, and previous therapies.

The most important point is to make the patient and family aware of and prepared for the possibility of visible bleeding. If catastrophic bleeding is anticipated, dark-colored (preferably the color red) linen, towels, and basins should be available at bedside to make bleeding less obvious.

For control of anxiety, IV or SC midazolam should be available, as well as family members who are trained in administration.

Local measures to control bleeding include the following:
- Packing
  - Nose, rectum, vagina
- Compressive dressings
  - Transparent films, hydrogel dressings, hydrocolloid dressing
- Topical hemostatics
  - Fibrin sealants
- Proper positioning
  - Lateral decubitus on the side of bleeding for patients with hemoptysis or hematemesis
- Astringents
  - Silver nitrate, aluminum ammonium sulfate, or aluminum potassium sulfate

Treatment modalities for bleeding include the following:
- Radiation therapy
  - Gynecological, lung, and superficial skin tumors
- Palliative transcatheter chemoembolization
- Endoscopy
  - Injection of sclerosing agents
  - Ligation
  - Laser coagulation

Systemic measures include the following:
- Vitamin K
- Vassopresin
- Antifibrinolytic agents
  - Transexaminic acid
  - Aminocaproic acid
- Octreotide for GI bleeding from varacies
- Platelet transfusion
  - Thrombocytopenia
  - Platelet dysfunction
- Fresh frozen plasma
  - Coagulopathies

When bleeding is catastrophic, palliative sedation for the patient should be provided in conjunction with psychosocial support for the family.

Superior vena cava syndrome

Superior vena cava (SVC) syndrome results from the impairment of blood flow through the SVC. It is usually caused by malignancies, the majority of which are due to non–small-cell lung cancer.[5] Other etiologies include small-cell lung cancer, germ cell tumors, lymphoma, thymoma, esophageal cancer, and mediastinal or lung metastasis from other tumors.

Recently, nonmalignant conditions resulting in SVC syndrome have arisen secondary to the increased use of intravascular devices.

Clinical presentation

Increased venous pressure secondary to SVC syndrome may result in symptoms of edema of the head, neck, and arms. These pressures often develop over a period of 2 weeks.

Clinical features may include cyanosis and distended subcutaneous vessels of the neck. Cough, hoarseness, stridor, and dysphagia may occur secondary to edema, occluding the airways or esophagus. Cerebral edema may result in head discomfort, confusion, and coma that can be fatal.

In severe cases, hemodynamic compromise can occur. In addition, pleural effusions are common in cancer patients with SVC syndrome.

Diagnosis

When SVC syndrome is suspected on the basis of clinical signs and symptoms, CT scan with contrast, or MRI for patients allergic to contrast, are the most useful imaging studies. Once SVC syndrome has been confirmed by imaging, it is critical to obtain a tissue diagnosis in patients with suspected malignancies for guiding future treatment.

In patients with pleural effusion, thoracentesis with cytological analysis should be considered. Bronchoscopy, transthoracic needle aspiration biopsy, mediastinoscopy, and mediastinotomy are used to obtain a tissue diagnosis.

Management

The management of SVC syndrome depends on the etiology, severity of symptoms, and the patient's goals of therapy. When there is enough collateral blood flow with minimal symptoms, the patient might not require further treatment.

Systemic chemotherapy could be the initial treatment of choice for sensitive tumors such as lung cancer (small cell and non-small cell), lymphoma, and germ cell tumors. When SVC syndrome is caused by a tumor that is refractory to chemotherapy, radiation therapy may be considered.

Percutaneous placement of an intravascular stent is another possible intervention. Stent placement can be done before a tissue diagnosis has been obtained and is a useful procedure for patients with severe symptoms such as dyspnea. Stent placement should also be considered for patients with mesothelioma, which tends to be refractory to chemotherapy and radiation therapy.

Complications of stent placement for treatment of SVC syndrome include infection, pulmonary embolus, stent migration, hematoma formation at the insertion site, perforation, bleeding, and, rarely, death. Anti-coagulation is often recommended after stent placement.

A multidisciplinary approach to treatment planning should be considered. The presence of SVC syndrome often does not affect the prognosis, which is directly related to the tumor type and stage of the cancer.

Spinal cord compression

Introduction

Cancer patients may develop spinal cord compression, which can result in pain, incontinence of bowel or bladder, and paraparesis or paralysis. Breast, prostate, and lung cancer account for the majority of spinal cord compression cases. Breast and lung cancers cause thoracic lesions whereas colon and pelvic malignancies involve the lumbosacral spine.

Clinical presentation

The most common clinical presentation of spinal cord compression is back pain, which can be localized, referred, and/or radicular in nature.

Complications of cauda equina syndrome result in decreased sensation over the buttocks, thighs, and perineal region and may result in decreased sphincter tone, urinary retention, and overflow incontinence.

Spinal cord compression presents with radiculopathy, sensory changes, weakness, autonomic dysfunction (i.e., urinary retention), and loss of sphincter tone, resulting in stool incontinence.

Diagnosis

Delay in diagnosis of spinal cord compression can lead to increased morbidity and mortality. When spinal cord compression is suspected, gadolinium-enhanced MRI of the whole spine should be urgently obtained and is considered the gold standard.

Management

A multidisciplinary team approach is critical to formulate the treatment for patients with spinal cord compression,[6] A surgical team, radiation oncologist, rehabilitation practitioner, and a palliative medicine consultant may be involved.

Treatment should be customized according to the patient's disease status, prognosis, performance status, and comorbidities and the severity of symptoms.

Glucocorticoid therapy

The general consensus is that glucocorticoid therapy is beneficial. While the optimal dose of steroid therapy is unknown, an initial bolus of dexamethasone 10 mg IV followed by a scheduled dose between 6 and 10 mg every 6 hours is commonly initiated.

After completion of radiation therapy, it is recommended that the dose be tapered to the smallest amount that maintains neurological benefits while minimizing side effects.

For patients who need prolonged glucocorticoid therapy, prophylaxis to prevent *Candida* and *Pneumocystis jiroveci* infections should be considered.

Radiation therapy

Cancer metastasis to the vertebral column can be painful and may result in various degrees of spinal cord compression. Radiation therapy has been shown to provide pain relief and preserve the ability to ambulate and maintain sphincter function.

Serious complications that may occur include myelosuppression and radiation myelopathy.

Longer courses of radiation therapy have not been shown to be superior to a short course, but patients receiving a shorter course experience increased recurrence.

High-precision radiotherapy techniques have been developed that are used for primary treatment and for recurrence of disease while minimizing radiation exposure to surrounding tissue.

Depending on the prognosis, the radiation oncologist can formulate a treatment regimen that is consistent with the patient's goals of care.

Surgery

Surgical decompression with reconstruction can provide benefit including pain control and preserving neurological function for patients with spinal cord compressions. Currently, the optimal treatment with surgical decompression and reconstruction followed by radiation therapy vs. radiotherapy alone is unclear.

Surgery for patients with progressive neurological deficits, vertebral column instability, or radioresistant tumors and patients with persistent pain despite radiotherapy has been recommended.

Most surgeons agree that a patient's life expectancy should be greater than 3 months, before undergoing any invasive surgical procedures.

Rehabilitation

Rehabilitation has been shown in observational studies to improve quality of life, improve mood, and provide better pain control in patients with spinal cord compressions. Paraplegic patients are taught how to manage bowel or bladder incontinence and transfer safely, and ambulatory patients receive assistance with their strength and mobility.

In addition, family support needs to be incorporated into a debilitated patient's bowel and bladder care, provision of nutritional needs, and daily hygiene regimens.

Palliative care

Regardless of whether radiation or surgery is offered for treatment of spinal cord compression, patients should be provided medical treatment and psychosocial support to assist with coping with the loss of independence or function.

For patients with a poor prognosis, palliative care consultants can assist with the transition from disease-orientated therapy to treatment focused on symptom control and improving quality of life.

Seizures

Introduction

Seizures in the palliative care setting may be seen in patients with a primary brain tumor, a metastatic brain lesion, metabolic abnormalities, a central nervous system infection, or drug toxicity or withdrawal.

Presentation

Seizures can be either focal or generalized, and not all seizures present with convulsions but can also present with altered mental status. Focal seizures can develop into a generalized seizure.

Status epilepticus, an emergent condition, is defined as a single seizure activity lasting more than 5 minutes or repeated seizures over a period of more than 30 minutes without full recovery of neurological function in between.

Work up

Electroencephalography (EEG) may be useful if the diagnosis is in doubt (e.g. nonconvulsive seizure) but is not routinely needed for patients who give a clear history of seizures or those without suggestive symptoms.

Management

The management of seizures in the palliative care setting is similar to that for non-cancer patients.[7]

Benzodiazepines

The most commonly used benzodiazepine for seizures is lorazepam. The mean time of lorazepam to achieve clinical effect is 3 minutes and the half-life is 10–15 hours. A dose of 2 mg should be given intravenously and can be repeated up to total dose of 0.1 mg/kg. It should be infused no faster than 2 mg/minute.

Because of its high lipid solubility, diazepam enters the brain rapidly, but its half-life is 15–30 minutes, thus its anticonvulsant effect is very brief and a second dose may be necessary after only 20–30 minutes. The recommended dose is 10 mg in adults.

Phenytoin/fosphenytoin

Traditionally, treatment with benzodiazepine is followed by phentytoin therapy. Recommended dosage is 15–20 mg/kg, not more than 50 mg/minute. The advantage of phenytoin therapy is that it is nonsedating.

Fosphenytoin is metabolized into phenytoin by the liver. The initial dose is the same as for phenytoin, although, it can be given faster than phenytoin, at 100–150 mg/minute.

Valproic acid

Valproic acid can be used as an alternate tp phenytoin or fosphenytoin. The dose is 6 mg/kg/minute up to a total dose of 30 mg/kg, followed by a maintenance dose of 1–2 mg/kg/hour.

Newer agents

To avoid interactions with other medications such as chemotherapy agents or antibiotics, newer agents, such levatiracetem, pregabalin, lamotrigine, and toprimate, are used because they do not induce hepatic cytochrome P450 enzymes. These agents could be used as a maintenance agent once seizure is under control.

Clinical pearls

- A high index of suspicion for hypercalcemia is necessary, as symptoms are nonspecific.
- Screen for hypercalcemia by checking ionized calcium level, as formulas to correct serum calcium levels are not reliable.
- Hydration and bisphosphonates are the main treatment of hypercalcemia.
- Anticipation of bleeding catastrophes in cancer patients is critical to minimize distress for patients and their family.
- A CT scan of the chest or an MRI is indicated to diagnose SVC syndrome.
- A gadolinium-enhanced MRI of the whole spine is the gold-standard test to diagnose spinal cord compression.
- Cancer patients may have nonconvulsive epilepsy when having altered mental status.

References

1. Stewart AF (2005). Hypercalcemia associated with cancer. *N Engl J Med* 352:373–379.
2. Saunders Y, Ross JR, Broadley KE, et al. (2004). Systematic review of bisphosphonates for hypercalcaemia in malignancy. *Palliat Med* 18(5):418–431.
3. Gagnon B, Mancini I, Pereira J, Bruera E (1998). Palliative management of bleeding events in advanced cancer patients. *J Palliat Care* 14:50–54.
4. Prommer E (2005). Management of bleeding the terminally ill patient. *Hematology* 10:167–175.
5. Wilson L, Detterbeck F, Yahalom J (2007). Superior vena cava syndrome with malignant causes. *N Engl J Med* 356:1862–1869.
6. Abrahm J, Banffy M, Harris M (2008). Spinal cord compression in patients with advanced metastatic cancer: "all I care about is walking and living my life". *JAMA* 299:937–946.
7. Knake S, Hamer H, Rosenow F (2009). Statue epilepticus: a critical review. *Epilepsy Behav* 15:10–14.

Other symptoms: xerostomia, hiccups, pruritis, pressure ulcers and wound care, lymphedema, and myoclonus

Paul W. Walker, MD

Introduction

This chapter includes "orphan" symptoms that usually get less attention than do more common symptom such as pain or nausea. These symptoms may have mutiple etiologies and often have a long list of possible remedies or limited options, reflecting our lack of understanding and our limitation in management.

Xerostomia

The complaint of dry mouth, xerostomia, is a common one in palliative care but is often perceived by clinicians as less serious than pain or other symptoms. It is important not to make light of its impact on the patient, as xerostomia can result in difficulty in mastication and swallowing and with speech. Also, there is increased risk of dental caries, periodontal disease, candidiasis, and changes in taste sensation.

In patients with advanced cancer, the prevalence of xerostomia is reported at between 30% and 97%.[1] The two main mechanisms underlying most cases include indirect alteration in the nervous tone supplying the salivary glands (e.g., as caused be medication) or destruction of the salivary tissue (e.g., radiotherapy). Causes of this condition are many but for the most part can be divided into three groups: medications, radiotherapy, and systemic diseases that cause decreased salivary flow.

Drug classes that can cause this problem include anticholinergics and antihistamines (e.g., scopolamine, diphenhydramine, oxybutynin, meclizine), psychotropics (e.g., amitiptyline, desipramine, lorazepam, hydroxyine, trazadone), opioids (e.g., codeine, fentanyl, tramadol, oxymorphone, hydromorphone), cardiovascular medications (e.g., hydrochlorothiazide, metoprolol, doxazosin, fosinopril, felodipine), and sympathetic agonists (e.g., albuterol, meta-proterenol, carbidopa-levodopa, selegiline).

Radiotherapy treatments for head and neck cancers commonly result in prolonged xerostomia. The list of medical conditions that can produce dry mouth is long but include rheumatic disorders such as Sjogren's syndrome, sarcoidosis, diabetes mellitus, graft-versus-host disease, and anxiety or depression. Dehydration can cause dry mouth, as can mouth breathing that occurs in the terminal phase of illness.

Management consists of evaluating for reversible causes, which includes a careful evaluation of the patient's drug regimen for medications that can be contributing to dry mouth and determining if they can be changed or the dose reduced.

Providing careful medical management for systemic conditions that can cause xerostomia (e.g., diabetes mellitus or chronic inflammatory rheumatic disorders) is prudent. Regular oral hygiene is important and use of a fluoride-containing toothpaste and regular dental brushing helps reduce caries, periodontal disease, and halitosis.

What remains are strategies for improving oral moisture.[2,3] These include frequent sips of fluid, ice, or popsicles; water spray; use of saliva substitutes; chewing sugarless gum; or sucking on sugar-free candy. Maintaining room humidity may also be helpful. Meal-time strategies aimed at providing moist and soft foods and avoiding dry foods are advised.

Pilocarpine is a muscarinic agonist with effects on the beta-adrenergic receptors of the sweat and salivary glands. It has been studied for treatment of radiation and drug-induced xerostomia with positive results. Pilocarpine must be used with caution, as glaucoma and cardiac disturbances can occur. The most common side effect with this agent is sweating, but also lacrimation and dizziness. The usual dose of pilocarpine for this indication is 5 mg PO tid.

Some studies report effective use of acupuncture and hypnosis.

Hiccup

Hiccup, or singultus, is an infrequent but troublesome symptom for which there are few research studies. It is defined as repeated, involuntary, spasmodic, diaphragmatic, and inspiratory intercostal muscle contrations with early glottic closure terminating inspiration.

Presently there is no known physiological function of the hiccup in the adult, and its existence is ascribed to coordination of fetal respiration or some persistent evolutionary reflex. Its neural mechanism is attributed to an afferent limb consisting of the phrenic and vagus nerves and the sympathetic chain (T6–T12), a central mediator between the cervical spine (C3–5) and the brainstem, and an efferent limb consisting mainly of the phrenic nerve.

The pathophysiology of the hiccup reflex is poorly understood. Pathological presentations are attributed to disturbances affecting one of the components of this reflex.

Although the list of conditions that have been associated with hiccup is extensive, they may be grouped into four categories: 1) disturbances affecting the phrenic or vagus nerve, 2) disturbances of central neurological control, 3) those produced by toxic and metabolic disturbances or drugs, and 4) psychogenic causes.

The perceived most frequent cause is gastroesophageal reflux disease (GERD) and gastric distention. Corticosteroids and benzodiazepines are the two drugs most associated with causing hiccup.

Males may be afflicted with hiccup up to 5 times more than women.

Persistent or recurrent hiccups lasting up to 48 hours are considered *acute,* those lasting longer than 48 hours are termed *persistent,* and those lasting longer than 2 months are *intractable.* The adverse effects can be multiple, including fatigue, significant discomfort, insomnia, depression, difficulty with speech and oral intake, weight loss, and decrease in quality of life.

Management is first directed at evaluating the possible underlying cause and taking corrective action, if possible.[4,5] To this end, the history and physical examination are important, and investigations such as laboratory, imaging, and endoscopic studies need to be considered.

Decreasing or discontinuing corticosteroids and benzodiazepines can be an important intervention.

Often the cause is unknown or cannot be rectified. In these cases, there is little from research studies to direct management; most guidelines suggest empiric management based on case studies or postulated mechanisms of action.

Traditional folk remedies may be tried and have little harm but unlikely to improve persistent hiccups. Such maneuvers include pharyngeal and gag reflex stimulation, vagal maneuvers, and breath-holding, among a long list of many others reported throughout history.

Drug treatments are many and varied. An "add-on therapy" approach is recommended given the likelihood of multiple etiologies and the difficulty of this clinical situation. The commonly suggested approach is to start with metoclopramide (10 mg q4h IV or SC) and a proton pump inhibitor (PPI), because GERD plays an important role in many patients.

If this is not effective and renal function is adequate, baclofen (5 mg tid, increased by 5 mg/dose every 3 days to a maximum of 80 mg/day) may be added and titrated upward, while watching for the side effects of sedation, vertigo, ataxia, slurred speech, and weakness.[6] This agent is an analog of gamma-aminobutyric acid (GABA) and is inhibitory at the spinal level. It has been used successfully in the palliative care population for this indication, with many case studies and a small randomized, double-blind, placebo-controlled crossover study to support its use.

Gabapentin (100–300 mg tid starting dose) may be the next agent to consider adding, again considering renal function.

Chlorpromazine (25 mg PO tid) or haloperidol (3–5 mg PO/SC tid) are the next-considered agents to add on.

Nifedipine (30–60 mg/day) or sertraline are further medications to be considered.

Acupuncture and vagal nerve stimulation are final options to consider. Phrenic nerve ablation is the treatment of last resort because of the risk to pulmonary function.

Pruritis

Pruritis is an unpleasant sensation that elicits a desire to scratch or itch. When experienced chronically, pruritis becomes a severely distressing and troublesome symptom.

Current pathophysiological models hold this symptom distinct from pain, and is transmitted via distinct neural pathways. Histamine appears to be an important mediator of itch in many conditions. Also, centrally acting mu-opioid agonists can mediate pruritis.[7]

Unfortunately, there is a paucity of research into this complex symptom. Treatments based on randomized controlled trials are rare.

A large number of diseases may present with itch as an important symptom. It is often helpful to think of these in four broad groups with some examples listed below.

Dermatological diseases

These include a common cause such as dry skin (xerosis). Examples of other skin conditions include scabies, urticaria, atopic dermatitis, dermatitis herpetiformis, bullous pemphigoid, miliari, and pediculosis, among many others.

Systemic conditions

This is a large group including malignancy, drug reactions, hepatic disorders, renal disorders, autoimmune diseases, endocrine, hematopoietic and infectious diseases, including HIV disease.

Disorders of the central or peripheral nervous system

These include peripheral neuropathy, depression, multiple sclerosis, and brain tumor.

Psychogenic

Psychogenic disorders in which pruritis can occur include delusions of parasitosis, neurodermatitis, and anxiety.

Evaluation of the patient who presents with pruritis should include a careful history probing for use of topical or ingested agents that could induce pruritis. Ask about new drugs or therapies instituted in the weeks prior to the itch. Determine whether there is a history of excessive bathing, other family members with itch, or symptoms of neurological or psychiatric diseases.

A physical examination with careful attention to inspection of the skin can reveal a classic dermatological diagnosis, such as xerosis or urticaria.

Dermatological consultation is often helpful if lesions are hard to classify. This may result in recommendations for skin biopsies or special examinations for fungal infections or scabies.

Laboratory investigations screening for systemic conditions that cause pruritis is useful if no etiology is apparent after the history-taking and physical examination. It is important to screen for hepatogenic and nephrogenic pruritis, as these make up a large proportion of cases of systemic pruritis.

Treatment is most effective when a specific cause is diagnosed and an effective treatment is available.[8,9] Any new medications likely to cause pruritis should be stopped, if possible.

General measures are appropriate in most all cases. These include avoiding topical products with fragrance or alcohol and limiting bathing to once per day as a gentle wash with a non-soap, low-pH cleanser. Emollients should be applied in most cases after bathing and frequently throughout the day to improve the skin barrier.

The list of possible systemic treatments for pruritis is extensive. The rational for using a particular therapy should relate to the etiology involved. While the many choices of agents may seem baffling, there are some recommended drug choices:

- Hepatogenic pruritis: mirtazapine (15–30 mg/day), butorphanol (1–4 mg intranasally every day)
- Nephrogenic pruritis: ultraviolet B (UVB) phototherapy (3 times per week), mirtazapine.
- Dermatological pruritus: hydroxyzine (25–100 mg q8h), doxepin (10–50 mg/hour).
- Psychogenic pruritus: mirtazapine, paroxetine (20–50 mg every day).

Other agents that may be useful for hepatic or nephrogenic pruritus include cholestyramine, ondansetron, and naltrexone. Thalidomide (HIV, uremia), gabapentin (neurological), charcoal (uremia), and rifampin (hepatic) have been reported to be helpful as well.

Pressure ulcers and wound care

Wounds presenting in the severely ill patient need to be evaluated for the underlying cause in order to direct management properly. Wounds in this population are commonly due to pressure ulceration, malignancy, venous stasis, arterial insufficiency, infection, or surgical dehiscence.

In the terminally ill, goals of care need to be established, as healing of the wound may not always be realistic. The goals of providing comfort and improving quality of life, promoting healing, and limiting wound progression as well as preventing further wound development may be appropriate for many patients.

Pressure ulcers are caused by compression of cutaneous and subcutaneous tissue between a bony prominence and a support surface. This results in ischemia and tissue necrosis.[10,11] Other forces that can traumatize these tissues include friction and shearing of the skin along the bed-sheets or other surfaces.

Factors that cause immobility are important in the development of these wounds. It is common to find patients at higher risk for these lesions as their illness progresses and they become less mobile.

Typical areas for the development of pressure ulcer are the sacrum, trochanter, ischial tuberosity, posterior heel, elbow, scapula, and occipital region. These areas deserve careful inspection in the routine care of the severely ill patient.

If a wound is evident, strategies for treating the lesion need to be instituted, including increasing the patient's mobility with frequent position changes and turning the patient. It is sometimes helpful to determine what the patient's position was that caused a lesion in a particular area and to inform the patient and caregiver of this as well as consider alternative positioning strategies. The assessment of a physical or occupational therapist can greatly assist with this process.

It is important to remember that unrelieved pressure on the area is the cause of a pressure ulcer[12]; the single most important strategy is the relief of that pressure. Special pressure-reducing mattresses or wheelchair cushions (e.g., Roho) can be helpful in relieving pressure in vulnerable areas.

Attention to dressings is also important. Consultation with a wound-ostomy care (WOC) nurse is useful, as these practitioners are familiar with the variety of dressings and their uses.

The principle of moist wound healing, one of the prime functions of an appropriate dressing, is important in treating this condition. The wound should not be allowed to become dry. Excess exudates can be managed with special dressings such as alginate, hydrofiber, or foam dressings.

It is important to protect the wound and normal skin from the maceration caused by incontinence. Cleansing the wound with a noncytotoxic cleaner such as normal saline, Ringer's lactate, or sterile water between dressing changes is recommended.

Assessment of the wound for infection by observing for inflammation, purulent discharge, and odor can result in effective treatment with antimicrobials, either topically or systemically.

In patients whose wound healing is possible, nutrition should be optimized. Nutritional strategies are feasible, and a dietician's expertise can be useful in developing these for individual patients.

Debridement improves healing and reduces infection. Surgical, enzymatic, and hydrotherapy techniques for debridement should be considered. For difficult situations, vacuum-assisted closure or surgical closure with a flap may be warranted.

General wound management includes consideration of radiotherapy for managing malignant wounds.

Topical sprinkling of crushed metronidazole tablets can decrease wound odor resulting from anaerobic bacteria. Lidocaine gel and compounded morphine gel are topical agents that may be considered when addressing local wound pain.

Lymphedema, edema, and anasarca

Lymphedema is swelling caused by failure of the lymphatic system to adequately drain lymph fluid[13–15]. This occurs secondary to disease (e.g., cancer) or as a result of surgery or radiotherapy of the draining lymph system. The involved limb is at risk for cellulitis because of the accumulation of protein-rich interstitial fluid. Chronic lymphedema results in inflammation that produces fibrosis and sclerosis.

Treatment for breast cancer with surgery and radiotherapy is a common cause of upper limb lymphedema. Surgery or involvement of the inguinal lymph nodes with cancer often results in lower extremity lymphedema.

Symptoms of limb heaviness, discomfort, decreased range of motion, body image concerns, and decreased quality of life are common. The presentation of an acute unilateral limb swelling requires the exclusion of deep venous thrombosis and cellulitis.

Management of lymphedema is optimized by using the skills of a lympedema therapist, who is usually a physiotherapist, nurse, or kinesiologist who has undergone special training. These therapists use a combination of skin care, manual lymph drainage (specialized massage), compression bandaging, pneumatic compression with electric pumps, education, and exercise, termed *combined/complex decongestive therapy* (CDT).

Compression garments are fitted to the limb for maintenance of the reduction in swelling.

Pharmacological therapy has not been effective. Diuretics are ineffective and place the patient at risk for electrolyte imbalance and hypotension. Placement of an IV or SC site in the affected limb is best avoided because of the risk of infection.

Previously, exercise was thought to worsen this condition, but recent evidence shows that even vigorous exercise does not worsen swelling.

Edema refers to excess fluid in body tissue. *Anasarca* describes generalized edema. Both conditions occur commonly in the terminally ill, with lower extremity edema being very frequent in advanced-cancer patients. In these cases other factors in addition to impaired lymphatic drainage occur, such as hypoalbuminemia or obstruction of the inferior vena cava.

Therapy with diuretics rarely results in significant reduction in swelling and is complicated by the complications of these drugs. Elevation of the affected limb, massage drainage, and compression bandaging remain the most effective strategies.

Body-image concerns of the patient and caregivers' distress are often addressed to the clinician and require appropriate discussion and reassurance.

External lymph drainage, a technique developed by Lawrence Clein,[14] is an exciting new development for symptomatic management at the end of life that requires further study, as it is supported by only a small number of case reports at present.

Scrotal edema can be very uncomfortable and can be reduced by scrotal elevation (a small towel or face cloth placed under the scrotum), a customized scrotal support, or bicycle shorts.

Myoclonus

Myoclonus is defined as sudden, brief, involuntary contractions of a muscle or a muscle group.[16] Progression to seizure can occur if the condition escalates. The complete pathophysiological mechanism has not been determined.

It is usually classified as physiological, essential, epileptic, or symptomatic. The latter category is of most concern in palliative care.

Toxic-metabolic syndromes such as renal and hepatic disease are etiologies, as are neurodegenerative disorders such as Parkinson's disease, Alzheimer's disease, Huntington's disease, and Lewy body dementia. Posthypoxic syndromes and drug-induced myoclonus also occur.

Medications associated with myoclonus include opioids, antipsychotics, antidepressants (TCAs and SSRIs), anticonvulsants, antibiotics, calcium channel blockers, and antiarrhythmics.[17]

Opioid-induced neurotoxicity (OIN) is a syndrome that occurs frequently in the palliative setting, where opioids are regularly administered.[17] Myoclonus is one of the most common manifestations of OIN and can alert the clinician to this syndrome. Accumulation of opioid metabolites is the perceived mechanism causing OIN.

Management is directed at reversing this mechanism by decreasing the opioid dose or, alternatively, by opioid rotation to an alternative opioid. Clonazepam (starting at 0.5 mg twice daily) and midazolam are agents that can reduce myoclonus if opioid reduction or rotation is ineffective.

For other conditions causing myoclonus, management consists of treating the underlying disorder or augmenting the GABAergic deficiency. Agents often used include clonazepam (often the drug of choice), valproic acid, and barbiturates.

Clinical pearls

- Eliminating the causative drug may reduce xerostomia.
- Many patients presenting with hiccup benefit from treatment of GERD.
- In the workup of pruritis, it is important to screen for hepatic and renal disease.
- The most important strategy in the management of pressure ulcers is the relief of pressure on the wound.
- Do not use diuretics to manage lymphedema.
- Consider opioid-induced neurotoxicity as a common cause of myoclonus.

References

1. Dion D, Lapointe B (2005). Mouth care. In MacDonald N, Oneschuk D, Hagen N, Doyle D (Eds), *Palliative Medicine: A Case-Based Manual*, 2nd ed, Oxford, UK: Oxford University Press, pp. 317–331.
2. Fusco F (2006). Mouth care. In Bruera E, Higginson IJ, Ripamonti C, von Gunten C (Eds), *Textbook of Palliative Medicine*. Oxford, UK, Hodder Arnold Publishers, pp. 773–779.
3. Lalla RV, Peterson DE (2009). Oral symptoms. In Walsh TD, Caraceni AT, Fainsinger R, Foley K, et al. (Eds.), *Palliative Medicine*. Philadelphia: WB Saunders, pp. 937–946.
4. Smith HS (2009). Hiccups. In Walsh TD, Caraceni AT, Fainsinger R, Foley KM, et al. (Eds.), *Palliative Medicine*. Philadelphia: WB Saunders, pp. 894–898.
5. Thomas T, Wade R, Booth S (2006). Other respiratory symptoms (cough, hiccup, and secretions). In Bruera E, Higginson IJ, Ripamonti C, von Gunten C (Eds), *Textbook of Palliative Medicine*. Oxford, UK: Hodder Arnold Publishers, pp. 663–672 .
6. Ramierz FC, Graham DY (1992). Treatment of intractable hiccup with baclofen: results of a double-blind randomized, controlled, cross-over study. *Am J Gastroenterol* 87(12):1789–1791.
7. Summey BT. Pruritus (2009). In Walsh TD, Caraceni AT, Fainsinger R, Foley K, et al. (Eds.), *Palliative Medicine*. Philadelphia: WB Saunders, pp. 910–913.
8. Pittelkow MR, Loprinzi CL (2004). Pruritus and sweating in palliative medicine. In Doyle D, Hanks G, Cherny N, Calman K (Eds.), *Oxford Textbook of Palliative Medicine*. New York: Oxford University Press, pp. 573–587.
9. Fleischer AB, Dalgleish D (2002). Pruritus. In Berger AM, Portenoy RK, Weissman DE (Eds.), *Principles and Practice of Palliative Care and Supportive Oncology*. Philadelphia: Lippincott Williams & Wilkins, pp. 299–306.
10. Schulz VN, Kozell KM, Martins LM (2009). Pressure ulcers and wound care. In Walsh TD, Caraceni AT, Fainsinger R, Foley K, et al. (Eds.), *Palliative Medicine*. Philadelphia: WB Saunders, pp. 478–484.
11. Froiland KG (2006). Pressure ulcers/wounds. In Bruera E, Higginson IJ, Ripamonti C, von Gunten C (Eds.), *Textbook of Palliative Medicine*. Oxford, UK: Hodder Arnold Publishers, pp. 768–772.
12. Reddy M, Gill SS, Kalkar SR, et al. (2008). Treatment of pressure ulcers: a systematic review. *JAMA* 300(22):2647–2662.
13. Towers A (2009). Lymphedema. In Walsh TD, Caraceni AT, Fainsinger R, Foley K, et al (Eds.), *Palliative Medicine*. Philadelphia: Saunders, pp. 474–478.
14. Clein LJ. Edema (2009). In Walsh TD, Caraceni AT, Fainsinger R, Foley K, et al (Eds.), *Palliative Medicine*. Philadelphia: WB Saunders, pp. 881–886.
15. Guo Y, Konzen B (2006). Lymphedema. In Bruera E, Higginson IJ, Ripamonti C, von Gunten C (Eds.), *Textbook of Palliative Medicine*. Oxford, UK, Hodder Arnold Publishers, pp. 787–796.
16. Groninger H, Muir JC (2009). Seizures and movement disorders. In Walsh TD, Caraceni AT, Fainsinger R, Foley K, et al (Eds.), *Palliative Medicine*. Philadelphia: WB Saunders, pp. 961–965.
17. Lawlor P, Lucey M, Creedon B (2009). Opioid side effects and overdose. In Walsh TD, Caraceni AT, Fainsinger R, Foley K, et al (Eds.), *Palliative Medicine*. Philadelphia: WB Saunders, pp. 1411–1416.

Chapter 17

Management of cancer treatment–related adverse effects

David Hui, MD

Introduction

A growing proportion of advanced-cancer patients seen by palliative care clinicians are on antineoplastic agents, including chemotherapy, hormonal therapy, and targeted agents. This can be attributed to the increasing availability of therapeutic options, as well as to earlier palliative care referral for symptom control.

While antineoplastic agents may improve patients' symptoms through tumor shrinkage or stabilization, they can also be associated with significant adverse effects. Thus, palliative care specialists caring for patients with advanced cancer should be familiar with the management of common side effects associated with these agents.

This chapter provides a brief review of the clinical management of a number of common adverse effects related to antineoplastic agents, including febrile neutropenia, cytopenia, chemotherapy-induced nausea and vomiting (CINV), oral mucositis, diarrhea, drug rash, and peripheral neuropathy.

Cancer-related fatigue, another side effect frequently experienced by cancer patients on treatment, is discussed in Chapter 5.

A detailed discussion of all adverse effects associated with each anti-neoplastic agent is beyond the scope of this chapter. Readers are referred to other resources for further information (e.g., Micromedex, Up-To-Date).

Clinical pearl

• Effective management of adverse effects related to antineoplastic agents requires a sound understanding of the common and serious side effects related to each drug, frequent symptom assessments, patient education, and early initiation of treatment.

Cytopenia and febrile neutropenia

In this section, some of the common management strategies for chemotherapy-induced bone marrow toxicities (Table 17.1) and febrile neutropenia are highlighted.

Anemia

Patients with significant anemia (hemoglobin [Hb] <8.0 g/dL) may benefit from packed red blood cell (RBC) transfusions. For patients with underlying ischemic heart disease or pulmonary disorders, the threshold for transfusion may be lower (e.g., Hb <9.0 g/dL).

Erythropoiesis-stimulating agents such as epoetin-alfa and darbepoetin are generally not given and should be avoided in patients with advanced cancer who are not on chemotherapy.

Erythropoiesis-stimulating agents are associated with not only a risk of thromboembolism but also increased mortality, which is thought to be related to stimulation of tumor growth.[1]

Neutropenia

Neutropenia (absolute neutrophil count [ANC] <1000/mm³) on its own is not life threatening, but it may predispose patients to febrile neutropenia and overwhelming sepsis.

Granulocyte colony–stimulating factor (GCSF) should generally not be used to treat neutropenia in the absence of fever, although it has a role in primary or secondary prophylaxis for patients at risk of developing febrile neutropenia.

Febrile neutropenia

Febrile neutropenia is one of the most common oncological emergencies, defined as the presence of fever >38.3°C (or >38°C for >1 hour) and neutrophil count <500/mm³ (or <1000/mm³ and expected to decrease further). Any patient who develops fever while on chemotherapy should be assumed to have febrile neutropenia unless proven otherwise—complete blood count (CBC) with differential and cultures should be done urgently.

Once febrile neutropenia is confirmed, broad-spectrum antibiotics should be initiated immediately while waiting for culture results.[2]

Table 17.1 National Cancer Institute common terminology criteria for adverse events, version 3.0: hematological toxicities[4]

Grade	Hemoglobin	Neutrophil count	Platelet count
1	<LLN–10.0 g/dL	<LLN–1500/mm³	<LLN– 75,000/mm³
2	<10.0–8.0 g/dL	<1500–1000/mm³	<75,000– 50,000/mm³
3	<8.0–6.5 g/dL	<1000–500/mm³	<50,000– 25,000/mm³
4	<6.5 g/dL	<500/mm³	<25,000/mm³

LLN, lower limit of normal.

Patients at low risk for complications (i.e., no significant signs or symptoms of infection, no comorbidities, ANC >100/mm³, and reliable for follow-up) may be treated on an outpatient basis with oral antibiotics, such as amoxicillin-clavulanate 500 mg PO q8h plus ciprofloxacin 500 mg PO bid for 7–10 days.

High-risk patients should be admitted and given intravenous (IV) antibiotics. Common antibiotic regimens include ceftazidime 2 g IV q8h, imipenem 500 mg IV q6h, and piperacillin/tazobactam 4.5 g IV q8h ± gentamicin 2–2.5 mg/kg IV q8h. It is important that clinicians check renal function and local susceptibility pattern before prescribing these drugs.

Vancomycin 1 g IV q12h should be added if line infection is suspected.

Antifungals should be considered if fever persists for more than 5 days.

GCSF should given to patients at high risk of developing complications.[3] Patients with febrile neutropenia should avoid being in direct contact with other infected individuals or fresh flowers, which are laden with bacteria; however, contact isolation is generally unnecessary.

Thrombocytopenia

Platelet transfusions should be considered for patients with a platelet count <20,000/mm³ or those with thrombocytopenia and clinically significant active bleeding.

Clinical pearls

- Any patients who developed a fever while on chemotherapy should be assumed to have febrile neutropenia unless proven otherwise.
- Avoid erythropoietin use, as it is associated with an increased risk of thromboembolism and mortality in advanced-cancer patients.

Chemotherapy-induced nausea and vomiting

Chemotherapy-induced nausea and vomiting (CINV) is one of the most common side effects (20–50%) experienced by cancer patients and is frequently ranked as the top symptom affecting quality of life during treatment.[5] Clinicians tend to underestimate patients' experience of CINV, particularly the delayed phase.

Prevention is key in the management of CINV. This requires appropriate identification of emetogenic risk and use of antiemetic prophylaxis. Significant advances in the management of CINV include use of corticosteroids, serotonin receptor antagonists, and, most recently, neurokinin 1 (NK-1) receptor antagonists.

In addition to prevention and treatment of CINV, it is important to assess hydration status, food intake, and other common treatment-related complications (e.g., mucositis, diarrhea) (see Table 17.2) and to initiate proper therapies, when appropriate.

Patients on chemotherapy may have nausea and vomiting from causes other than CINV, including bowel obstruction, hypercalcemia, brain metastasis, and opioids. Chapter 10 provides further management strategies for nausea and vomiting in palliative care patients not on chemotherapy.

Table 17.2 National Cancer Institute common terminology criteria for adverse events, version 3.0: nausea and vomiting[4]

Grade	Nausea	Vomiting
1	Loss of appetite without alteration in eating habits	1 episode in 24 hours
2	Oral intake decreased without significant weight loss, dehydration or malnutrition; IV fluids indicated <24 hours	2–5 episodes in 24 hours; IV fluids indicated <24 hours
3	Inadequate oral caloric or fluid intake; IV fluids, tube feedings, or total parenteral nutrition (TPN) indicated ≥24 hours	≥ 6 episodes in 24 hours; IV fluids, or TPN indicated ≥24 hours
4	Life-threatening	Life-threatening

Types of CINV

- *Acute emesis* happens within 24 hours of chemotherapy administration. It usually begins in 1 to 2 hours and peaks at 4 to 6 hours.
- *Delayed emesis* happens after 24 hours of chemotherapy administration and can last for 4 days or more. It is most commonly associated with cisplatin but may also occur with carboplatin, cyclophosphamide, and anthracyclines.
- *Anticipatory emesis* is a conditioned response in patients who experienced severe nausea with previous cycles of chemotherapy. This typically begins 3 to 4 hours prior to chemotherapy initiation.

Emetogenic levels of antineoplastic agents

- *High risk* (>90% risk of CINV in the absence of antiemetic prophylaxis)—carmustine, cisplatin, cyclophosphamide (>1500 mg/m^2), dacarbazine, dactinomycin, mechlorethamine, streptozocin
- *Moderate risk* (31–90% risk)—carboplatin, cyclophosphamide ≤1500 mg/m^2), cytarabine (>1000 mg/m^2), daunorubicin, doxorubicin, epirubicin, idarubicin, ifosfamide, irinotecan, oxaliplatin
- *Low risk* (10–30% risk)—bortezomib, cetuximab, cytarabine ≤1000 mg/m^2), docetaxel, etoposide, fluorouracil, gemcitabine, ixabepilone, lapatinib, methotrexate, mitomycin, mitoxantrone, paclitaxel, pemetrexed, temsirolimus, topotecan, trastuzumab
- *Minimal risk* (<10% risk)—bevacizumab, bleomycin, busulfan, cladribine, fludarabine, vinblastine, vincristine, vinorelbine, rituximab

Clinical pearl

- Prevention is key in management of CINV. Identify the emetogenic risk category and prescribe prophylaxis accordingly.

Management of chemotherapy-induced nausea and vomiting

Selection of antiemetic agents for prophylaxis should be based on the highest emetogenic level among the intravenously administered antineoplastic agents (see Table 17.3).

Table 17.3 Prevention and treatment of acute and delayed CINV: a practical approach[6]

	Any high-risk agents or AC chemotherapy	Any moderate-risk agents	Any low-risk agents	Minimal-risk agents
1. 5HT3 antagonist (choose one)				
Dolasetron (Anzemet)	100 mg PO/IV on day 1	100 mg PO/IV on day 1, then 100 mg PO days 2–3	—	—
Granisetron (Kytril)	1 mg IV or 2 mg PO on day 1	1 mg IV or 2 mg PO on day 1, then 1 mg PO bid on days 2–3	—	—
Ondansetron (Zofran)	8–12 mg IV or 16–24 mg PO on day 1	8 mg IV or 8 mg PO bid on day 1, then 8 mg PO bid on days 2–3	—	—
Palonosetron (Aloxi)	0.25 mg IV on day 1	0.25 mg IV on day 1	—	—
Tropisetron (Navoban)	5 mg PO/IV on day 1	5 mg PO/IV on day 1, then 5 mg on days 2–3	—	—
2. Dexamethasone	12 mg PO/IV on day 1, then 8 mg PO days 2–4	12 mg PO/IV on day 1, then 8 mg PO or 4 mg PO bid days 2–3	8 mg PO/IV day 1	—
3. Aprepitant (Emend)	125 mg PO on day 1, then 80 mg PO days 2–3	—	—	—
4. As needed for breakthrough CINV (choose one or more)				
Metoclopramide (Reglan)	5–10 mg PO/IV q4h PRN			
Prochlorperazine (Compazine)	5–10 mg PO/IV q4h PRN			

Oral mucositis

Oral mucositis, defined as inflammation and ulceration of membranous mucosa, can occur throughout the gastrointestinal tract (see Table 17.4). It is very common among cancer patients, with an incidence of 20–40%.

Risk factors for mucositis include chemotherapy (e.g., 5-fluorouracil, cytarabine, methotrexate, bleomycin, capecitabine, chlorambucil, doxorubicin, etoposide and vinblastine), radiation to the head and neck region, specific cancer primaries (requiring above treatment modalities), younger age, poor oral hygiene, smoking, and alcohol use.

Severe cases (grades 3–4) can lead to complications such as severe pain, bleeding, and superinfections (bacteremia, febrile neutropenia) and may result in hospitalization.

For patients on chemotherapy, the presence of oral mucositis may indicate that other parts of the alimentary tract are involved. Thus, one should always assess for the presence of diarrhea, abdominal pain, nausea, and vomiting. Patients should be encouraged to ensure good oral intake and oral hygiene.

Management of oral mucositis

Prevention is key to the management of mucositis. A number of resources are available on this topic.[7] For patients on 5-fluorouracil, edatrexate, or high-dose melphalan, cryotherapy with ice chips is reasonably tolerable, easily assessable, and cheap. Treatment of established oral mucositis consists of the following.

Hydration and oral hygiene

Maintenance of good oral hygiene and adequate hydration is essential.
- Use of a soft tooth brush for at least 90 seconds twice daily
- Daily flossing

Table 17.4 National Cancer Institute common terminology criteria for adverse events, version 3.0: oral mucositis[4]

Grade	
1	Minimal symptoms, normal diet; minimal respiratory symptoms but not interfering with function
2	Symptomatic but can eat and swallow modified diet; respiratory symptoms interfering with function but not interfering with activities of daily living (ADL)
3	Symptomatic and unable to adequately aliment or hydrate orally; respiratory symptoms interfering with ADL
4	Symptoms associated with life-threatening consequences

- Denture care (where applicable)
- Bland rinses include 0.9% saline, baking soda, or salt and baking soda solution (mix 1 teaspoon of baking soda and one-half teaspoon of salt in 1 L of water). The patient should take a tablespoon every 4 hours, swish for at least 30 seconds, and spit out rinse right afterward.

Analgesia

Topical analgesia may be useful for short-term pain relief of mucositis.
- Different preparations of Magic (or Miracle) mouthwashes may vary, but they generally consist of lidocaine for pain control. One example is a 100 mL solution of hydrocortisone 25 mg, glycerin 95% 2 mL, normal saline 52 mL, lidocaine 2% 25 mL, and nystatin 2083,300 IU or 20.833 mL. Use 10 mL swish and spit q4h to q6h.
- Morphine sulfate 2 mg/mL in 15 mL of water, swish and spit, q4h to q6h
- Lidocaine viscous 2% 10 mL, swish and spit, q4h PRN

Pharmacological treatment

- Systemic opioids remain the mainstay in management of pain associated with mucositis (e.g., morphine 5 mg PO q4h PRN, titrating up as needed). For patients who cannot tolerate the oral route, patient-controlled analgesia (PCA) with parenteral opioids may be considered.
- Current guidelines from the Multinational Association of Supportive Care in Cancer (MASCC) and European Society for Medical Oncology (ESMO) recommend against the use of chlorhexidine mouthwash in the prevention and treatment of mucositis.

Infections

- For patients with oral candidiasis, treatment with nystatin 500,000 IU swish and swallow qid, clotrimazole troches, or fluconazole should be considered.
- Acyclovir or valacyclovir may be given for suspected herpes simplex virus (HSV) infection after cultures have been taken.

Clinical pearls

- Patients with painful oral mucositis should be prescribed adequate analgesia (topical agents or systemic opioids), and monitored for dehydration.
- CINV, oral mucositis, and chemotherapy-induced diarrhea often co-exist. When one of these is present, inquire about the others.

Chemotherapy-induced diarrhea (CID)

Chemotherapy-induced diarrhea (Table 17.5) occurs in 20–40% of cancer patients on treatment and is commonly associated with fluoropyrimidines (5-fluorouracil and capecitabine) and irinotecan. Other causative agents include cisplatin, docetaxel, paclitaxel, doxorubicin, cyclophosphamide, methotrexate, cytosine arabinoside, and topotecan. Targeted agents such as imatinib, erlotinib, sunitinib, and sorafenib may also cause diarrhea.

The pathophysiology of CID is incompletely understood. CID may be caused by treatment-induced intestinal mucosal damage, leading to reduced transit time and decreased water absorption.

Other factors such as alteration in intestinal microflora may also play a role. Irinotecan causes both an early secretory and delayed severe diarrhea in up to 60–80% of patients. This is partly related to its active metabolite SN30, which causes damage of the intestine.

Management of chemotherapy-induced diarrhea

A clinical practice guideline is available for CID[8]:

* First-line treatment—loperamide 4 mg PO, followed by 2 mg every 2 hours (or 4 mg every 4 hours) until 12 hours has elapsed without any diarrhea
* Second-line treatment—octreotide 100–150 mcg SC as needed. Octreotide is a somatostatin analog that slows intestinal transit and decreases fluid secretion into the small intestine.
* For irinotecan-induced diarrhea, neomycin, pentoxifylline, kampo medicine, and chrysin represent a number of potential treatment options; however, the evidence supporting their use remains limited.

It is also important to ensure adequate hydration and to assess for other symptoms such as oral mucositis, nausea, and vomiting. Remember to hold all laxatives in patients who have diarrhea.

Table 17.5 National Cancer Institute common terminology criteria for adverse events, version 3.0: diarrhea[4]

Grade	
1	Increase of <4 stools per day over baseline; mild increase in ostomy output compared to baseline
2	Increase of 4–6 stools per day over baseline; IV fluids indicated <24 hours; moderate increase in ostomy output compared to baseline; not interfering with ADL
3	Increase of < 7 stools per day over baseline; incontinence; IV fluids ≥ 24 hours; hospitalization; severe increase in ostomy output compared to baseline; interfering with ADL
4	Life-threatening consequences (e.g., hemodynamic collapse)

Treatment-related skin lesions

Dermatological complications of antineoplastic agents include alopecia, palmar plantar erythrodysesthesia, xerosis, skin rash, hair and nail changes, and phototoxicity. In this section, discussion is focused on palmar plantar erythrodysesthesia and rash related to epidermal growth factor receptor (EGFR) inhibition.

Palmar plantar erythrodysesthesia

Palmar plantar erythrodysesthesia,[9] also known as hand-foot syndrome (Table 17.6), is commonly associated with capecitabine, 5-fluorouracil, docetaxel, doxorubicin (including liposomal formulation), and cytarabine. Multi-kinase inhibitors such as sorafenib and sunitinib can also be associated with a hand-foot skin reaction, which tends to be more localized and hyperkeratotic than classic palmar planter erythrodysesthesia.

Early recognition and modification of treatment regimen are key to managing this syndrome. Supportive measures to keep skin moist and intact include topical Bag Balm and petroleum jelly.

Pyroxidine 100–300 mg PO daily may be useful for treatment and/or prevention of hand-foot syndrome. Appropriate analgesia should be given if pain becomes an issue. The role of systemic or topical corticosteroids remains undefined.

Skin lesions associated with EGFR inhibition

Targeted agents that inhibit the EGFR pathway, including erlotinib, gefitinib, cetuximab, and panitumumab, are commonly associated with a rash involving the face, chest, and upper back. This reaction typically peaks after 1–2 weeks of therapy.

It is papulopustular or macropapular in nature and frequently gets mistaken as an acneiform eruption. Importantly, the presence of skin rash is a predictive marker of treatment response to EGFR inhibitors.

The following proposed classification is based on symptom severity[10]:

- *Mild toxicity:* generally localized papulopustular reaction that is minimally symptomatic, with no sign of superinfection, and no impact on daily activities

Table 17.6 National Cancer Institute common terminology criteria for adverse events, version 3.0: hand-foot syndrome[4]

Grade	Criteria
1	Minimal skin changes or dermatitis (e.g., erythema) without pain
2	Skin changes (e.g., peeling, blisters, bleeding, edema) or pain, not interfering with function
3	Ulcerative dermatitis or skin changes with pain interfering with function

- *Moderate toxicity:* generalized papulopustular reaction, accompanied by mild pruritus or tenderness, with minimal impact on daily activities and no signs of superinfection
- *Severe toxicity:* generalized papulopustular reaction, accompanied by severe pruritus or tenderness, that has a significant impact on daily activity and has the potential for superinfection or has become superinfected.

Patients with EGFR inhibitor–associated skin rash should be advised to avoid sun exposure. Specific management is based on rash severity[10]:

- *Mild toxicity:* consider observation alone, topical hydrocortisone 1–2.5% cream, or clindamycin 1% gel. Continue EGFR inhibitor at same dose and monitor carefully.
- *Moderate toxicity:* topical hydrocortisone 2.5% cream or clindamycin 1% gel or pimecrolimus 1% cream, plus either doxycycline 100 mg PO bid or minocycline 100 mg PO bid. Continue EGFR inhibitor at the same dose and monitor carefully.
- *Severe toxicity:* topical hydrocortisone 2.5% cream or clindamycin 1% gel or pimecrolimus 1% cream, plus either doxycycline 100 mg PO bid or minocycline 100 mg PO bid. Consider dose reduction of EGFR inhibitor and monitor carefully.

Treatment-induced peripheral neuropathy

Peripheral neuropathy is one of the major adverse effects associated with antineoplastic agents, including taxanes (docetaxel, paclitaxel), platinum agents (oxaliplatin, cisplatin, carboplatin), vinca alkalodis (vincristine, vindesine, vinblastin, vinorelbine), epothilones (ixabepilone, patupilone), thalidomide, lendalidomide, and bortezomib.

Cisplatin and carboplatin are mainly associated with sensory neuropathy, whereas the rest may also have a motor component.[11] Oxaliplatin is associated with both acute neuropathy (cold hypersensitivity and muscle contractions) and chronic sensory peripheral neuropathy that is closely associated with the cumulative dose.

Risk factors for development of peripheral neuropathy include high treatment dose, prior or concurrent use of neurotoxic agents, and pre-existing neuropathy due to comorbidities such as diabetes.

Severe peripheral neuropathy has a negative impact on quality of life (see Table 17.7) and is an important dose-limiting toxicity that frequently results in early termination of cancer treatments.

Management of peripheral neuropathy

If patients develop significant peripheral neuropathy (grade 2 or above), dose reduction or delay or discontinuation of treatment may be required. Early diagnosis can minimize development of more neurotoxicity. The neuropathy may not improve (and may sometimes worsen) until several weeks or months after discontinuation of the antineoplastic agent. In some cases, the neurotoxicity may be irreversible.

Table 17.7 National Cancer Institute common terminology criteria for adverse events, version 3.0: neuropathy[4]

Grade	Sensory neuropathy	Motor neuropathy
1	Asymptomatic; loss of deep tendon reflexes or pares-thesia (including tingling) but not interfering with function	Asymptomatic, weakness on exam/testing only
2	Sensory alteration or paresthesia (including tingling), interfering with function but not with ADL	Symptomatic weakness interfering with function, but not interfering with ADL
3	Sensory alteration or paresthesia interfering with ADL	Weakness interfering with ADL; bracing or assistance to walk (e.g., cane or walker) indicated
4	Disabling	Life-threatening; dis-abling (e.g., paralysis)

Specific prophylactic strategies for oxaliplatin-induced peripheral neuropathy include stop-and-go administration schedules and neuromodularlory agents such as Ca/Mg infusions. For neuropathic pain, gabapentin, carbamazepine and venlafaxine have also been used with variable success.

References

1. Bohlius J, Schmidlin K, Brillant C, Schwarzer G, Trelle S, Seidenfeld J, Zwahlen M, Clarke M, Weingart O, Kluge S, Piper M, Rades D, Steensma DP, Djulbegovic B, Fey MF, Ray-Coquard I, Machtay M, Moebus V, Thomas G, Untch M, Schumacher M, Egger M, Engert A (2009). Recombinant human erythropoiesis-stimulating agents and mortality in patients with cancer: a meta-analysis of randomised trials. *Lancet* 373(9674):1532–1542.

2. Hughes WT, Armstrong D, Bodey GP, Brown AE, Edwards JE, Feld R, Pizzo P, Rolston KV, Shenep JL, Young LS (1997). Guidelines for the use of antimicrobial agents in neutropenic patients with unexplained fever. Infectious Diseases Society of America. *Clin Infect Dis* 25(3):551–573.

3. American Society of Clinical Oncology (1994). Recommendations for the use of hematopoietic colony-stimulating factors: evidence-based, clinical practice guidelines. *J Clin Oncol* 12(11): 2471–2508.

4. National Cancer Institute (2006). National Cancer Institute Common Terminology Criteria for Adverse Events (CTCAE) v3.0. Retrieved May 2009 from http://safetyprofiler-ctep.nci.nih.gov/CTC/CTC.aspx.

5. Hesketh PJ (2008). Chemotherapy-induced nausea and vomiting. *N Engl J Med* 358(23): 2482–2494.

6. Kris MG, Hesketh PJ, Somerfield MR, Feyer P, Clark-Snow R, Koeller JM, Morrow GR, Chinnery LW, Chesney MJ, Gralla RJ, Grunberg SM (2006). American Society of Clinical Oncology guideline for antiemetics in oncology: update 2006. *J Clin Oncol* 24(18):2932–2947.

7. Keefe DM, Schubert MM, Elting LS, Sonis ST, Epstein JB, Raber-Durlacher JE, Migliorati CA, McGuire DB, Hutchins RD, Peterson DE; Mucositis Study Section of the Multinational Association of Supportive Care in Cancer and the International Society for Oral Oncology (2007). Updated clinical practice guidelines for the prevention and treatment of mucositis. *Cancer* 109(5):820–831.

8. Benson AB, Ajani JA, Catalano RB, Engelking C, Kornblau SM, Martenson JA Jr, McCallum R, Mitchell EP, O'Dorisio TM, Vokes EE, Wadler S (2004). Recommended guidelines for the treatment of cancer treatment-induced diarrhea. *J Clin Oncol* 22(14):2918–2926.

9. Nagore E, Insa A, Sanmartín O (2000). Antineoplastic therapy–induced palmar plantar erythrodysesthesia ('hand–foot') syndrome. Incidence, recognition and management. *Am J Clin Dermatol* 1(4):225–234.

10. Lynch TJ Jr, Kim ES, Eaby B, Garey J, West DP, Lacouture ME (2007). Epidermal growth factor receptor inhibitor–associated cutaneous toxicities: an evolving paradigm in clinical management. *Oncologist* 12(5):610–621.

11. Behin A, Psimaras D, Hoang-Xuan K, Leger JM (2008). Neuropathies in the context of malignancies. *Curr Opin Neurol* 21(5):534–539.

Radiotherapy and palliative care

Elizabeth A. Barnes, MD, FRCPC

Introduction

Radiotherapy (RT) plays an important role in the multidisciplinary management of patients with cancer. Approximately half of all RT treatment is given with palliative and not curative intent. Local RT is used in the palliative setting to relieve symptoms resulting from tumor mass effect.

The goal of palliative RT is to use a short treatment schedule to provide effective and durable symptom relief with minimal treatment-related side effects.

Typically, one RT treatment (fraction) is given per day, 5 days a week (Monday through Friday). Small doses per fraction (2 Gy or less) reduce the risk of late toxicity and are used in the curative setting.

For symptom palliation, a high total dose is not required and palliative fractionation schedules can therefore be shorter, thus minimizing patient visits to the cancer center. Commonly used palliative RT regimes include 8 Gy in a single fraction, 20 Gy in 5 fractions, and 30 Gy in 10 fractions.

Treatment-related side effects are defined as acute (≤90 days after treatment start) or late (>90 days). As RT is a local treatment, side effects depend on the area treated. A description of the common acute side effects from palliative RT and management is given in Table 18.1.

Table 18.1 Acute side effects from local palliative radiotherapy and their management

Site	Symptom	Management
Head and neck	Mucositis	Soft diet, viscous xylocaine PRN, treat infection
Chest	Dysphagia	Soft diet, viscous xylocaine PRN, treat infection
Abdomen	Nausea and vomiting	Antiemetics (ondansetron)
Pelvis	Diarrhea	Low fiber diet, imodium or lomotil as required
Skin	Erythema	Skin hygiene (mild soap and water)
	Dry desquamation	Moisturizer (plain, non-scented, lanolin-free hydrophilic cream), hydrocortisone for pruritis
	Moist desquamation	Topical antibiotics, moist wound dressings

Late toxicity is usually not a problem in the palliative setting, given the low total dose used and the limited life expectancy of this population.

Palliative RT is usually very effective for relieving pain, bleeding, and other symptoms due to tumor mass effect. Treatment is usually well tolerated with minimal acute side effects.

Indications for palliative RT are summarized and details on the most common clinical scenarios are given in Box 18.1.

Box 18.1 Common indications for palliative radiotherapy

Pain
- Bone metastases, lung tumor invading chest wall, tumor mass compressing nerve or soft tissue

Neurological symptoms
- Spinal cord compression, brain metastases

Bleeding
- From gynecological, GI, GU, lung, or skin tumors

Obstruction
- Esophageal, airway, ureteric, or rectal obstruction from tumor mass
- Superior vena cava obstruction

Skin ulceration and fungation
- Skin cancer or other tumors eroding through the skin

Bone metastases

Indications

Bone metastases are common in patients with advanced cancer and are the most common cause of cancer pain. RT is a very effective modality for palliating painful bone metastases.

Dose

There has been some controversy over the optimal dose fractionation schedule, with numerous randomized trials published on the subject since the 1980s. The latest meta-analysis (2007) reviewed 16 randomized trials of single- (SF) vs. multiple-fraction (MF) RT for palliation of painful uncomplicated bone metastases.[1]

No significant difference was found in pain relief between SF and MF RT. For intent-to-treat patients, the overall response rates for pain were 58% (SF) and 59% (MF), and complete response rates were 23% (SF) and 24% (MF). No difference was found between the two arms in the rates of acute toxicity, pathological fracture, or spinal cord compression. The retreatment rate was 2.5-fold higher after SF RT (20% vs. 8% for MF).

The results from this meta-analysis confirm conclusions from previous clinical practice guidelines and consensus documents stating that SF RT should be the standard of care, for patient convenience, cost-effectiveness, and resource implications for the given RT department.

However, a 2009 international survey of patterns of practice of American, Canadian, Australian, and New Zealand radiation oncologists found that most of these clinicians continued to prescribe MF for bone metastases.[2] Membership affiliation, country of training, location of practice, and practice type independently predicted use of SF. This finding suggests that factors other than the medical literature influence the prescription of RT for bone metastases.

Contraindications to radiotherapy

Patients with inherited hypersensitivity syndromes such as ataxia-telangiectasia can have severe abnormal tissue reactions. Another contraindication is previous RT to a site where normal tissue tolerance would be exceeded with retreatment. Relative contraindications include collagen vascular diseases.

Retreatment can be considered for patients who experience initial pain relief followed by a relapse, have incomplete pain relief, or experience no pain relief after the initial treatment. An ongoing phase III international randomized trial of SF vs. MF for re-irradiation of painful bone metastases is being conducted to determine the optimal dose fractionation regime for retreatment.

For diffuse bony metastatic disease, half-body irradiation (HBI) and systemic radionuclides can be used to simultaneously target all bony lesions. HBI encompasses either the upper half (base of skull to iliac crest) or lower half (iliac crest to ankles) of the body in a single large RT field.

Systemic radionuclides are deposited at the site of osteoblastic bony metastases, mirroring the uptake seen on bone scan. Radionuclides have been studied mainly in patients with prostate cancer, as bone metastases are osteoblastic (rather than the osteolytic or mixed metastases seen with other primary tumors).

The acute gastrointestinal toxicity associated with HBI requires pre-medication and IV hydration, and there are concerns of late toxicity to visceral structures. The use of systemic radionuclides is limited by cost and availability. Both HBI and systemic radionuclides are associated with transient myelosuppression, which delays the use of chemotherapy.

Prophylactic surgical fixation should be considered for good-performance status patients with bone lesions at high risk of fracture. Postoperative RT is routinely given and has been shown to improve functional status, decrease pain, and reduce the risk of refracture.

Lesions at high risk of fracture include those with >50% cortical destruction of a long bone; femoral lesions >25 mm in the neck; subtrochanteric, intertrochanteric, or supracondylar regions; and diffuse lytic involvement of a weight-bearing bone that is especially if painful.

An analysis of femoral metastases from the Dutch Bone Metastasis Study[2] found that the risk of fracture was mostly dependent on the amount of axial cortical involvement. These investigators recommended prophylactic fixation for lesions >30 mm, or in nonsurgical candidates MF RT to decrease fracture occurrence.

Spinal cord compression (SCC) involves compression of the dural sac and contents (spinal cord and/or cauda equina) by an extradural tumor mass. If left untreated, progressive pain, motor and sensory loss, and sphincter dysfunction result.

A pooled analysis found that after RT, 95% of patients who were ambulatory pretreatment retained ambulation, compared with 63% of patients requiring ambulation assistance, 36% of paraparetic patients, and 13% of paraplegic patients. Corticosteriods are initiated for symptomatic patients, followed by either surgery and/or RT.

A randomized trial published in 2005 compared decompressive surgery followed by RT to RT alone in patients with satisfactory medical status and one level of cord compression.[3] This study met early stopping criteria because of significantly improved outcomes in the surgery arm, with 101 patients randomized. Significantly more patients randomized to the surgical arm were able to walk (84% vs. 57%) and regained the ability to walk (62% vs. 19%).

However, there were many criticisms of this study, including the long time for accrual (10 years), patients in the RT-alone arm having worse outcomes than historical controls, and 40% of randomized patients having spinal instability.

Spinal instability or bone compression should be an indication for surgery, rather than RT, as neurological outcomes are improved. A number of different radiation fractionation regimes are used in clinical practice.

Preliminary results from a nonrandomized trial of short- vs. long-course RT confirm the results from previous retrospective studies showing that local control was better after long-course RT, but functional outcomes and survival were no different.

Brain metastases

Brain metastases occur in approximately 20–40% of cancer patients and are associated with major neurological morbidity; prognosis is often limited to 2–4 months. Treatment typically consists of corticosteroids to reduce peritumoral edema, followed by whole brain radiotherapy (WBRT). The goal of WBRT is to provide neurological symptom relief, allow corticosteriod tapering, and possibly improve survival.

However, prospective observational studies of patients who have undergone WBRT have shown that patient- and observer-related symptoms, including quality of life and neurological symptoms, often deteriorate after treatment. Patients with poor performance status and rapidly progressive extracranial disease may not derive a clinical benefit from WBRT.

Quality of Life After Radiotherapy and Steroids (QUARTZ) is a Medical Research Council phase III trial currently being conducted in the United Kingdom and Australia. Patients with inoperable brain metastases from non–small-cell lung cancer have been randomized to supportive care (steroids) alone vs. supportive care (steroids) plus WBRT. The primary outcome is patient-assessed quality-adjusted life years, and secondary endpoints are overall survival, Karnofsky Performance Scale (KPS), and neurological symptoms.

From 30 to 40% of patients present with a single brain metastasis. For this population with good performance status and minimal or no evidence of extracranial disease, surgical excision followed by WBRT has been shown to improve survival over that with WBRT alone.[4] The use of post-operative WBRT after surgical excision of a single metastasis has been shown to improve local control.

After WBRT, a stereotactic radiosurgery boost for good-performance status patients has been shown to improve survival for those with a single brain metastasis and to improve functional autonomy for those with 2–3 metastases.[5]

A 2004 practice guideline report found no benefit with respect to survival or symptom control for WBRT doses higher than 20 Gy in 5 fractions or 30 Gy in 10 fractions.[6]

The acute side effects of WBRT include fatigue, alopecia, and erythema of the scalp. Long-term toxicity is limited and rarely a concern for these patients with limited life expectancy.

Lung cancer

Lung cancer is one of the most common causes of cancer death worldwide. More than two-thirds of patients with non–small-cell lung cancer present with incurable locally advanced or metastatic disease. The overall prognosis is poor, with a median survival of less than 1 year.

Thoracic symptoms can be effectively palliated with local RT, with up to 90% of patients obtaining relief from hemoptysis and chest pain, and up to 65% obtaining relief from cough and dyspnea.

In a systemic review of 13 randomized controlled trials examining fractionation regimes involving 3473 patients,[7] for specific symptom-control end points, lower-dose (LD) RT was comparable to higher-dose (HD) [(biological effective dose (BED) $\geq$35 Gy(10)].

Four trials reporting a total symptom score rather than individual symptoms found significantly greater improvement in the HD than in LD arm. One-year survival was significantly greater after HD than after LD RT, 26.5% vs. 21.7%. The authors concluded that consideration should be given for delivering $\geq$35 Gy(10) BED, but this must be weighed against increased esophagitis and greater time investment for the patient.

Pelvic disease

Locally advanced and recurrent pelvic malignancies arising from gastrointestinal, gynecological, or genitourinary sites can result in many disabling symptoms. These include hemorrhage, necrotic vaginal discharge, pain (due to adenopathy, tumor invasion of bone, lumbosacral plexus, and soft tissue), lower extremity edema, fistula formation, gastrointestinal tract obstruction, and renal failure due to bilateral ureteric obstruction.

Palliative RT is commonly useful for patients with invasive bladder cancer, who are often elderly, are smokers, and have medical comorbidities. One randomized trial compared the efficacy and toxicity of two palliative RT regimes (35 Gy in 10 fractions vs. 21 Gy in 3 fractions on alternate days over 1 week) and found no difference between regimes, with a 68% overall improvement in bladder symptoms at 3 months and late bowel toxicity rate of <1%.[8]

Individual symptomatic improvement at 3 months was 88% for hematuria, 82% for frequency, 72% for dysuria, and 64% for nocturia and was maintained in many patients for the duration of their survival (median survival was 7.5 months). Other groups have looked at delivering 5–6 weekly fractions of 6 Gy and also found effective symptom palliation.

Recurrent ovarian cancer is typically treated with chemotherapy. However, RT can offer excellent symptom palliation even in patients with platinum-resistant disease. A review of 53 patients found a symptom response rate of 100%, with a complete response (CR) of 68%. The CR rates were 88%, 65%, and 36% for the symptoms of bleeding, pain, and "others," respectively, and the median duration of response was 4.8 months (range: 1–71 months).[9]

Patients with locally advanced, recurrent, or metastatic rectal cancer can suffer from severe pelvic pain and bowel obstruction. Palliative chemoradiotherapy with concurrent 5-fluorouracil (5-FU) provided symptom relief in 94% of patients, with a 1-year colostomy-free survival rate of 87%.[10] A BED ≥35 Gy was associated with higher pelvic control.

A systematic review to find the most effective dose fractionation regime for symptom relief in patients with pelvic recurrence from colorectal or rectal cancer found there were only retrospective series in the literature.[11] Although there was a suggestion of a more favorable response with higher doses, the authors concluded that well-designed randomized studies with symptom control end points were needed to determine if a dose–response relationship exists.

Emerging technologies

Conformal and intensity-modulated RT is beginning to play an important role in palliative and curative RT. These treatment modalities have the ability to conform the radiation dose to the tumor while minimizing dose, and thus toxicity, to surrounding normal tissue. This offers the potential for dose escalation, which may be useful when higher rates of local tumor control translate into increased symptom palliation.

Conformal RT can be useful in the setting of retreatment where it is often important to avoid retreating normal tissue. An extreme application of this technology is stereotactic body RT (SBRT), in which a three-dimensional frame of reference is used to accurately localize the tumor. As setup uncertainty and tumor movement are significantly reduced, the margin around the tumor can be reduced, which allows one to deliver a high dose per fraction to the target.

A prospective study of "curative-intent" SBRT for patients with ≤ 5 metastatic lesions using 50 Gy in 10 fractions found a 2-year local control rate of 67%; however, no symptom control end points were reported. SBRT is also being used for spinal and paraspinal metastases. The hypothesis is that a high dose will lead to higher rates of local control and pain. However, no randomized control trials with conventional RT have been conducted.

Conclusion

Palliative RT provides effective and efficient palliation of symptoms due to locally advanced or metastatic disease experienced at the end of life. Side effects are minimal, and the time to symptom response is rapid; for painful bone metastases or bleeding, response can be seen within a week.

Rapid-access palliative radiotherapy clinics have been established in many Canadian cancer centers and offer radiation treatment planning and delivery in the same day, reducing the number of visits the patient needs to make to the cancer center.

Clinical pearls

- A single fraction of RT can often palliate distressing symptoms due to local disease.
- Palliative RT may not be suitable for patients with uncontrolled pain, severe orthopnea, or delirium, as they must lie still, supine, and unattended for 10–15 minutes for planning and treatment.
- The acute side effects of palliative RT are usually mild and transient.
- Spinal cord compression should be ruled out in patients presenting with rapid-onset lower extremity neurological changes.

References

1. Chow E, Harris K, Fan G, Tsao M, Sze WM (2007). Palliative radiotherapy trials for bone metastases: a systematic review. *J Clin Oncol* 25:1423–1436.
2. Fairchild A, Barnes E, Ghosh S, et al. (2009). International patterns of practice in palliative radiotherapy for painful bone metastases: evidence-based practice? *Int J Radiat Oncol Biol Phys* 75(5):1501–1510.
3. Patchell RA, Tibbs PA, Regine WF, et al. (2005). Direct decompressive surgical resection in the treatment of spinal cord compression caused by metastatic cancer: a randomised trial. *Lancet* 366:643–648.
4. Patchell RA, Tibbs PA, Walsh JW, et al. (1990). A randomized trial of surgery in the treatment of single metastases to the brain. *N Engl J Med* 322:494–500.
5. Andrews DW, Scott CB, Sperduto PW, et al. (2004). Whole brain radiation therapy with or without stereotactic radiosurgery boost for patients with one to three brain metastases: phase III results of the RTOG 9508 randomised trial. *Lancet* 363:1665–1672.
6. Tsao MN, Lloyd NS, Wong RK, Rakovitch E, Chow E, Laperriere N, Supportive Care Guidelines Group of Cancer Care Ontario's Program in Evidence-based Care. Radiotherapeutic management of brain metastases: a systematic review and meta-analysis. Cancer Treat Rev. 2005;31:256–273.
7. Fairchild A, Harris K, Barnes E et al. (2008). Palliative thoracic radiotherapy for lung cancer: a systematic review. *J Clin Oncol.* 26:4001–4011.
8. Duchesne GM, Bolger JJ, Griffiths GO, et al. (2000). A randomized trial of hypofractionated schedules of palliative radiotherapy in the management of bladder carcinoma: results of medical research council trial BA09. *Int J Radiat Oncol Biol Phys* 47:379–388.
9. Choan E, Quon M, Gallant V, Samant R (2006). Effective palliative radiotherapy for symptomatic recurrent or residual ovarian cancer. *Gynecol Oncol* 102:204–209.
10. Crane CH, Janjan NA, Abbruzzese JL, et al. (2001). Effective pelvic symptom control using initial chemoradiation without colostomy in metastatic rectal cancer. *Int J Radiat Oncol Biol Phys* 49:107–116.
11. Wong R, Thomas G, Cummings B et al.(1996).The role of radiotherapy in the management of pelvic recurrence of rectal cancer. Can J Oncol. 1996 Feb;6 Suppl 1:39–47.

Hospice approach to palliative care, including Medicare hospice benefit

Joan K. Harrold, MD, MPH
Charles F. von Gunten, MD, PHD

Hospice care in the United States

Hospice care is palliative care at the end of life. Hospices differ as to how early in the course of an illness they provide care, so it is important to know the scope and timing of services provided by your local hospices. Nearly all hospices, however, provide care for patients with life expectancies of 6 months or less.

In the United States, 80% of hospice care is paid for by Medicare, the federal system of health care coverage for the elderly and the disabled. The Medicare Hospice Benefit (MHB) pays for comprehensive medical, nursing, counseling, and bereavement services to terminally ill patients and their families[1] (Box 19.1). These services are provided by an interdisciplinary team that meets at least biweekly to review the plan of care and its effectiveness in advancing the goals expressed by the patient, family, and other caregivers. The services can be provided in the patient's home, a nursing home, inpatient hospice unit, and a hospital.

Although hospice provides end-of-life care, referral for hospice care does not shorten life expectancy. For certain diagnoses, hospice enrollment is associated with longer survival times.

Box 19.1 Medicare hospice benefit

Covered services (100%—no co-pay)

- Nursing care: to provide intermittent (usually 1–3 times/week) assessment, support, skilled services, treatments, and case management services
- 24-hour availability for assessment and management of changes, crises, and other acute needs
- Social work: supportive counseling, practical aspects of care (other community services), and planning (health care surrogates, advance directives)
- Counseling services: including chaplaincy
- Home health aid and homemaker services
- Speech therapy, nutrition, physical therapy (PT), and occupational therapy (OT) services
- Bereavement support to family after the death
- Medical oversight of plan of care (POC) by hospice medical director
- All medications and supplies for management and palliation of the terminal illness (hospices may collect a small co-pay for medications)
- Durable medical equipment (e.g., hospital bed, commode, wheelchair, etc.)
- Short-term general inpatient care for problems that cannot be managed at home, such as pain, dyspnea, delirium, acute skilled needs
- Short-term respite to permit family caregivers to take a break
- Continuous care at home for short episodes of acute need

Services not covered by Medicare hospice benefit

- Continuous nursing or nurse aid care
- Medications unrelated to the terminal illness
- Physician visits for direct medical care (billed to Medicare separately)
- Residential (non-acute) care in a facility

Referring for hospice care

Referral for hospice care is appropriate when the patient has a limited prognosis and the most important goals are comfort and symptom management.

The number one complaint about hospice care from patients and families is that no one told them about it sooner. The second most common complaint is that no one told them about the practical benefits; there was too much talk about the philosophy of care and not enough about who would help and how.

When patients elect coverage using the MHB, the hospice agency becomes responsible for coordinating and paying for all treatments and medications related to the primary hospice diagnosis. Patients can continue to receive care for diseases unrelated to the terminal illness (e.g., dialysis for renal failure if the patient is dying of cancer, cataract removal) using regular Medicare coverage.

Most Medicaid and commercial insurers use the Medicare Hospice Benefit Model for coverage of hospice care.

Medicare hospice benefit eligibility

To pay for hospice care, Medicare requires both the attending physician and hospice physician to certify that the patient has a life expectancy of 6 months or less if the disease or condition runs its normal course. If patients improve or resume disease-directed therapy with the primary goal of extending life expectancy, they can be discharged and resume services later without penalty.

Individual patients can continue to be eligible if they live longer than 6 months as long as the physician believes death is more likely than not within 6 months. The patient does not need a do-not-resuscitate (DNR) order to be eligible for hospice care. There is no limit to the number of days a patient can receive hospice care. There is no penalty if the patient outlives the diagnosis.

Prognosis

Physicians overestimate prognosis when compared with actual survival by a factor of 3 or greater. Prognostication may be more accurate for cancer because of the pattern of decline that precedes death (Box 19.2).

Although trajectories of other terminal conditions are less well defined, there are a variety of factors to consider and resources to use when assessing prognosis and considering hospice referral (Box 19.3).

Some factors are reviewed by Medicare and deemed decisive when determining eligibility. Because the prognostic utility of these factors changes according to advances in medical research, they may be insufficient to guide timely planning by patients and families.

Box 19.2 Cancer: prognostic factors

General
- Performance status:
  - Karnofsky ≤50, ECOG ≤3
  - Most of the time in bed or lying down

Signs associated with prognosis ≤6 months
- Malignant pericardial or pleural effusions
- Malignant ascites
- Multiple brain metastases
- Carcinomatous meningitis
- Malignant bowel obstruction
- Serum albumin <2.5 mg/dL
- Hypercalcemia (except in newly diagnosed breast cancer or myeloma)

Cancers associated with prognosis ≤6 months
- Metastatic lung cancer
- Unresectable pancreas cancer
- Progressive metastatic breast or prostate cancer with poor or decreasing functional status
- Metastatic solid tumor, acute leukemia, or high-grade lymphoma forgoing chemotherapy

Box 19.3 Non-cancer prognostic factors

Heart disease
- Functional capacity, comorbidities, recent cardiac hospitalization, systolic blood pressure <100 mmHg and/or pulse >100 bpm, cachexia, anemia, hyponatremia, elevated BUN and/or creatinine ≥1.4 mg/dL, left ventricular ejection fraction ≤45%, ventricular dysrhythmias (treatment resistant); Seattle Heart Failure Model

Lung disease
Ambulatory patients
- FEV_1, age, exercise capacity, low body mass index (BMI), low PaO_2, subjective estimates of dyspnea

Hospitalized patients
- Age, functional status, comorbidities, severity of illness (APACHE II score), need for mechanical ventilation, hypoxia, hypercarbia, low serum albumin, low hemoglobin

Dementia
- Age, comorbidities, cardiac dysrhythmias, peripheral edema, aspiration, bowel incontinence, recent weight loss, dehydration, fever, pressure ulcers, seizures, shortness of breath, dysphagia, low oral intake, not awake for most of the day, low BMI, recent need for continuous oxygen, recent hospitalization for pneumonia or hip fracture

Box 19.3 (*Contd.*)

Renal disease
- Age, functional status, comorbidities, albumin <3.5 g/dL, refusal or discontinuation of dialysis

Liver disease
- Age, comorbidities, ascites, encephalopathy, bilirubin, albumin, prolonged prothrombin time, hepatorenal syndrome, hepatocellular carcinoma, rate of clinical decompensation; MELD Score

Plan of care (POC)

The hospice program approves, coordinates, and pays for services that are reasonable and necessary for palliation and/or management of the terminal illness. The POC is based on the patient's diagnosis and needs, orders of the attending physician, and, as necessary, collaboration with the hospice medical director.

Physician role

The attending physician is indicated by the patient at the time of enrollment. Sometimes the patient will select a hospice physician for this role.

The attending physician is responsible for working with the hospice team to determine appropriate care. Direct patient care services by the attending physician are billed to Medicare in the usual fashion.

Places of care

Home

The majority (95%) of hospice care takes place in the home because that's where patients say they want to be. Hospice team members visit the patient and family on an intermittent basis. Care continues as long as the patient remains eligible and wants the care. Medicare rules do not require a primary caregiver in the home.

Nursing home or other long-term care facility

This is the patient's home, and the patient's "family" frequently includes the staff. Hospice care is specialty care provided in addition to usual nursing home care.

Hospice inpatient unit

Dedicated units that are free-standing or within other facilities such as nursing homes or hospitals are sometimes available. Permitted length of stay varies, as some are for residential care and others for short-term acute care.

Hospital

Occasionally, pain and other symptoms or other conditions related to the terminal illness cannot be managed at home and the patient is admitted to an inpatient hospital or other contracted inpatient facility for more intensive management. The inpatient facility must have a contract with the hospice program.

Payment to the hospice

Medicare pays for covered services using a per diem capitated arrangement in one of four categories:

- *Routine home care:* care at home or nursing home
- *Inpatient respite care:* care in an inpatient setting (usually a nursing home or inpatient hospice unit) for up to 5 days to give family caregivers a break
- *General inpatient care:* acute inpatient care for conditions related to the terminal illness (e.g., pain and symptom control, caregiver breakdown, impending death and the patient doesn't want to die at home)
- *Continuous home care:* provides acute care at home with around-the-clock care for a crisis that might otherwise lead to inpatient care

Payment to attending and consulting physicians

Direct patient care services by the attending physician for care related to the terminal illness are covered by Medicare, but not under the Medicare Hospice Benefit.

If the attending physician is not associated with the hospice program, the physician bills Medicare Part B in the usual fashion. The bill must indicate that the physician is not associated with the hospice program or the claim may be denied.

If the attending physician is associated with the hospice program or is a consultant, the physician submits the bill to the hospice program, which in turn submits the claim to Medicare under Part A. The physician is reimbursed on the basis of a contract with the hospice program.

Discussing hospice care

One of the biggest barriers to timely referral for hospice care is physician discomfort with the discussion.[2–7]

Clinical pearls

• Discuss hospice care in the context of the larger goals of care, using a step-wise approach.

1. Establish the setting

Ensure comfort and privacy; sit down next to the patient. Ask if family members or others should be present. Introduce the subject with a phrase such as "I'd like to talk with you about our overall goals for your care."

2. What does the patient understand?

Ask open-ended questions to elicit patient understanding about their current health situation. It is important to get the patient talking; if the doctor is doing all the talking, it is unlikely that the rest of the conversation will go well. Consider starting with phrases such as "What do you understand about your current health situation?" **or** "What have the doctors told you about your cancer?"

Listen for phrases like "I know I'm going to die of this cancer." **or** "I know I don't have much time left" **or** "I know the cancer is getting worse." If the patient does not know or appreciate their current status, this is the time to review that information.

3. What does the patient expect?

Next, ask the patient to consider the future. Examples of ways to start this discussion are "What do you expect in the future?" **or** "What goals do you have for the time you have left—what is important to you?" This step allows you to listen while the patient describes a real or imagined future. Most patients with advanced cancer use this opening to voice their thoughts about dying—typically mentioning comfort, family, and home as their goals of care. If there is a sharp discontinuity between what you expect and what the patient expects, this is the time to clarify.

Listen carefully to the patient's responses; most patients have thought a lot about dying, they only need permission to talk about what they have been thinking. Setting up the conversation in this way allows the physician to respond with clarifying and confirming comments, such as "So what you're saying is, you want to be as independent as possible and stay out of the hospital" **or** "What you've said is, you don't want to be a burden on your family."

Use the opportunity to teach the patient about what to expect if they express inaccurate or exaggerated fears—pain can be controlled; they can avoid returning to the emergency department or hospital. Consider asking what other experiences they have had. Some have seen (or read or heard about) "bad" deaths that can be prevented by modern care.

4. Discuss hospice care

Use language that the patient will understand, and give information in small pieces. Never say, "There's nothing more we can do." "Nothing" is euphemistic and easily misinterpreted. To a patient, "nothing" means abandonment.

Consider summarizing the patient's goals as part of introducing a discussion of hospice care. For example: "You've told me you want to be as independent and comfortable as possible. Hospice care is the best way I know to help you achieve those goals."

Listen carefully to the response. Many patients have distorted views of hospice care. Others have never heard the term. Ask what the term means to them. Patients frequently describe hospice as a place to go to die or what you do when you give up. Respond by asking why they think that. Probe for previous experiences or how they developed their point of view.

Respond by describing hospice as a program that helps the patient and family achieve the goals the patient just described. It's a team of people that help the doctor meet the patient's and family's physical, psychological, social, and spiritual needs.

Offer to ask someone from the hospice to come by to give information. You don't have to be the expert. Tell the patient you can talk again after they have more information.

Offer your recommendation: "From what you've told me, I think it would be best if we got the hospice involved" **or** "I always recommend the hospice to get involved for my patients at this stage of their illness."

Reassure the patient and family that, if they get better, or if there is a new treatment discovered, they can be discharged (or graduate) from hospice care to receive that care. Nationally, 10% of hospice patients are discharged alive.

5. Respond to emotions
Strong emotions are expected when discussing death. Typically, the emotional response is brief. The most profound initial response a physician can make is silence, providing a reassuring touch, and offering tissues. The most frequent mistake is to talk too much.

6. Establish a plan
Clarify the plan. For example: "I'll ask the hospice to come by to talk with you, and then you and I can talk again."

Common questions and dilemmas

- My patient has end-stage disease and wants CPR. Can I still refer him to hospice?
  - Yes. A DNR order is not required to be eligible for hospice care. Since CPR is unlikely to be successful, however, discuss your patient's goals for such treatment. If he still wants CPR, revisit the plan after hospice care has been established. If he wanted CPR because going to the hospital for care was his only experience, the patient may have different goals once he has experienced care in his home.
- My patient has a prognosis of 4–6 months, but her symptoms are controlled. When should I make the referral to hospice?
  - Now. Your patient and her family can get to know the hospice team, begin to establish trust, and be monitored for new or worsening symptoms before a crisis occurs. They will also receive emotional and spiritual support, coordination of care and resources, and preparation for what to expect with disease progression.
- The hospice does not cover the pain medication that my patient is taking unless other medication has failed him. What do I do?
  - Call the hospice medical director and discuss the treatment plan. Ask him or her if other medications were ineffective prior to hospice care. If not, ask why the hospice prefers certain medications as first-line therapy.
- If I refer my patient to hospice, will I still be her doctor or will the hospice physicians take over her care?
  - The patient chooses the physician to manage her care. If you are willing to do so, your patient can choose to have you as her attending physician. Some physicians prefer to have the hospice physician manage or comanage their patients. Let the hospice know if you prefer that model so that your patient can make an informed choice.
- My patient has a prognosis of about 6 months, but she may need chemotherapy or radiation therapy to help manage her symptoms. Will hospice cover the treatments?
  - Hospice coverage may vary according to the goals of care, expected effectiveness, and resources. Many hospices will cover treatments that are expected to significantly reduce symptoms. Some hospices will cover all treatments as long as they are unlikely to increase the patient's life expectancy past 6 months. Most hospices will help assess if the benefits outweigh the burdens relative to the patient's life expectancy. Larger programs with more resources may be able to cover treatments that smaller programs cannot. If radiation therapy or chemotherapy is indicated, call the hospice medical director and discuss the treatment plan.
- I want to prescribe a treatment for my patient, but the hospice does not cover it and recommends that he revoke the MHB. What does that mean?
  - Your patient can revoke the MHB if he wants to use his regular Medicare benefits to cover his care. This is not a decision to be taken lightly, as the patient forfeits all of his hospice services when he revokes the MHB unless he re-elects to use the MHB in the

future. He should not revoke just for the treatments and then re-elect the MHB in between, as this is inconsistent with the intent of the MHB. If you believe that the treatment should be included in the hospice coverage, call the hospice medical director and discuss the treatment, goals of care, and reasons that it is not covered.

- The hospice says that my patient has an extended prognosis and no longer qualifies for hospice services. What happens now?
  - If a patient no longer has a life expectancy of 6 months or less given the natural course of the disease process, he or she cannot be certified as eligible for the MHB. The hospice is expected to establish a discharge plan with the patient to ensure that care needs can be met in other ways.
- My patient has improved since she was referred to hospice. Why doesn't the hospice discharge her?
  - Some patients appear to "improve" after admission to hospice because symptoms are managed, support is provided, and care needs are met. These improvements do not change the patient's eligibility for hospice care. Other patients have illnesses marked by fluctuations and exacerbations. If the patient's death appeared imminent but the patient rallied, the longer-term prognosis may still be poor and consistent with eligibility.
- My patient lives in a nursing home. Why would he need hospice, too?
  - Hospice care augments the care to residents living the end of their lives in nursing homes. Hospice provides expertise in pain and symptom management, coverage of medications and other treatments, additional care for complex needs, and support for family members and other caregivers. The nurses, aides, counselors, and volunteers from hospice work with the staff of the nursing home to provide comprehensive end-of-life care, increased presence to comfort patients and families, and support and recognition of the efforts of nursing home staff as they face the death of a resident to whom they may have become attached.
- My patient only has days to live. Isn't it too late for hospice care?
  - Although patients are eligible for hospice care with a life expectancy of 6 months or less, referral at any time has been shown to benefit patients and families.[8,9] In addition to helping during an often difficult time, bereavement support will also be offered to your patient's family.
- My patient is likely to die during this hospital admission. Can hospice still help her?
  - Many hospices provide end-of-life care in hospitals as general inpatient care. Although you may be managing physical symptoms quite well, the additional presence of hospice staff may be especially helpful to patients and families coping with death and dying in the hospital setting.

References

1. Centers for Medicare and Medicaid Services (2003). Medicare Hospice Benefits. Publication No. CMS 02154. Revised July 2003.
2. Emanuel LL, von Gunten CF, Ferris FD (Eds.) (1999). The EPEC Curriculum. The EPEC Project. Retrieved January 31, 2009, from www.epec.net.
3. End of Life/Palliative Education Resource Center (EPERC). Fast facts and concepts. Retrieved January 31, 2009, from www.eperc.mcw.edu/ff_index.htm.
4. Diem SJ. Lantos JD. Tulsky JA (1996). Cardiopulmonary resuscitation on television. Miracles and misinformation. *N Engl J Med* 334(24):1578–1582.
5. Junkerman C, Schiedermayer D (1998). *Practical Ethics for Students, Interns and Residents*, 2nd ed. Hagerstown, MD: University Publishing Group.
6. Council on Ethical and Judician Affairs, American Medical Association (1999). Council report: medical futility in end-of-life care. *JAMA* 281:937–941.
7. Buckman R (1992). How to Break Bad News: A Guide for Health Care Professionals. Baltimore: Johns Hopkins University Press.
8. Taylor DH, Ostermann J, Van Houten CH, et al. (2007). What length of hospice use maximizes reduction in medical expenditures near death in the US Medicare program? *Soc Sci Med* 65(7):1466–1478.
9. Connor SR, Pyenson B, Fitch K, et al. (2007). Comparing hospice and nonhospice patient survival among patients who die within a three-year window. *J Pain Symptom Manage* 33(3):238–246.

Psychosocial and cultural considerations in palliative care

V.S. Periyakoil, MD

Common psychological issues in palliative care patients

There is often a complex interplay of medical and psychosociocultural issues in the setting of any chronic and/or serious life-limiting illness. While the conventional biomedical model works very well for any acute illness, it often minimizes and tends to ignore the role of these issues in patient health care and well-being.

A stance that focuses narrowly on only the biological aspects and ignores the underlying psychosociocultural aspects will lead to poor care outcomes resulting in both increased patient and family distress and clinician frustration.

This chapter discusses common psychosociocultural issues in a palliative care and provides key clinical pearls regarding assessment and management as well as resources for further self-directed learning.

Preparatory grief

Preparatory grief[1] is the normal grief reaction to perceived losses experienced by persons who are dying. Persons who are dying prepare for their death by mourning the losses implicit in death. The anticipated separation from loved ones is an obvious one. Simple pleasures of living may also be grieved.

People may reflect on their past and relive great moments and disappointments, as well as mourn missed opportunities. Looking to the future, they may grieve the loss of much-anticipated experiences, such as a child's graduation or the birth of a grandchild.

Distinguishing[1-3] between grief and depression in patients who are dying can be difficult. Many of the signs and symptoms traditionally used to diagnose depression are also present in patients who are grieving (see Fig. 20.1).

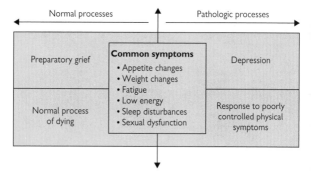

Fig. 20.1 Overlap of processes in patients with advanced disease. Reprinted with permission from Periyakoil VS, Hallenbeck JL (2002). Identifying and managing preparatory grief and depression at the end of life. *Am Fam Physician* 65(5):883–890.

Clinical pearls
- Many patients with serious life-limiting illness will experience grief.
- Grief, a normal part of the dying process, responds well to support.
- Grief can mimic depression and the two should be differentiated, as the management is different.

Depression

Major depression is defined[4] by persistent low mood, or anhedonia (pervasive loss of interest or pleasure), that lasts for 2 weeks or more and is accompanied by at least 4 of the 9 following symptoms: sleep disruption (especially early-morning insomnia), weight loss or change in appetite, psychomotor

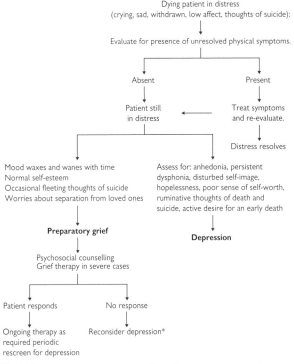

Fig. 20.2 Differentiating preparatory grief from depression in patients with terminal illness. Reprinted with permission from Periyakoil VS, Hallenbeck JL (2002). Identifying and managing preparatory grief and depression at the end of life. *Am Fam Physician* 65(5):883–890.

retardation or agitation, fatigue or loss of energy, feelings of worthlessness or excessive guilt, diminished ability to think or concentrate, and recurrent thoughts of death or suicidal ideation.

False positives are very common in a palliative care setting (see Fig. 20.2), as the illness per se can cause many of the somatic (appetite, weight, sleep, libido, energy changes) and affective (sadness, fleeting thoughts of death or suicide, crying, limiting social activities).

Clinical pearls
- Depression is NOT a normal part of the terminal illness process.
- Presence of hopelessness, helplessness, worthlessness, pervasive loss of pleasure, and persistent dysphoria are signs of depression in palliative care patients, and their presence should trigger an in-depth screening.
- Anxiety and depression usually coexist in a palliative care setting.
- Depression is underdiagnosed and undertreated. Depression can and should be treated. Treatment will improve the quality of life of palliative care patients.
- Medication choice in treating depression in a palliative care setting is determined by patient prognosis, drug–drug interactions, and medication side effects. Selective serotonin reuptake inhibitors (SSRIs) are the drug of choice for depression in palliative care patients and are usually well tolerated. SSRIs have a latency of onset of a few weeks and are not useful in patients with an anticipated life span of hours to days.
- Common SSRIs used include citalopram 20–60 mg/day, escitalopram 10–20 mg/day, fluoxetine 20–60 mg/day, fluvoxamine 50–150 mg bid, paroxetine 20–50 mg/day, and sertraline 50–200 mg/day. These medications typically take at least 4–6 weeks for full effect. This late onset of action is particularly problematic for patients with advanced illness and an expected prognosis of days to weeks.
- Common SSRI side effects include nausea, diarrhea, headache, insomnia, anxiety, anorexia, dizziness, tremor, sweating, and sexual dysfunction.
- Depressed patients with anticipated prognosis of days to weeks can be treated with psychostimulants such as methylphenidate.

Anxiety

About 18% of American adults have anxiety disorders. *Anxiety* is a state of apprehension and fear resulting from the perception of a current or future threat to oneself.

At least 25% of cancer patients and 50% of patients with congestive heart failure (CHF) or chronic obstructive pulmonary disease (COPD) experience significant anxiety. Anxiety[5,6] is often seen secondary to poorly managed acute or chronic pain, dyspnea, nausea, and other distressing symptoms.

Anxiety can also be precipitated by medications such as corticosteroids, psychostimulants, and some antidepressants, as well as by withdrawal of alcohol, opioids, benzodiazepines, nicotine, clonidine, antidepressants, and corticosteroids. In addition, death anxiety and existential and psychosocial concerns about dying, disability, loss, legacy, family, finances, and religion or spirituality can also precipitate anxiety.

Anxiety is a predominant symptom of the following psychiatric disorders that are common in palliative care patients.

Generalized anxiety disorder (GAD)

Anxiety and fear occur commonly in the dying patient. However, disabling anxiety and/or panic is not a normal aspect of the dying process.

Patients with GAD can't seem to shake their worries, which are usually also accompanied by physical symptoms, especially fatigue, headaches, muscle tension, muscle aches, difficulty swallowing, trembling, twitching, irritability, sweating, and hot flashes.

Further, panic disorder (PD) diagnosis in the patient's caregiver can be associated with patient GAD, and patient GAD can be associated with caregiver PD.

Panic disorder

A *panic attack*[7,8] is defined in the *Diagnostic and Statistical Manual of Mental Disorders, fourth edition (DSM-IV)* as a discrete period of intense fear or discomfort, in which four (or more) of the following symptoms develop abruptly and reach a peak within 10 minutes: palpitations, pounding heart or accelerated heart rate, sweating, trembling or shaking, sensations of shortness of breath or smothering, feeling of choking, chest pain or discomfort, nausea or abdominal distress, feeling dizzy, unsteady, lightheaded, or faint, derealization or depersonalization, fear of losing control or going crazy, and fear of dying.

Derealization is a sensation of feeling estranged or detached from one's environment. *Depersonalization* is an altered and unreal perception of self, feelings, and/or situation (described by one patient as "feeling like you are on the outside looking in").

Clinical pearls

- Panic disorder is more common in palliative care patients with chronic dyspnea.
- Medical management is influenced by anticipated lifespan and severity of panic symptoms.
- SSRI monotherapy or SSRI therapy augmented with low-dose benzodiazepines for a period of 3 to 4 weeks followed by SSRI monotherapy (taper off benzodiazepines after 3 weeks) is indicated in patients with an anticipated lifespan of at least several weeks.
- SSRIs can exacerbate anxiety in some patients during the first few days of therapy. Consider adding benzodiazepines as needed for the first few weeks in such cases.
- Benzodiazepine monotherapy should be considered in patients with an anticipated lifespan of days to weeks.

Posttraumatic stress disorder (PTSD)

An estimated 25% of patients with a past history of traumatic life events can develop posttraumatic stress disorder (PTSD). Traumatic events that trigger PTSD[9,10] include exposure to robbery; physical assault; sexual assault; natural disasters; fires or arson; exposure to environmental hazards; tragic death of a close friend or family member by means of accident, suicide, or homicide; cancer diagnosis; motor vehicle crash; and war combat.

PTSD is an anxiety disorder that can develop when a person has experienced, witnessed, or was confronted with an event(s) that involved actual or threatened death or serious injury, or a threat to the physical integrity of self or others.[4]

PTSD can manifest as anxiety, agitation, nightmares, and hyperarousal.

Clinical pearls
- A simple four-item screen helps identify PTSD (see Table 20.1)
- SSRIs are the drug of choice for PTSD. While the FDA has approved both sertraline and paroxetine for PTSD, other SSRIs like citalopram are effective and well tolerated.
- SSRIs help palliate all symptom groups (re-experiencing, avoidance, hyperarousal) of PTSD.
- TCAs are second line for treatment of PTSD and are thought to alleviate intrusive symptoms, anxiety, depression, and insomnia.
- Serotonin–norepinephrine reuptake inhibitor (SNRI) antidepressants, such as venlafaxine and nefadazone, are effective in treating PTSD.

Advance directives

An advance directive (AD) is a form that documents the patient's expressed wishes about what kind of care they would like to have if they become incapable of making medical decisions (when in a coma or due to dementia). The advance directive should guide the physicians and family when making health-care decisions on behalf of the patient.

Advance directives can take many forms and, more importantly, the laws about advance directives are different in each state. Physicians must have a good understanding of the local institutional policy as well as the state laws governing care.

Clinical pearls
- A living will is one type of advance directive that describes the kind of medical treatments or life-sustaining treatments a patient would want if they were to become seriously or terminally ill. A living will does not let the patient name a surrogate decision maker.
- A durable power of attorney (DPA) for health care is another kind of advance directive. A DPA documents the person(s) chosen by the patient to make health-care decisions on their behalf in event they become incapable of making such decisions. A DPA becomes active

Table 20.1 PTSD Screening Questionnaire

In your life, have you ever had any experience that was so frightening, horrible, or upsetting that, *in the past month, you* …

1. Have had nightmares about it or thought about it when you did not want to?

2. Tried hard not to think about it or went out of your way to avoid situatios that reminded you of it?

3. Were constantly on guard, watchful, or easily startled?

4. Felt numb or detached from others, activities, or your surroundings?

screen is positive if patient answers "yes" to any two of the four questions.

any time a patient is unable to make medical decisions. A DPA is generally more useful than a living will. But a DPA may not be a good choice if the person doesn't have another person they can trust to make these decisions for them.

- Physician Orders for Life-Sustaining Treatment (POLST): A POLST[11] form is a brightly colored medical order form used to write orders indicating life-sustaining treatment wishes for seriously ill patients. The POLST accomplishes two major purposes: 1) it turns treatment wishes of an individual into actionable medical orders, and 2) it is portable from one care setting to another.
- The POLST form remains with a patient if they are moved between care settings, regardless of whether the patient is in the hospital, at home, or in a nursing home. The POLST is legally used in some states in the United States, and in these states, when a patient has a completed POLST form, the form must be honored by all health-care providers.

Cultural issues

Culture has a great influence on how people make health-care decisions and on their preferences for care interventions, including advance-care planning as well as heroic life-prolonging measures. It also has a huge influence on rituals related to death and dying and after-death care.

Clinical pearls

- Racial differences persist[12–14] in all of health care, including end-of-life care. Ethnicity has been shown to be a marker of common cultural beliefs and values that, in combination, influence decision making at the end of life.
- Review of racial variations in hospice use indicates that minorities use services disproportionately less than white patients, even after researchers control for specific sociodemographic and clinical characteristics.
- Another study[14] showed that, compared with white patients, black and Hispanic patients are less likely to consider themselves terminally ill and more likely to want intensive treatment and less likely to have advance-care planning.

Explanatory model

Sometimes patients and families from diverse cultural backgrounds have very different ways of understanding their illness, its consequences, and how it needs to be treated—i.e., a different "explanatory model of illness" as described by Kleinman.[15] This is especially true for recent immigrants and those who are not acculturated to mainstream American culture and are still unfamiliar with Western biomedicine.

Eliciting the patient's understanding of their illness process in a culturally competent manner will help the clinician better understand the patient's stance and be better able to tailor health care interventions, avoid frustration, and promote adherence to the care plan.

See Box 20.1 for trigger questions that help elicit the explanatory model.

Nondisclosure and the concept of protective truthfulness

In some cultures and ethnic minorities, the family may request nondisclosure of terminal illness—i.e., they may request that the physician withhold the diagnosis from the patient (e.g., "Doctor, please don't tell my father that he has cancer. If he finds out that he has cancer, he will lose all hope and just give up and die").

Requests for nondisclosure may cause clinicians considerable distress and ethical conflict. Some may feel that it is the patient's right to know their diagnosis and that withholding diagnostic and prognostic information is ethically questionable.

In addition, physicians may feel that it is not possible to obtain informed consent for interventions like chemotherapy and radiation therapy if the patient does not know her diagnosis.

Box 20.1 provides points that can guide the clinician in dealing with requests for nondisclosure.

Box 20.1 Explanatory model of illness

Often patients from different cultural backgrounds may have very specific beliefs about why and how they contracted an illness. Beliefs can vary from the mundane to the very unusual (e.g., a patient may believe that an illness is due to being possessed by evil spirits).

To understand the patient's perception, it is helpful to ask the following *what, why, how, and who* questions:

- **What** do you call the problem?
- **What** do you think the illness does?
- **What** do you think the natural course of the illness is?
- **What** do you fear?
- **Why** do you think this illness or problem has occurred?
- **How** do you think the sickness should be treated?
- **How** do want us to help you?
- **Who** do you turn to for help?
- **Who** should be involved in decision making?

Reprinted with permission from Kleinman A, et al. (1978). Culture, illness and cure: clinical lesions from anthropologic and cross-cultural research. *Ann Intern Med* 88:251–258.

Clinical pearls

- Request for nondisclosure are usually motivated by the concept of "protective truthfulness," i.e., truth-telling is thought to be an insincere and potentially harmful act if a patient were to lose hope and confidence in life after learning of their disease. Thus the intent of the family is to protect the patient and to not harm the patient.
- When the family asks you to withhold the truth, the explanatory model of open-ended questions can be used to elicit their concerns:
  - Why do you want me to withhold the information?
  - What are you concerned about?
  - What do you think will happen if the patient were to hear the truth?
- Discuss with the family how you are going to approach the patient and what you are going to talk about.
- Approach the patient and explore the sensitive subject gently. For example, "Mr. Patel, I understand from your family that you do not want to know the details about your illness and that you want them to make decisions for you regarding your health care." If the patient requests not to know and wants the family to make decisions, this is ethically acceptable, as he or she is exercising autonomy by choosing not to know.
- Reassure the patient that anytime they want to know more information, you are always available to discuss their medical situation.
- Autonomy, the right to exercise free will, can be invoked by the patient when not wanting to know diagnostic and prognostic information related to the illness—i.e., the patient has the right to refuse to learn about the diagnosis and defer all decision making to the designated decision maker.

Working with medical interpreters

Communicating with patients and families with limited English proficiency is particularly challenging. Lack of adequate communication could lead to loss of critical information, resulting in suboptimal care and poor patient and family satisfaction.

In communicating with patients with limited English proficiency, physicians must use a professional medical interpreter. Such services are and should be available in all health-care systems (some systems have interpreters on staff and others use commercial telephone-based interpreter services).

Clinical pearls

• Family members should not serve as interpreters. The gold standard is to use a professional medical interpreter.

• Interpreters should be from the same culture as the patient. Interpreters not only translate the patients' words but also interpret them within the cultural context. They should serve as cultural brokers and translate the concept and meaning from the patient's language into English.

• The professional medical interpreter should similarly interpret the physician's explanations and proposed interventions and explain these to the patient and family.

• Professional medical interpreters are bound by the standard Health Insurance Portability and Accountability Act (HIPPA) regulations and should treat all information learned as confidential.

• The professional medical interpreter should *not* influence the opinion and actions of the patient.

• When communicating through a professional medical interpreter, use short, simple sentences (avoid jargon), ask them to translate a few sentences at a time, frequently check in with them, and debrief with them after the interaction. This will help foster accuracy and collegiality.

References

1. Periyakoil VS, Hallenbeck JL (2002). Identifying and managing preparatory grief and depression at the end of life. *Am Fam Physician* 65(5):883–890.

2. Periyakoil VS, Kraemer HC, Noda A, Moos R, Hallenbeck J, Webster M, Yesavage JA (2005). The development and initial validation of the Terminally Ill Grief or Depression Scale (TIGDS)" *Int J Methods Psychiatr Res* 14(4):202–212.

3. Periyakoil VS (2005) Is it grief or depression? 2nd edition. Retrieved December 28, 2010, from http://www.eperc.mcw.edu/display/router.aspx?docid=72296&

4. American Psychiatric Association (1994). *Diagnostic and Statistical Manual of Mental Disorders.* 4th ed. Washington, DC: American Psychiatric Association.

5. Stoklosa J, Patterson K, Rosielle D, Arnold R (2007). Anxiety in palliative care: causes and diagnosis. Fast Facts and Concepts. 186. Retrieved December 28, 2010, from http://www.eperc.mcw.edu/fastfact/ff_186.htm

6. National Institute of Mental Health (2007). When Worry Gets Out of Control: Generalized Anxiety Disorder. Retrieved November 8, 2008, from http://www.nimh.nih.gov/health/publications/generalized-anxiety-disorder.shtml

7. Periyakoil VS, Skultety K, Sheikh J (2005). Panic, anxiety and chronic dyspnea at the end of life. *J Palliat Med* 8(2):453–459.

8. Periyakoil VS (2005). Panic disorders at the end of life. Fast Facts and Concepts #145. November, 2005. Retrieved December 28, 2010, from http://www.eperc.mcw.edu/fastfact/ff_145.htm

9. Feldman DB, Periyakoil VS (2006). Posttraumatic stress disorder at the end of life. *J Palliat Med* 9(1):213–218.

10. Prins A, Ouimette P, Kimerling R, Cameron RP, Hugelshofer DS, Shaw HJ, Thraikill A, Gussman FD, Sheikh JI (2003). The Primary Care PTSD Screen (PC-PTSD): development and operating characteristics. *Prim Care Psychiatry* 9:9–14.

11. Physician Orders for Life-Sustaining Treatment Paradigm (POLST). Retrieved November 8, 2008, from http://www.ohsu.edu/ethics/polst

12. Johnson KS, Kuchibhatla M, Tulsky JA (2008). What explains racial differences in the use of advance directives and attitudes toward hospice care? *J Am Geriatr Soc* 56(10):1953–1958.

13. Cohen LL (2008). Racial/ethnic disparities in hospice care: a systematic review. *J Palliat Med* 11(5):763–768.

14. Smith AK, McCarthy EP, Paulk E, Balboni TA, Maciejewski PK, Block SD, Prigerson HG (2008). Racial and ethnic differences in advance care planning among patients with cancer: impact of terminal illness acknowledgment, religiousness, and treatment preferences. *J Clin Oncol* 26(25):4131–4137.

15. Kleinman A (1978). Culture, illness and cure: clinical lesions from anthropologic and cross-cultural research. *Ann Intern Med* 88:251–258.

Additional resource

Periyakoil VS, Stanford End of Life Curriculum. Retrieved November 8, 2008, from http://endoflife.stanford.edu

Spiritual issues in palliative care

Christina M. Puchalski, MD, FACP
Betty Ferrell, PhD, RN, FAAN
Edward O'Donnell, MA

Introduction

Since the inception of hospice and the development of palliative care, spirituality has been recognized as an essential element of palliative care. Saunders described the concept of "total pain" as encompassing spiritual distress as well as psychosocial and physical distress.[1] Her model was eventually described as the biopsychosocial-spiritual model, which is the framework for palliative care.[2] The model emphasizes the totality of a patient's experience in the context of their illness and/or dying.

While the primary diagnosis may be cancer, for example, the span of the clinician's assessment of that patient includes the physical signs and symptoms of the cancer, the patient's emotional response to the illness, the social ramifications of the cancer on the patient and their family and friends, and, finally, the spiritual issues that may present as a result of the illness. Integrating all dimensions of a patient's experience with illness is key to patient-centered care.

Spirituality as part of patient-centered care, particularly in palliative care, is supported by ethical as well as empirical literature.[3–6] Studies have demonstrated that spiritual care affects health-care outcomes including quality of life,[7–9] will to live,[9,10] survival,[11,12] and coping.[13]

Surveys demonstrate that patients want their spiritual issues formally addressed in the clinical setting[14,15] and want their spiritual needs attended to by health-care professionals.[16,17]

In hospital settings, the degree to which spiritual needs of patients are attended to is the strongest predictor of patient satisfaction with care and with patient perception of quality of care.[18] Studies have also indicated that spiritual or religious beliefs can impact end-of-life decision-making.[19]

The Picker Institute has noted that respecting patients' beliefs and values may improve patients' health-care outcomes and is critical to the practice of patient-centered care.[20]

The National Consensus Project for Quality Palliative Care (NCP), a coalition of leading palliative care organizations in the United States, represents the nation's 4700 hospices, 9000 hospice and palliative care nurses, 1400 hospital-based palliative care programs, and 4000 members of American Academy of Hospice and Palliative Medicine. In 2004, the NCP developed guidelines to strengthen new and existing palliative care services.[21] The guidelines were updated in 2009.[22]

Spiritual care is one of the eight distinct domains within the NCP guidelines, and spiritual and existential concerns are mentioned throughout as aspects of pain, psychological concern, and grief.

The National Quality Forum (NQF), one of the leading forces in health care, accepted the NCP domains and created preferred practices to operationalize the NCP guidelines.[22,23] These preferred practices are all relevant to clinical practice (see www.nationalconsensusproject.org).

The NQF framework presents 38 best practices across the eight domains of the NCP framework. These practices are evidence based or endorsed through expert opinion and apply to both hospice and palliative care provided across settings.[23] The NCP guidelines are a significant contribution in acknowledging the importance of spiritual care in palliative medicine and provide a foundation for the broader integration of spirituality into medical care.

Despite these guidelines, the implementation of spiritual care is not uniform in palliative or other care settings. Reasons for this include confusion over the definition of spirituality, lack of resources and tools, inadequate professional education, and lack of practical implementation tools. The variability in approaches to spirituality in palliative care underscores the need to articulate a definition of spirituality and to set common guidelines for spiritual care as a dimension of palliative care.

In 2009, Puchalski and Ferrell co-led a national Consensus Conference to develop recommendations for implementing the spiritual care domain of the NCP guidelines for palliative care. The project was a collaboration between the George Washington Institute for Spirituality and Health and the City of Hope National Medical Center. Forty leaders in palliative care and spiritual care who were from various disciplines were invited to develop specific and practical recommendations for the implementation of interdisciplinary spiritual care in palliative care, which was defined as starting from initial diagnosis of a serious or chronic illness.

Specific recommendations as well as models for spiritual care implementation and interdisciplinary spiritual care education were developed. The resultant recommendations were then reviewed nationally and approved through a consensus process and published for widespread dissemination as a consensus document, titled "Improving the Quality of Spiritual Care as a Dimension of Palliative Care."[24] More detailed information is published in a handbook of spiritual care in palliative care.[25]

As part of this initiative, resources for spiritual care are available on a national repository for spirituality and health, called SOERCE, on the Web site of the George Washington Institute for Spirituality and Health (www.gwish.org). The goal of this seminal work is to provide resources and tools for increased integration of spiritual care into palliative care and into medical care in general.

Implementing spirituality in clinical settings

The key to implementing spirituality in clinical settings is to have a practical model for implementation that allows all clinicians to recognize and integrate patients' spiritual issues into the treatment or care plan. A key outcome of the Consensus Conference was the development of a spiritual care implementation model (Fig. 21.1).

This model, which is based on a generalist–specialist model in which board-certified chaplains are recognized as the spiritual care experts, includes the following features:

- All patients receive a spiritual screening, history, and assessment by the appropriate health-care professional.
- Spiritual screenings are admissions questions to screen for spiritual distress; screening is limited to two questions: Is spirituality or religion important for you? Are your spiritual or religious beliefs helping you right now? A yes/no combination to these questions triggers a referral to a board-certified chaplain.
- Spiritual histories are more detailed and done by clinicians who determine treatment or care plans. The spiritual history can be taken by means of a tool, such as the FICA (Faith, Importance, Community, Action),[26] HOPE (sources of Hope, Organized religion, Personal spirituality and Practices, Effects on medical care and End-of-life issues),[27] or SPIRIT (Spiritual belief system, Personal spirituality, Integration with a spiritual community, Ritualized practices and restrictions, Implications for medical care, and Terminal events planning) instruments.[28] All of these tools were developed for clinicians.
- Spiritual diagnoses are made by clinicians, ideally in an interdisciplinary team setting with the input of board-certified chaplains, who will also integrate spirituality into the treatment and care plan.
- There is an ongoing follow-up and modification of the plan, as needed.
- Clinicians receive professional training in practicing spiritual care.

Once the clinician obtains the information from the history, he or she integrates it into the treatment plan. This includes making a diagnosis of spiritual distress or pain, or identification of spiritual issues or spiritual goals, if appropriate, and determining and implementing the appropriate spiritual interventions.

There are two possible pathways once a diagnosis is made: the simple and complex. For simple issues, such as a patient wanting to learn about yoga or meditation, the clinician can make the appropriate referral or course of action.

For more complex spiritual and religious issues, such as the need for forgiveness and/or reconciliation of self or others, severe existential distress, or lack of connection or love of others or God, referral to a chaplain

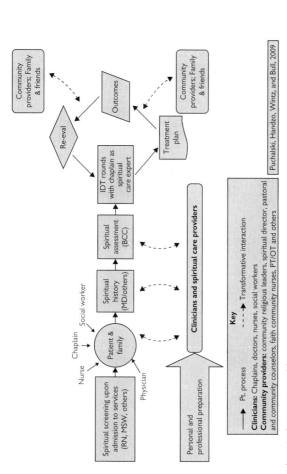

Fig. 21.1 Spiritual care implementation model.
Reprinted with permission from Puchalski CM, Ferrell B, Virani R, et al. (2009). Improving the quality of spiritual care as a dimension of palliative care: the report of the Consensus Conference. *Journal of Palliative Medicine* 12(10):885–904. The publisher for copyrighted material is Mary Ann Liebert, Inc., publishers.

and other spiritual care professionals is critical. Each of these elements is discussed in depth in the title report of the Consensus Conference, which includes decision-tree algorithms (Fig. 21.2).

In the final analysis, the spiritual care model is a relational model in which the patient and clinicians work together in a process of discovery, collaborative dialogue, treatment, and ongoing evaluation and follow-up.

Thus, an integral part of this model is ongoing professional development of the clinician in their ability to provide compassionate, patient-centered care. This would include attention to the spiritual needs of the health-care professional as related to their call to serve others in an altruistic, compassion-based model of professional practice.

Clinicians should also attend to their biopsychcosocial-spiritual issues with the goal of having balance in their lives and healthy approaches to stress management and to the issues that arise in caring for seriously ill patients.

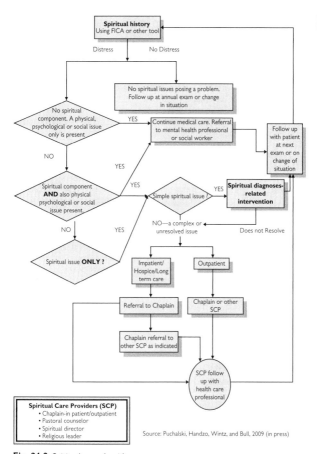

Fig. 21.2 Spiritual care algorithm.
Reprinted with permission from Puchalski CM, Ferrell B, Virani R, et al. (2009). Improving the quality of spiritual care as a dimension of palliative care: the report of the Consensus Conference. *Journal of Palliative Medicine* 12(10):885–904. The publisher for copyrighted material is Mary Ann Liebert, Inc., publishers.

Spiritual issues and diagnosis

Spirituality may be defined as that part of the person that seeks meaning in life and finds coherence in the midst of disorder and purpose in his or her life. Spirituality has been described as the essence of the human being, the search for meaning and purpose,[29] the expression of connection to others, God, or the transcendent or sacred,[24] and the basis for the healing relationships that clinicians form with patients.[30] The definition agreed upon for palliative care in the Consensus Conference is as follows: "Spirituality is the aspect of humanity that refers to the way individuals seek and express meaning and purpose, and the way they experience their connectedness to the moment, to self, to others, to nature, and to the significant or sacred."[24]

There is some concern in the field about labeling spiritual issues as "diagnosis." Spiritual or religious concerns are thought to be so integral to a person's being that caution has been raised about labeling spirituality as pathology, as this is an aspect of a human being and not a disorder.[31]

Yet spirituality and religion in the context of illness may also present as distress. Religion may have negative effects on health[13] and spirituality in general may result in distress, pain, or suffering.[32] In this context, we would argue that spiritual or existential issues may in some circumstances be classified as diagnosis, in those cases where patients are experiencing distress or where beliefs may be impacting health adversely.

Spiritual issues include the following:
• Despair and hopelessness
• Lack of meaning and purpose
• Grief and loss
• Guilt and shame
• Anger
• Abandonment by God or others
• Isolation
• Reconciliation
• Concerns about relationship with deity
• Conflicted or challenged beliefs

Each of these spiritual issues may present as part of a person's life but not as causing distress or not even affecting the illness with which the patient presents.

For example, patients may be experiencing demoralization, finding no meaning or purpose in their lives. This may be experienced as part of a transition in life, such as during a divorce, illness, or as a mid-life crisis. A patient may simply be questioning meaning in life as a reflective process. This would be identified as a spiritual issue that may or may not be affecting the presenting medical or health problem.

On the other hand, a patient may experience deep suffering and distress from a lack of meaning in life. We would suggest that in times when meaningless produces pain, suffering, or distress, it should be identified as a diagnosis and treated as a symptom equal to physical pain.

Forgiveness or reconciliation might be understood as a spiritual or religious practice, but in certain contexts the inability to forgive might impact the illness or the person in such as a way as to cause severe distress or suffering or even be a contributing cause of clinical depression.

It is important that clinicians be able to differentiate the full spectrum of how spirituality presents in patients' lives in the context of their illness and how it presents in the clinical environment. Integral to this process of differentiation is working with board-certified chaplains who are trained in distinguishing spiritual pathology from normal spiritual developmental issues.

Spiritual development issues

Spiritual growth and development is a lifelong journey. Spiritual development often parallels emotional development.[33] In childhood, the main psychosocial tasks include development of trust, autonomy, and initiative. Spiritually, children start making meaning of a world that is new to them, a world that is gradually becoming part of their life.

Religion often plays a role at this time if the family is religious. This is a time of extrinsic religiosity, a time when children are exposed to rituals and religious customs of the family. Clinically, this might be manifested as a clear, concrete vision of what life after death may mean, as, for example, a picture of heaven with a grandfather-like God.

In adolescence, the primary psychosocial task is to form identity. Spiritually, the adolescent begins to accept conventional ways of finding meaning in life but also begins to question what has been offered to them by parents and teachers. It is a time of movement from extrinsic to intrinsic faith. Clinically, a dying adolescent might struggle with what they believe but might revert back to what the conventional beliefs are if they have not determined what their own beliefs are.

Early adulthood is a time of establishing a career and intimate relationships. Spiritually, the young adult develops a personal faith or way of making meaning in life by reflecting on what has been passed on to them and determining what elements of this faith or meaning-making they will integrate as their own. This is often called a time of *intrinsic faith*.

A young adult who has established his or her own faith will use that as a foundation for dealing with illness. But many people sacrifice attention to spiritual development in favor of intellectual and career development. So in times of crisis they may revert back to childhood faith, sometimes called "foxhole faith."

In adulthood, generativity is the key psychosocial task, one of establishing oneself securely in one's professional and family or relational life. At this time, spirituality is expressed in the integration into oneself of much that was suppressed or unrecognized in the interest of a career or family. Some refer to this stage as *holistic spirituality*. It may be a deep time of searching for what is meaningful beyond the external.

Spirituality may be expressed in religious terms but also in nature, beauty, pets, people, or other beliefs. Clinically, illness may actually push an adult onto a spiritual path, especially if the illness prevents the person from working or from doing the things that were meaningful.

As people grow older, they often become satisfied with the achievement of career goals and find a deep sense of meaning for life in their self and the world. This is also a time of acknowledging loss and disappointments, of navigating the joys as well as the sorrows of life.

Many arrive at a place of peace and understanding regarding the universal value and goodness of life and of all that constitutes' one's world. The adult who goes through this part of spiritual growth comes to an acceptance of the paradoxes of life.

Clinically, this journey may be intensified in illness, particularly in end-of-life care, and some patients may not arrive at this peace. In this situation, one goal of care would be to provide the support and environment for people to explore these deep issues of existence and find some peace or acceptance of their life.

Spiritual development often does not move along in a linear fashion.[34] Also, spiritual growth many times does not parallel professional or personal development. Illness or dying may be the triggers for deeper questioning.

But if people have not had the opportunity to focus on spiritual developmental issues, they may experience spiritual distress in the context of illness and may need to revert to their childhood spirituality for support. The beliefs and practices they valued as children may not support them or help them in their time of illness and stress.

Awe is the primary spiritual attitude that children experience. But when a religious dimension is added to the child's life, it can either foster or diminish that spiritual awakening. Religion fosters this awakening if ritual and dogma support a growing awareness of the transcendent, so that the growth of awe in the life of the child is nourished and encouraged. Religion can diminish or retard spiritual development in the childhood stage if it is rule centered or emphasizes a punishment-and-reward approach to dealing with the transcendent.[34]

Neglect or abuse can also dampen or destroy a child's enthusiasm for the transcendent. This can be evident in the way people handle illness, stress, or dying.

If people's sense of the transcendent has been nurtured, they are likely to have positive religious coping. If they have had a rule-centered approach, it is more likely that they will experience negative religious coping. Pargament et al.[13] have demonstrated this pattern in their work on religious coping.

People who have a partnership relationship with God or find support in their religious communities have better psychological coping than those who see the illness as a punishment from God.

Spiritual diagnosis

While there has been some attempt to develop diagnosis codes for spiritual issues that impact health (e.g., National Comprehensive Cancer Network), this is still an area that needs further work. In the Consensus report we set up a potential model for framing these issues within clinical care. In general, a spiritual issue becomes a diagnosis if the following criteria are met:

- A spiritual issue leads to distress or suffering. Examples include lack of meaning, conflicted religious beliefs, and inability to forgive.
- A spiritual issue is the cause of psychological or physical diagnosis such as depression, anxiety, or acute or chronic pain. Examples include severe meaninglessness that leads to depression or suicidal ideation, or guilt that leads to chronic physical pain.
- A spiritual issue is a secondary cause or affects the presenting psychological or physical diagnosis—for example, hypertension that is difficult to control because the patient refuses to take medications because of religious beliefs.

Treatment or care plans

Palliative care is based in the biopsychosocial-spiritual model of care.[2] Thus, spiritual treatment or care plans should be developed by an interdisciplinary team, with the board-certified chaplain as the expert in spiritual care, and should be documented in the framework of the whole patient.

For example, if a patient expresses a lack of meaning and purpose in his or her life, the spiritual issue or diagnosis would be meaninglessness or demoralization. The primary care clinician would make that diagnosis and then discuss the management of that with the interdisciplinary team, specifically the chaplain. If there is no team or no chaplain, as in outpatient settings, the clinician would determine the appropriate treatment modality.

In Table 21.1, possible treatment options are listed. These include continued presence and support from the clinician, referral to an outpatient spiritual care professional such as a chaplain or pastoral counselor, meaning-centered group therapy, reflection and journaling, or other spiritual support group.

In diagnosing and documenting spiritual issues, it is important to also recognize that the spiritual issue may be affecting the physical, emotional, or social domains. So a patient who finds no meaning in life may experience greater physical pain, may feel unengaged from treatment and be noncompliant, or may have depressive symptoms or be isolated from their community of support.

In documentation therefore, the assessment and plan should include the diagnosis and plans for all four domains as illustrated in Table 21.1.

Table 21.1 Examples of spiritual health interventions

Therapeutic communication techniques	• Compassionate presence • Reflective listening, query about important life events • Support patient's sources of spiritual strength • Open-ended questions to illicit feelings • Inquiry about spiritual beliefs, values, and practices • Life review, listening to the patient's story • Continued presence and follow-up
Therapy	• Guided visualization for "meaningless pain" • Progressive relaxation • Breathing practice or contemplation • Meaning-oriented therapy • Referral to spiritual care provider as indicated • Use of story telling • Dignity-conserving therapy
Self-care	• Massage • Reconciliation with self or others • Spiritual support groups • Meditation • Sacred or spiritual readings or rituals • Yoga, Tai Chi • Exercise • Art therapy (music, art, dance)Journaling

Case example: assessment and plan

Mrs. M. is a 78-year-old female who has had a recent stroke, which has left her with mild cognitive impairment, as well as some loss of motor function. Her source of meaning was being a political activist and making a difference in people's lives. She feels useless now and without meaning and purpose. Her support group is other homeless activists.

Physical	s/p CVA, rehab, speech therapy, Plavix, resume enalapril and monitor blood pressure
Emotional	Referral to counselor for support, however, patient declined
Social	Explore possible other work with activist group; encourage patient to explore options with her group. Social worker to record patient's life story and help her explore themes.
Spiritual	Referral to chaplain; patient willing to explore meaning issues; continued supportive care and listening, explore what gave meaning in past and how that can occur with present physical limitations, referral to social work for narrative medicine as above

Demonstration projects: INSPIR

Integrating spirituality in hospital settings

This successful study involved training interdisciplinary teams of health-care professionals in five hospitals. Each site had 1 year to develop and pilot spiritual care interventions specifically focused on training providers to do a spiritual history. Part of the training included how to provide spiritual care.

Program evaluation included quantitative patient and provider outcome measurements at 3, 6, and 12 months. The pilot studies demonstrated that health-care professionals find greater meaning at work and have a greater ability to provide compassionate care if they address patients' spiritual issues and focus on whole-person care and have the opportunity to focus on their own spirituality and call to service within the professional context.

Results of the study included culture changes in test units, improved patient satisfaction with care, increased staff satisfaction, lower burnout, and lower turnover.

These pilot studies also provide examples of practical tools used for spiritual care and enhance the knowledge of best practices in clinical environments.[17] Some examples of these tools are listed in Box 21.1.

Box 21.1 Tools for integrating spirituality into clinical settings

- Education for staff: brown bag lunches, workshops, grand rounds (didactic, experiential), in-service talks
- Team activities: huddle, group activities centered around spirituality and compassionate care
- Art work, posters, inspirational quotes on hospital walls and in staff lounges
- Rituals in clinical practice (e.g., moment of silence when a patient dies, journal at bedside of patient where staff can write comments, thoughts, blessings), rituals to honor transitions (birth, death of patients, or transitions for staff)
- Recognition of excellence in spiritual care (beads, certificates)
- Institutionalized spiritual assessment, interdisciplinary spiritual histories, spiritual screening
- Reminders of calling to profession (chimes, rituals, reinforcement from administration)
- Accountability measures for spiritual care

Conclusion

Patients with chronic and serious illness have spiritual needs that can impact their care and affect health outcomes. While there are national guidelines requiring that spiritual care be provided for seriously ill patients, surveys demonstrate that most patients do not have their spiritual issues addressed in their care.

Based on a national consensus process, a model has been developed for the implementation of spiritual care within a medical model that can be implemented in palliative care settings and in settings where seriously ill patients are treated. This model includes the identification or diagnosis of spiritual issues as well as integration of patients' spirituality into the treatment or care plan in conjunction with board-certified chaplains who function as the spiritual care experts.

Integral to this model is the recognition that clinicians should also attend to their own spiritual needs as related to their professional work of service. Examples of practical tools in hospital settings can be used to further create more holistic hospital and clinical settings for both the patient and clinician.

References

1. Smith WJ (2009). Dame Cecily Saunders: the mother of modern hospice care passes on. *The Weekly Standard*, March 27.
2. Sulmasy, DP (2002). A biopsychosocial-spiritual model for the care of patients at the end of life [see comment]. *Gerontologist*, 42(Spec No. 3):24–33.
3. Sulmasy DP (1999). Is medicine a spiritual practice?. *Acad Med* 74(9):1002–1005.
4. Astrow AB, Puchalski CM, Sulmasy DP (2001). Religion, spirituality, and health care: social, ethical, and practical considerations. *Am J Med* 110(4):283–287.
5. Ferrell BR, Coyle N (2008). The nature of suffering and the goals of nursing. *Oncol Nurs Forum* 35(2):241–247.
6. Puchalski CM, Lunsford B, Harris MH, Miller RT (2006). Interdisciplinary spiritual care for seriously ill and dying patients: a collaborative model. *Cancer J* 12(5):398–416.
7. Cohen SR, Mount BM, Tomas JJ, Mount LF (1996). Existential well-being is an important determinant of quality of life. Evidence from the McGill quality of life questionnaire. *Cancer* 77(3):576–586.
8. Roberts JA, Brown D, Elkins T, Larson DB (1997). Factors influencing views of patients with gynecologic cancer about end-of-life decisions. *Am J Obstet Gynecol* 176(1 Pt 1):166–172.
9. Tsevat J, Sherman SN, McElwee JA, Mandell KL, Simbartl LA, Sonnenberg FA, et al. (1999). The will to live among HIV-infected patients. *Ann Intern Med* 131(3):194–198.
10. Yi MS, Mrus JM, Wade TJ, Ho ML, Hornung RW, Cotton S, et al. (2006). Religion, spirituality, and depressive symptoms in patients with HIV/AIDS. *J Gen Intern Med* 21(Suppl. 5):S21–S27.
11. Kimmel PL, Emont SL, Newmann JM, Danko H, Moss AH (2003). ESRD patient quality of life: symptoms, spiritual beliefs, psychosocial factors, and ethnicity. *Am J Kidney Dis* 42(4):713–721.
12. Koenig HG, McCullough ME, Larson DB (2001). *Handbook of Religion and Health.* New York: Oxford University Press.
13. Pargament KI, Smith BW, Koenig HG, Perez L (1998). Patterns of positive and negative religious coping with major life stressors. *J Sci Study Relig* 37(4):710–724.
14. McCord G, Gilchrist VJ, Grossman SD, King BD, McCormick KE, Oprandi AM, et al. (2004). Discussing spirituality with patients: a rational and ethical approach. *Ann Family Med* 2(4):356–361.
15. Ehman JW, Ott BB, Short TH, Ciampa RC, Hansen-Flaschen J (1999). Do patients want physicians to inquire about their spiritual or religious beliefs if they become gravely ill?. *Arch Intern Med* 159(15):1803–1806.
16. Balboni TA, Vanderwerker LC, Block SD, Paulk ME, Lathan CS, Peteet JR, et al. (2007). Religiousness and spiritual support among advanced cancer patients and associations with end-of-life treatment preferences and quality of life. *J Clin Oncol* 25(5):555–560.
17. Puchalski CM, McSkimming S (2006). Creating healing environments. *Health Prog* 87(3):30–35.

18. Astrow AB, Wexler A, Texeira K, Kai He M, Sulmasy DP (2007). Is failure to meet spiritual needs associated with cancer patients' perceptions of quality of care and their satisfaction with care? *J Clin Oncol* 25(36):5753–5757.

19. Phelps AC, Maciejewski PK, Nilsson M, Balboni TA, Wright AA, Paulk ME, et al. (2009). Religious coping and use of intensive life-prolonging care near death in patients with advanced cancer. *JAMA* 301(11):1140–1147.

20. Institute for Alternative Futures (2004). Patient-centered care 2015: Scenarios, vision, goals & next steps. Alexandria, VA: The Picker Institute. Retrieved from http://www.altfutures.com/pubs/Picker%20Final%20May%2014%202004.pdf

21. National Consensus Project for Quality Palliative Care (2004). Clinical practice guidelines for quality palliative care, executive summary. *J Palliat Med* 7(5):611–627. Retrieved from http://search.ebscohost.com/login.aspx?direct=true&db=aph&AN=14963387&site=ehost-live

22. National Consensus Project for Quality Palliative Care (2009). Clinical practice guidelines for quality palliative care, 2nd ed. Retrieved from http://www.nationalconsensusproject.org

23. National Quality Forum (2006). A national framework and preferred practices for palliative and hospice care quality. Washington, DC: National Quality Forum. Retrieved from http://qualityforum.org/publications/reports/palliative.asp

24. Puchalski C, Ferrell B, Virani R, Otis-Green S, Baird P, Bull J (2009). Improving the quality of spiritual care as a dimension of palliative care: the report of the Consensus Conference. *J Palliat Med* 12(10):885–904.

25. Puchalski C, Ferrell B (Eds.) (2010). *Making Health Care Whole: Integrating Spirituality into Healthcare.* West Conshohocken, PA: Templeton Press.

26. Puchalski C, Romer AL (2000). Taking a spiritual history allows clinicians to understand patients more fully. *J Palliat Med* 3(1):129–137.

27. Anandarajah G, Hight E (2001). Spirituality and medical practice: using the HOPE questions as a practical tool for spiritual assessment [see comment]. *Am Fam Physician* 63(1):81–89.

28. Maugans TA (1996). The SPIRITual history. *Arch Fam Med* 5(1):11–16.

29. Frankl VE (1963). *Man's Search for Meaning.* New York: Washington Square Press, Simon & Schuster.

30. Association of American Medical Colleges (1999). Report III. Contemporary issues in medicine. Medical School Objectives Project (MSOP III). Washington, DC: AAMC. Retrieved from https://services.aamc.org/Publications/showfile.cfm?file=version89.pdf&prd_id=200&prv_id=241&pdf_id=89

31. Griffith JL, Griffith ME (2002). *Encountering the Sacred in Psychotherapy: How to Talk with People about Their Spiritual Lives.* New York: Guilford Press.

32. Doka, K. J., & Morgan, J. D. (1993). *Death and Spirituality.* Amityville, NY: Baywood.

33. Kelcourse (2004). *Human Development and Faith.* A multi-authored textbook for use in human development courses. St. Louis: Chalice Press.

34. Fowler, J. (1995). *Stages of Faith: The Psychology of Human Development and the Quest for Meaning.* San Francisco: HarperSanFrancisco.

The palliative care team

Eduardo Bruera, MD

Introduction

Since its origins in the United Kingdom in the 1960s to the further development of this field in Canada in the 1970s and the United States in the 1980s, palliative care has evolved and developed a series of principles and practices.

Modern palliative care programs have three major principles:

1. *Multidimensional assessment and management.* This includes the presence of structures, processes, and outcomes needed to address multiple physical symptoms, psychosocial and spiritual distress, and functional, financial, and family concerns.

2. *Interdisciplinary care.* Modern palliative care is recognized as a team effort including not only physicians and nurses but also social workers, pastoral care, occupational therapy, physiotherapy, pharmacy, counselors, dieticians, and volunteers who work in an integrated fashion for the delivery of assessment and management of patients and families.

3. *Emphasis on caring for patients and their families.* Palliative care teams recognize that the overwhelming majority of the physical and emotional care is delivered by the family and that delivering care at the end of life to a loved one puts an enormous physical, emotional, financial, and existential burden on family members. Palliative care programs consider families the unit of care.

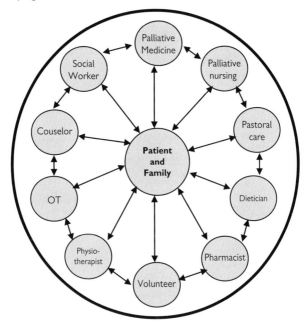

Fig. 22.1 The palliative care team. OT, occupational therapy.

Fig. 22.1 summarizes the interdisciplinary nature of care delivered by the palliative care team.

The palliative medicine specialist

In 2008, the United States established hospice and palliative medicine as a formal medical subspecialty after lengthy but ultimately highly successful negotiations led by the American Board of Hospice and Palliative Medicine and the American Academy of Hospice and Palliative Medicine. Palliative medicine was established as a medical specialty in the United Kingdom in 1987 and since then this specialty and/or subspecialty status has been formally established in Canada, Australia, a significant number of European countries, and even several developing countries.

The body of knowledge of palliative medicine is by nature multidimensional. Figure 22.2 summarizes the contribution of different medical and nonmedical fields to palliative medicine.

Pioneers in the field of palliative medicine had to search for information from all of these disparate fields to acquire the necessary knowledge for effectively practicing as clinical and/or academic specialists.

Fortunately, in recent years, the field has developed peer-reviewed journals; national, regional, and international congresses; and a number of excellent textbooks that successfully summarize aspects of the body of knowledge consisting of different medical and nonmedical disciplines that is required of the palliative medicine specialist.

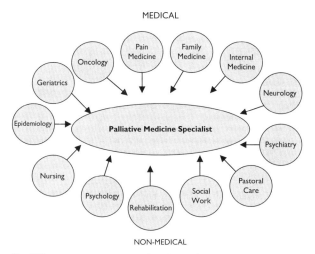

Fig. 22.2 Contributions to the body of knowledge of a palliative medicine specialist.

The palliative care team

While all the disciplines described in Figure 22.1 are required for the appropriate care of palliative care patients and their families, not all of these disciplines have the body of knowledge and expertise to specialize in the delivery of palliative care.

Palliative nursing has made considerable progress in recent years, including some specific board certification in many countries, publication of books on palliative nursing, and scientific meetings. Unfortunately, there has been limited success in other areas.

Therefore, the establishment and maintenance of a palliative care team requires much more emphasis on initial orientation and support of members than in other more established areas of health care.

Acute care hospitals

All of the disciplines are readily available in these hospitals. Therefore, ideally outpatient and inpatient programs should be placed geographically within acute care facilities in such a way as to enable allocation of a proportion of health-care professionals' time to the delivery of interdisciplinary palliative care.

Acute palliative care units

These are the most sophisticated and effective settings for the delivery of palliative care to highly distressed patients and families. In this setting, it is mandatory that the vast majority of patients and families receive assessment and management by all the major disciplines and that all the disciplines meet at least once per week for the purpose of discussing particularly complex problems and continuing education and support.

Consult teams

These teams see patients in settings where there is no palliative care unit. They are particularly at risk for professional burnout and achieving less successful outcomes. This situation is aggravated when physicians and nurses working on these teams have no access to an interdisciplinary palliative care team but instead have to interact with ad hoc professionals from areas in the hospital (e.g., for a patient on a surgical ward, the social worker, chaplain, case manager, physiotherapist, and pharmacist will be those assigned to surgery).

These well-intentioned professionals usually have no undergraduate or postgraduate palliative care training. This lack of training complicates communication and planning of care for complex situations such as somatization of physical symptoms, chemical coping, emotional distress, preexisting psychiatric or social problems for the patient or family, advance directives, and conflict among different health care teams.

Ideally, consult teams in acute care hospitals that have no palliative care units should develop Internet-based "virtual palliative care units" through which members of an interdisciplinary palliative care team can visit all patients and participate in the necessary assessment, management, family conferences, and discharge planning.

The two main limitations of such virtual units, compared to a palliative care unit, are the absence of a trained, full-time palliative care bedside nurse and the absence of administrative leadership, such as a unit manager capable of allocating resources and inpatient policies and procedures.

Outpatient palliative care

This can be challenging when patients in severe physical and psychosocial distress and their primary caregivers are asked to make multiple appointments to see members of an interdisciplinary team.

Outpatient palliative care clinics should be capable of delivering an assessment by many different disciplines in one single physical setting where patients have access to a full-size bed, proximity to a bathroom, and enough space in the consult room for some relatives to participate in the visit.

Outpatient facilities for palliative care patients should also have extra rooms where split visits can take place. This allows patients and relatives to meet separately with different members of the palliative care team, thereby optimizing the visit time for both patients and families and health care professionals.

Home palliative care

This is particularly challenging for interdisciplinary teams. Newly developed techniques, including lower-cost video conferencing, interactive voice response systems, and active telephone visiting, are increasing access to members of the team, such as social workers, counselors, pastoral care, and case management. Unfortunately, the vast majority of patients at home will have very limited access to members of an interdisciplinary team.

One of the challenges for the visiting nurses and physicians is to determine when a patient and family are not coping well at home and when much more intense interdisciplinary care is required. At that point, admission to an acute care hospital, acute palliative care unit, or inpatient hospice facility may be required, depending on the severity of the patient's and family's distress, to provide rapid and interdisciplinary resolution of the distress. Home or inpatient community-based care may be required depending on the level of patient needs and community-based support.

In addition to formal periodic communication such as team meetings, daily informal interaction among the different team members is important to coordinate efforts and, most importantly, to unify goals of care and interactions with patients, families, and primary referring health-care professionals.

Palliative care teams are only effective when regular and consistent communication and dialogue take place. This is what differentiates a successful interdisciplinary team from a multidisciplinary approach to patient care currently available in most acute care institutions and hospices.

Formal symptom assessment tools, joint charting of findings and recommendations by different members, and a strong commitment from all members of the team to communicate with other members of the team at any time when they make an important observational finding are key to successful outcomes.

The interdisciplinary team should regularly participate in educational activities, ideally based on clinical cases of difficult problems with patients, families, or referring health-care teams. These joint regular educational sessions are crucial to generating common understanding of the principles and practice of palliative care.

While continued review of all principles and practice is an important intellectual activity for all team members, it is equally important that the team maintain a very consistent message in the communication with every individual patient and/or family. This is the key to dramatically reducing distress and conveying to the patient and family that the team is well integrated and can effectively lead them through very difficult times.

Perhaps the most important member of an interdisciplinary palliative care team in an acute care facility is the bedside nurse. All clinical findings relating to the patient and family as well as all pharmacological and non-pharmacological interventions or investigations should be discussed at length with the bedside nurse, and his or her impressions about patient and family distress and coping should be assessed on a daily basis.

Interdisciplinary teams spend a limited amount of time with each admitted patient. The bedside nurse is in charge of the patient 24 hours a day, including off hours when no members of the interdisciplinary team are present. It is therefore crucial that the bedside nurse be made a pivotal member of the interdisciplinary care team for each admitted patient.

Family conference:
role in palliative care

Margaret Isaac, MD
J. Randall Curtis, MD, MPH

Introduction

Family conferences can be critical events in the course of an illness, often defining goals of care for the patient and shaping the experience of the family and surrogate decision-makers involved in a patient's care. Whether in the ICU, medical ward, clinic, or home setting, family conferences conducted by palliative care providers or other clinicians have an important role in patient care at the end of life.

Role of palliative care specialists in communication at the end of life

The presence of palliative care specialists in the hospital and other settings is becoming increasingly common, and involvement of interdisciplinary palliative care teams has been associated with improved patient satisfaction in both the home[1] and hospital[2] setting.

Role of families and surrogate decision-makers

Many patients at the end of life are unable to participate in their own medical decision-making, and clinicians often rely on surrogate decision-makers to assist in establishing a plan of care.

Not only is it an ethical obligation for physicians to share medical and prognostic information with surrogates, it is incumbent upon surrogate decision-makers to use the principle of substituted judgment in making decisions. In addition, even if patients have decisional capacity, many may want to involve their families in decision-making about end-of-life care.

Shared decision-making model

Shared decision-making has several defining characteristics: 1) involvement and participation of both a clinician and patient (and/or surrogate decision-maker); 2) information shared by the clinician, specifically treatment options and their relative risks and benefits; 3) information shared by the patient and/or surrogate decision-maker about values and goals of care; and 4) consensus between clinician and patient and/or surrogate on treatment decisions.[3]

Shared decision-making is only one of numerous models, others being parentalism, in which decisions are made unilaterally by clinicians, and informed consent, in which information regarding treatment options is given to the patient or surrogate, and decision-making is left entirely in their hands. Shared decision-making has been advocated by many as an optimal way to engage patients and families in medical decisions in the critical care setting.

That said, patients and family members vary widely in their desired level of involvement in medical decision-making. Assessing the degree to which patients' families and decision-makers want to be involved in medical decision making is critical in providing effective, appropriate, and patient- and family-centered end-of-life care.

Approach to communication during family conferences

Evidence-based approach to family conferences

Communication from clinicians during family conferences can have a significant impact on medical decision-making as well as on patient and family satisfaction. Specifically, statements that include affirmations of non-abandonment, assurances that the patient will not suffer, and support of families' decisions have been associated with higher family member satisfaction.[4]

Additionally, increased proportion of family speech has been associated with higher degrees of family satisfaction.[5] Table 23.1 details recommended components of effective family conferences, initially developed for the ICU, but also useful in the clinic and home settings.

The VALUE mnemonic has been proposed as an effective method in communicating with families in the ICU setting and has been shown to reduce family member symptoms of anxiety and depression after death of a loved one in an ICU. This approach is summarized in Figure 23.1.

Discussing prognosis

Clinicians have a responsibility to share prognostic information with patients and families, as this information can have an important impact on medical decision-making.[6] Recommendations include using quantitative estimates framed as information about groups of patients along with a description of the uncertainty involved in these estimates. It is also important to address the risk of long-term functional impairment, in addition to death, when discussing prognosis.

Table 23.1 Components of a family conference about end-of-life care

- Plan the specifics of location and setting: a quiet, private place.
- Introduce everyone present.
- Discuss the goals of the specific conference.
- Find out what the family understands.
- Review what has happened and what is happening to the patient.
- Discuss prognosis frankly in a way that is meaningful to the family.
- Acknowledge uncertainty in the prognosis.
- Review the principle of substituted judgment: "What would the patient want?"
- Make a recommendation about treatment.
- Support the family's decision.
- Make it clear that withholding life-sustaining treatment is not withholding caring.
- If life-sustaining treatments will be withheld or withdrawn, discuss what the patient's death might be like.
- Acknowledge strong emotions and use reflection to encourage patients or families to talk about these emotions.
- Tolerate silence.
- Ask if there are any questions.
- Ensure a basic follow-up plan and make sure the family knows how to reach you for questions.

Adapted from Curtis JR, Patrick DL, Shannon SE, et al. (2001). The family conference as a focus to improve communication about end-of-life care in the intensive care unit: opportunities for improvement. *Crit Care Med* 29:26–33.

V	Value family statements
A	Acknowledge family emotions
L	Listen to the family
U	Understand the patient as a person
E	Elicit family questions

Fig. 23.1 VALUE: 5-step approach to improving communication in the ICU.
From Lautrette A, Darmon M, Megarbane B, et al. (2007). A communication strategy and brochure for relatives of patients dying in the ICU. *N Engl J Med* 356:469–478.

Spirituality and religion

Spiritual and religious concerns are often prominent at the end of life, although many clinicians can feel uncomfortable discussing these topics. Because of the distinctively open relationship between a clinician and patient, clinicians often have a unique opportunity to explore these issues with patients and families.

Making appropriate referrals to spiritual-care providers can improve satisfaction on the part of patients and families. The FICA[7] mnemonic can assist clinicians in better understanding a patient's religious or spiritual background during family conferences (adapted from Puchalski):

F: Faith and Belief
  "Is Mr. X a spiritual or religious person?"
I: Importance
  "What importance does faith or belief have in Mr. X's life?"
C: Community
  "Is Mr. X a member of a spiritual or religious community?"
A: Address in Care
  "How would Mr. X like us to address these issues in his health care?"

Cross-cultural communication

Cultural competence in communication about palliative care

Discussing end-of-life care can be additionally complex with patients or families from diverse cultural backgrounds. Addressing cultural differences directly, using medical interpreters and cultural mediators, involving family in decision-making, and reconciling issues of informed refusal can all be helpful.[8]

Use of interpreters, cultural liaisons

Use of medical interpreters is critical in facilitating communication with patients and families who speak different primary languages than that of the clinicians. More than simply translating, interpreters can function as "cultural mediators," promoting understanding on both sides, provided that their role in the patient–clinician interaction is clear to all involved.

However, it is important to understand the limitations of working with medical interpreters and to follow basic best practices such as speaking slowly, confirming the patient's or family's understanding, meeting with the interpreter before the clinical encounter to brief the interpreter on topics to be discussed, and debriefing the interpreter after difficult discussions.[9]

Summary

Family conferences are a critical element in medical decision-making for seriously ill patients. By assessing the desired involvement in medical decision-making, using a shared decision-making model as a default, clinicians can provide effective guidance and support to patients and surrogate decision-makers.

Clinical pearls

- Families often play an important role in family conferences, even if patients have decisional capacity.
- Assess patients' desired level of involvement in medical decision-making.
- Effective communication in family conferences requires clinicians to adapt to family needs and respond accordingly.
- The practice of affirming and supportive statements and allowing patients and families to speak more in family conferences increases their satisfaction.
- Spirituality, religion, and culture need to be addressed directly with open-ended questions.
- Medical interpreters, when properly trained, can also act as cultural mediators in family conferences.

References

1. Brumley R, Enguidanos S, Jamison P, et al. (2007). Increased satisfaction with care and lower costs: results of a randomized trial of in-home palliative care. *J Am Geriatr Soc* 55:993–1000.
2. Gade G, Venohr I, Conner D, et al. (2008). Impact of an inpatient palliative care team: a randomized controlled trial. *J Palliat Med* 11:180–190.
3. Charles C, Gafni A, Whelan T (1997). Shared decision making in the medical encounter: what does it mean? (or it takes at least two to tango). *Soc Sci Med* 44(5): 681–692.
4. Stapleton RD, Engelberg RA, Wenrich MD, et al. (2006). Clinician statements and family satisfaction with family conferences in the intensive care unit. *Crit Care Med* 34:1679–1685.
5. McDonagh JR, Elliott TB, Engelberg RA et al. (2004). Family satisfaction with family conferences about end-of-life care in the intensive care unit: increased proportion of family speech is associated with increased satisfaction. *Crit Care Med* 32:1484–1488.
6. Murphy DJ, Burrows D, Santilli S, et al. (1994). The influence of the probability of survival on patients' preferences regarding cardiopulmonary resuscitation. *N Engl J Med* 330:545–549.
7. Puchalski CM (2002). Spirituality and end-of-life care: a time for listening and caring. *J Palliat Med* 5:289–294.
8. Kagawa-Singer M, Blackhall LF (2001). Negotiating cross-cultural issues at the end-of-life: "You got to go where he lives". *JAMA* 286:2993–3001.
9. Norris WM, Wenrich MD, Nielsen EL, et al. (2005). Communication about end-of-life care between language-discordant patients and clinicians: insights from medical interpreters. *J Palliat Med* 8:1016–1024.

Ethical aspects of palliative medicine

James D. Duffy, MD, FAAHPM, FANPA

Introduction

The clinical practice of palliative medicine is inherently fraught with very significant ethical issues. Patients suffering from incurable and/or chronic physical ailments inevitably face decisions about the goals for their medical care that are colored by the quality of their lives and the values that shape their decisions.

Every patient and family infuses their disease with meaning and constructs their own particular reality of their illness. As clinicians, we often play the role of journeymen as we accompany our patients along their unique path through suffering, not imposing our own agenda but providing a safe space in which our patients can construct their own meaning. Rather than constructing rigid rules, bioethics attempts to provide patients and their clinicians with a framework that outlines the parameters of their decision-making.

The modern palliative care clinician is working at the sharp edge between modern medicine's scientific breakthroughs and the practical concerns of patients to optimize the quality and quantity of their lives. A thorough understanding of bioethical principles is crucial as our field continues to advocate for the interests of our patients while optimizing the benefits of modern medical science.

Bioethical approaches can be broadly defined within four categories.

1. Principal-based

This (deontological) approach is sometimes described as "duty"- or "obligation"-based ethics and is founded on the principal that clearly defined ethical rules should bind our behaviors. This rule-based approach has significant utility in our complex medical environment because it allows clinicians to clearly assess and communicate the ethical justification for their actions.

The clinical utility of the four principles of deontological ethics (autonomy, justice, beneficence, and nonmaleficence) are discussed in greater detail in the next section.

2. Virtue-based

The modern term *ethics* is derived from the Greek word *ethikos*. Aristotle posited that positive moral virtue or intent is the most important determinant in deciding ethical behavior. According to Aristotle, virtue represents the balanced center between two extreme behaviors, e.g., pride represents the mean between vanity and humility. In this vein, modern palliative care clinicians strive to enhance their compassion as a motivation for their work.

Although a virtue-based ethical approach might have face validity within the context of the private patient–physician relationship, it is not robust enough to define behaviors within our complex modern medicolegal system.

3. Utilitarianism (Consequentialism)

This approach asserts that any action should be assessed in the overall context of whether it does more harm than good for all affected by the action.

While this approach may have utility in the context of broad public health decisions, it is less useful in bedside clinical decision-making.

4. Casuistry

Rather than relying on rules, rules, and theories, the casuist approach emphasizes the intimate understanding of a particular clinical situation and uses this information to shape decisions.

Four major principles of bioethics

Respect for autonomy

In the context of health care, *autonomy* describes the patient's right to act intentionally without any controlling influences that might mitigate against their free will. Respect for autonomy does not simply represent an attitude but requires actively acknowledging and supporting the patient's right to choices and actions based on their personal values and beliefs.

The respect for autonomy provides the basis for the concept of informed consent. In the context of palliative care, if the patient has decisional capacity, the clinician should actively attempt to both understand and support the patient's preferences—even when these might be contrary to the recommendations and/or wishes of health-care professionals and family.

The principle of nonmaleficence

The ethical principle of nonmaleficence requires that the clinician not *intentionally* harm or injure a patient, through acts of either commission or omission. This principle requires the clinician to be medically competent and able to meet clinical standards of care.

The legal term *negligence* describes harm caused by exposing the patient to unreasonable risk and/or careless behavior on the part of the clinician. In palliative medicine, the clinician often participates in the withholding or withdrawing of treatments.

However, if such actions are undertaken with the primary intention of reducing the patient's suffering and are consistent with the patient's stated preferences, then the action is not considered to be maleficent but rather beneficent.

In some situations, the palliative medicine clinician prescribes a treatment that has both a wanted and an unwanted effect—e.g., opiate analgesics produce pain relief but may also suppress respiratory drive and hasten the patient's demise. The ethical construct being invoked in such cases is the *principle of double effect*. The four characteristics of the principle of double effect are as follows:

1. The action must inherently be a neutral or beneficial act (e.g., prescribing an analgesic).
2. The primary intention for the action should be the beneficial effect, not the bad effect (e.g., the relief of pain).
3. The harmful means must not be the means of the good effect (shooting and killing a person is not an acceptable means of treating pain).
4. The beneficial effect of the action must outweigh the negative effect (the relief of the patient's overwhelming suffering is more beneficial than increasing their risk of pneumonia).

The principle of beneficence

The duty of the clinician is to be of a benefit to the patient. This principle applies to the patient, their family, and to society as a whole. Palliative medicine clinicians often encounter situations where there may be some uncertainty around what action or goal is of most benefit to the particular patient.

The clinician often has an important role in shaping and even directing the patient's decision about the relative benefit (and risk) of various medical decisions. It is imperative that the clinician strive to actively respect the patient's autonomy; however, patients and their families often look to the clinician to provide insights into these risks and benefits.

While the principle of autonomy would appear to prohibit "paternalism" on the part of the clinician, it is also clear that a clinician's honest and informed perspective can be of great benefit and can minimize a patient's ruminative and disabling ambivalence around ambiguous medical decision-making.

In clinical situations where the patient lacks decisional capacity and in the absence of a medical surrogate decision-maker, the clinician is justified in assuming a paternalistic role directed by a beneficent intention for the patient's well-being. Unfortunately, palliative medicine clinicians frequently encounter such situations and must always remain mindful of their responsibility to act with beneficent intention.

The principle of justice

Justice describes the "fair" distribution of goods in society and requires a "fair" method for allocating scarce resources. What constitutes a "fair distribution is ambiguous and largely determined by the social morality of a particular group. The principal of distributive justice is therefore shaped by many sociopolitical and religious influences, which may include each individual's need, effort, contribution, merit, and influence.

Since most chronically ill and dying patients lack the ability to advocate for themselves, palliative medicine clinicians must frequently act as advocates for their patients' needs. Issues relating to the right to avoid unnecessary suffering raise human rights as they pertain to end-of-life care and often necessitate that that the palliative medicine clinician assume an advocacy role that extends far beyond the bedside and sometimes into the political arena.

Decisional capacity and informed consent

The assessment of a patient's decisional capacity is crucial to the provision of effective and appropriate palliative care. Patients have the legal and ethical right to direct what happens to their bodies, and their physician has an ethical and legal responsibility to provide them with the information necessary to make an informed decision.

Informed consent is the process whereby a fully informed patient can actively and voluntarily participate in decisions regarding their health care. However, given their often significant cognitive deficits, patients receiving palliative care frequently lack the decisional capacity to make such an informed decision. It is the duty of the physician to fully ascertain whether the patient has the ability to become fully informed.

Although psychiatrists are frequently called upon to provide a clinical opinion regarding a patient's decisional capacity, every time any clinician makes a clinical decision, they have de facto made the determination of their patient's decisional capacity. Unfortunately, in practice, this means that a patient's decisional capacity is only questioned when they counter the recommendation of their clinician.

A patient is deemed to possess decisional capacity when they are considered capable of providing fully informed consent for a specific intervention (i.e., decisional capacity is always task specific and not a global construct).

The elements of a clinical determination of decisional capacity are the evaluation of the patient's ability to

- Understand what decision is being made.
- Understand the alternatives to the proposed intervention
- Understand the relevant risks, benefits, and uncertainties related to each alternative. The degree of understanding required will turn on the importance of the decision to be made. Since palliative medicine often involves life-and-death decisions, the clinician should expect the patient (or surrogate) to exhibit a high degree of understanding of the risks and benefits.
- Maintain consistent reasoning based on the patient's values and goals.
- Clearly communicate their decision.

How much medical information is sufficient?

Clinicians possess far more medical information than is necessary for their patient to be able to make an informed decision. One question that arises is just how much information does a patient need in order to be considered informed. Most states have legislation that determines the required standard for informed consent. This standard may be subsumed under one or more of three approaches:

- *The reasonable physician standard*—i.e., what would a competent physician tell the patient about the proposed medical intervention? This standard is predicated on the physician's perspective and may not therefore address the interests of the patient.

- *The reasonable patient standard*—i.e., what would the average patient need to know in order to be an informed participant in the decision? This standard is predicated on the "standard" patient and does not address the idiosyncratic needs and perspectives of the patient who is making the informed decision.
- *The specific patient standard*—i.e., what would this particular patient need to know and understand in order to make an informed decision? This standard is somewhat ambiguous and may sometimes be difficult to accomplish. However, it is likely to be the most effective strategy to ensuring that a patient is informed

If the patient is determined to be incapacitated and lacking the decisional capacity to make a particular medical decision to make health care decisions, a surrogate decision-maker must speak for the patient.

Different states have their own laws that define the hierarchy of appropriate surrogate decision makers (e.g., the patient's spouse is typically the first person who assumes the surrogate role). In the event of a medical emergency, if no appropriate surrogate decision-maker can be contacted, the physician is expected to act in the best interest of the patient.

Telling the truth and withholding information

Research indicates that the great majority of patients want their physicians to tell them the truth about their diagnosis, prognosis, and all therapeutic options. Any discussion of treatment planning and goals of care should always include a discussion with the patient about how much information they wish to receive.

Only fully informed patients are able to act as autonomous agents in their decision-making and make value-based decisions about their goals of care. These discussions should, however, always be sensitive to the particular sociocultural and religious beliefs of the patient.

In situations where the physician is unfamiliar with the social or religious perspectives of a patient, it is advisable to obtain consultation from a professional (e.g., chaplain or religious adviser) who can provide insight and guidance on these issues.

It is difficult to justify the deception of a patient under any circumstance unless this is in the context of a larger social context and belief system (e.g., some communities consider it damaging to tell the person information about the negative side effects of an intervention).

Advance directives and living wills

An *advance directive* (AD) is a document or recording in which a legally competent individual specifies their health-care preferences in the event that they are unable to participate in medical decision-making. Advance directives full under two broad categories: *instructive* (e.g., living wills, DNR directive) and *proxy* (e.g., designation of a durable power of attorney for health care).

The principle of advance directives is recognized in all 50 states. If the AD is constructed in accordance with the requirements of that particular state, it is considered legally binding. Advance directives should only be invoked when the patient lacks decisional capacity.

Unfortunately, since the AD is frequently written in ambiguous terms, the health-care team and family must frequently attempt to interpret the patient's stated preferences. In situations where the patient's family and decisional surrogates disagree with the patient's AD, the clinician should attempt whenever possible to assist the family in understanding the ethical and legal weight of the AD.

Only in situations where medical circumstances arise that were unpredictable to the patient (e.g., discovery of a new medical option) should the patient's surrogate be allowed to override the AD. In situations where the patient's family refuses to accept the patient's clearly stated AD, a hospital ethics committee should be requested.

Withholding and withdrawing life-sustaining treatments

A patient with decisional capacity has the legal and ethical right to accept and/or refuse any and all potentially life-sustaining treatments. Patients may have clearly communicated their preferences regarding withdrawing or foregoing treatment in their advance directive (e.g., living will, DNR).

Physicians are not required to, and should not, prolong a patient's stated wishes. It is important to recognize that the patient's decision to withdraw or forego life-sustaining treatments does not release the physician of the obligation to offer the patient effective palliative interventions.

There is no ethical distinction between withholding and withdrawing an intervention. Withdrawing unwanted treatment is entirely consistent with the four ethical principles of beneficence, nonmaleficence, autonomy, and justice.

It is important to remember that medical treatments in themselves are ethically neutral and their relative benefit can only be ascertained from the specific patient's particular diagnosis, prognosis, quality of life, goals of care, and beliefs and values.

In palliative care, issues relating to quality of life (rather than cure) are likely to frame the patient's decision. When the patient who has undergone treatment eventually dies from the underlying disease process, the physician is not morally responsible for that patient's death.

Concerns that an intervention will later be withdrawn should not preclude time-limited trials of a palliative treatment, e.g., treating a patient's metabolic abnormality to determine if it will enhance the patient's cognitive status and enhance their quality of life.

Decisions about the withdrawal of treatment are often framed by the patient's religious or spiritual belief system. In this regard, it is important to recognize that certain religions indicate that life be prolonged no matter what the quality. It is therefore important that the clinician clarify the patient's belief system as part of any conversation around the withdrawal of medical interventions.

Discussions with patients or their decisional surrogate on withdrawing and withholding treatments should include a review of the following:

- The patient's medical status and prognosis
- A review of any previous advance directives
- The benefits and burdens of specific interventions
- The patient's beliefs and values and how they are impinged upon by the various treatment options
- The proposed treatment plan and clarification that ineffective and/or unwanted interventions can be withdrawn at any time

It is crucial that all decisions regarding the withdrawal and withholding of treatment be clearly documented in the chart (including DNR forms) and that ALL members of the treatment team are clearly informed about the patient's preferences. Each facility or treatment team should establish effective and unambiguous methods for communicating such information (e.g., computer alerts, chart flags).

Clinical sites where the withdrawal of mechanical life support is implemented should establish effective and clearly defined guidelines for the procedures that minimize the patient's distress and are consistent with the doctrine of double effect (see above).

Withdrawing artificial nutrition and hydration

Artificial nutrition-hydration (ANH) is an invasive medical procedure that requires the placement of a tube into the gastrointestinal tract (e.g., PEG tube, nasogastric tube), into the vascular system, or below the skin. ANH does not include simple noninvasive assisted nutrition such as assistance with oral feeding.

The withdrawal or withholding of ANH remains a contentious issue. Patients' families and clinicians frequently equate nutrition with nurturance and caring. With the exception of total parenteral nutrition in cancer patients, there is very little empirical evidence to support the efficacy of ANH in improving the quality or quantity of a patient's life.

The absence of any clear risk associated with ANH compounds the ambiguity around its utility. The issue is even more complex in patients experiencing a persistent vegetative state; ANH may prolong the survival of patients who are unable to communicate their quality of life and preferences.

In response to increasing public debate and controversy over the issue of ANH, in 2006 the American Academy of Hospice and Palliative Medicine (AAHPM) issued a position statement,* discussed next.

Background

Artificial nutrition and hydration were originally developed to provide short-term support for patients who were acutely ill. When used in

---

*AAHPM. Statement on Artificial Nutrition and Hydration Near the End of Life. Approved by the Board of Directors, December 8, 2006. AAHPM reviews its position statements every 5 years for possible revision, if required by new and emerging evidence. Please see aahpm.org for the most current position statements.

patients near the end of life, the available data suggest these measures are seldom effective in preventing suffering or prolonging life.

Patients with advanced, life-limiting illness often lose the capacity to eat and drink and/or the interest in food and fluids. Ethical issues may arise when patients, families, or caregivers request ANH even if there is no prospect of recovery from the underlying illness.

AAHPM statement on ANH

"....The AAHPM endorses the ethically and legally accepted view that artificial nutrition and hydration, whether delivered parenterally or through the gastrointestinal tract via a tube, is a medical intervention. Like other medical interventions, it should be evaluated by weighing its benefits and burdens in light of the patient's clinical circumstances and goals of care.

ANH may offer benefits when administered in the setting of acute, reversible illness. Near the end of life, some widely assumed benefits of ANH, such as alleviation of thirst, may be achieved by less invasive measures including good mouth care or providing ice chips.

The potential burdens of ANH depend on the route used and include sepsis (with total parenteral nutrition) and diarrhea (with tube feeding). In addition, agitated or confused patients receiving ANH may suffer the indignity of physical restraints, which are often instituted to prevent them from removing a gastrostomy tube or central intravenous line.

The AAHPM advocates respectful and informed discussions of the effects of ANH near the end of life among physicians, other health care professionals, patients, and families, preferably before the patient is actively dying. Ideally, the patient will make his or her own decision about the use of ANH based on a careful assessment of potential benefits and burdens, consistent with legal and ethical norms that permit patients to accept or forgo any medical interventions.

Such choices are best made in concert with family and should be communicated to the patient's health-care proxy. For patients who are unable to make decisions, the evaluation of benefits and burdens should be carried out by the patient's designated surrogate or next of kin, using substituted judgment whenever possible, in accordance with local laws.

The AAHPM recognizes that for some patients and families, ANH is of symbolic importance, beyond any measurable effects on the patient's physical well-being. Such views should be explored, understood, and respected, in keeping with patient and family values, beliefs, and culture.

Good communication is necessary for caregivers to learn about patient and family fears about "starvation" and other expressed concerns. At the same time, communication is essential to clarify the patient's clinical condition and explain that inability to eat and drink can be a natural part of dying that is generally not associated with suffering.

In some situations, particularly if there is uncertainty about whether a patient will benefit from ANH, a time-limited trial may be useful. The caregiving team should explain that, as with other medical therapies, ANH can be withdrawn if it is not achieving its desired purpose.

Key elements

- Recognize that ANH is a form of medical therapy that, like other medical interventions, should be evaluated by weighing its benefits and burdens in light of the patient's goals of care and clinical circumstances.
- Acknowledge that ANH, like other medical interventions, can ethically be withheld or withdrawn, consistent with the patient's wishes and the clinical situation
- Establish open communication between patients and families and caregivers, to assure that their concerns are heard and that the natural history of advanced illness is clarified
- Respect patients' preferences for treatment, once the prognosis and anticipated trajectory with and without ANH have been explained."

Sedation at the end of life

Unfortunately, a significant percentage of patients experience severe or unbearable symptoms at the end of their lives. *Therapeutic sedation* (the term *terminal sedation* is discouraged) refers to the last-resort use of high-dose sedatives specifically to relieve the patient's extreme suffering.

Therapeutic sedation is limited to patients with a terminal prognosis (i.e., usually days to weeks) for whom other therapeutic interventions have proved ineffective in relieving their severe symptoms. Whenever the clinician is considering therapeutic sedation, it is important to include the family and surrogate decision-makers and to obtain a second opinion from another palliative medicine physician and relevant specialist.

It is also important to obtain the input from clinical staff involved in the immediate care of the patient and to obtain consent for their participation in this form of care.

In 2006, the American Academy of Hospice and Palliative Medicine published their statement on palliative sedation, discussed below.*

Background

Palliative care seeks to relieve suffering associated with disease. Unfortunately, not all symptoms associated with advanced illness can be controlled with pharmacological or other interventions. Patients need and deserve assurance that suffering will be effectively addressed, as both the fear of severe suffering and the suffering itself add to the burden of terminal illness.

AAHPM statement on palliative sedation

The AAHPM believes that distinctions must be made among the following uses of sedatives in medical practice.

Health-care providers serving patients near the end of life have a responsibility to offer sedatives in appropriate circumstances, usually targeted at specific symptoms ("ordinary sedation"). Palliative sedation (PS) is occasionally necessary to relieve otherwise intractable suffering, with the degree of sedation proportionate to the severity of the target symptom.

PS to unconsciousness should only be considered in the rare circumstance that thorough interdisciplinary assessment and treatment of a patient's suffering has not resulted in sufficient relief (or is associated with unacceptable side effects), and when sedation to unconsciousness is needed to meet the patient's goal of relief from suffering.

As with all treatment, the use of PS requires informed consent. Treatment of pain and other symptoms should be continued with PS, as sedation may decrease the patient's ability to communicate symptoms. PS should not be considered irreversible; reducing the sedation should be considered if clinical evaluation suggests that the symptom status may have changed.

* AAHPM. Statement on Palliative Sedation. Approved by the Board of Directors, September 15, 2006. AAHPM reviews its position statements every 5 years for possible revision, if required by new and emerging evidence. Please see aahpm.org for the most current position statements.

Ethical principles and legal rulings support the use of palliative sedation even to the level of unconsciousness to relieve otherwise refractory suffering. With regard to PS, the key ethical features are as follows:

- The clinician's intent is to relieve suffering;
- The degree of sedation must be proportionate to the severity of suffering; and
- The patient should give informed consent. If the patient is not capable of decision-making, the surrogate decision-maker should give informed consent consistent with the goals of care and values previously stated by the patient.

In clinical practice, PS usually does not alter the timing or mechanism of a patient's death, as refractory symptoms are most often associated with very advanced terminal illness. The possibility that PS might hasten death as an unintended consequence should be assessed by the health-care team in its consideration of PS, and then addressed directly in the process of obtaining informed consent.

Institutional bioethics committees may be consulted in cases where there is disagreement regarding the provision of PS.

Medical futility

Although the term is frequently invoked in medical discussions about goals of care, there is currently no universally accepted definition of the term *medical futility*. The ethical authority to render a medical intervention as medically futile rests with the medical profession as a whole and not with individual patients and/or clinicians.

Any discussion around medical futility must therefore be cognizant of generally accepted standards of medical care. Although the ethical principle of autonomy states that a patient has the right to choose from the available medical interventions, it does not entitle the patient (or their surrogate) to receive medical interventions that are considered by acceptable standards of medical care to be futile. It is important to remember that medical futility is not equivalent to rationing.

When considering the definition of medical futility, two approaches are employed:

- *Quantitative futility* applies to an intervention that has a very low likelihood of being effective (usually defined as less than 1%).
- *Qualitative futility* is where the intervention will not result in any improvement in the quality of a patient's life (e.g., improving the patient's physiological parameters without addressing the larger aspects of the patient's suffering).

When a patient and/or family members request a medical intervention that the physician considers to be futile, that physician should make every attempt to clearly communicate the treatment options available and their utility.

Language such as "giving up" and "a waste of time" should be avoided, and attempts to define the goals of care in terms of quality rather than quantity should be stressed. In situations where agreement cannot be reached, the physician should obtain a second opinion from an appropriate medical specialist and request a consultation from the ethics committee.

Physician-assisted suicide

The issue of physician-assisted suicide is controversial and complex, with opponents and proponents for the concept both presenting valid justifications for their position.

A meaningful review of these issues is beyond the scope of this brief text; however, the recent position statement by the American Academy of Hospice and Palliative Medicine includes the key principals.*

Background

Suffering near the end of life arises from many sources, including relentless pain, depression, loss of sense of self, loss of control and dignity, fear of the future, and/or fear of being a burden on others. A primary goal of the American Academy of Hospice and Palliative Medicine is to promote the development, use, and availability of palliative care to relieve patient suffering and to enhance quality of life while upholding respect for patients' and families' values and goals.

Excellent medical care, including state-of-the-art palliative care, can control most symptoms and augment patients' psychosocial and spiritual resources to relieve most suffering near the end of life. On occasion, however, severe suffering persists; in such a circumstance a patient may ask his physician for assistance in ending his life by providing physician-assisted death (PAD).

PAD is defined as a physician providing, at the patient's request, a lethal medication that the patient can take by his or her own hand to end otherwise intolerable suffering. The term *PAD* is used in this document with the belief that it captures the essence of the process in a more accurately descriptive fashion than the more emotionally charged designation *physician-assisted suicide*.

Subject to safeguards, PAD has been legal and carefully studied in Oregon since 1997. In all other states, PAD remains prohibited by law, although there is an underground practice that remains largely unstudied.

Situations in which PAD is requested are particularly challenging for physicians and other health-care practitioners because they raise significant clinical, ethical, and legal issues.

AAHPM statement on physician-assisted death

"… When a request for assistance in hastening death is made by a patient, the AAHPM strongly recommends that medical practitioners carefully scrutinize the sources of fear and suffering leading to the request with the goal of addressing these sources without hastening death.

A systematic approach is essential.

Evaluation of requests includes the following elements.

Determine the nature of the request.

Is the patient seeking assistance right now? Is he or she seriously exploring the clinician's openness to the possibility of a hastened death in the future? Is he or she simply airing vague thoughts about ending life?

*AAHPM. Statement on Physician-Assisted Death. Approved by the Board of Directors, February 14, 2007. AAHPM reviews its position statements every 5 years for possible revision, if required by new and emerging evidence. Please see aahpm.org for the most current position statements.

Clarify the cause(s) of intractable suffering.
Is there severe pain or another unrelieved physical symptom? Is the distress mainly emotional or spiritual? Does the patient feel he or she is a burden? Has the patient grown tired of a prolonged dying?

Evaluate the patient's decision-making capacity.
Does the patient have cognitive impairment that would affect their judgment? Does the patient's request seem rational and proportionate to the clinical situation? Is their request consistent with the patient's past values?

Explore emotional factors.
Do feelings of depression, worthlessness, excessive guilt, or fear substantially interfere with the patient's judgment?
   Initial responses to requests for hastened death include the following:
• Respond empathically to the patient's emotions.
• Intensify treatment of pain and other physical symptoms.
• Identify and treat depression, anxiety, and/or spiritual suffering when present.
• Consult with specialists in palliative care and/or hospice.
• Consult with experts in spiritual or psychological suffering, or other specialty areas depending on the patient's circumstances.
• Use a caring and understanding approach to encourage dialogue and trust and to ensure the best chance of relieving distress.
• Commit to the patient to work toward a mutually acceptable solution for his suffering.

When unacceptable suffering persists, despite thorough evaluation, exploration, and provision of standard palliative care interventions as outlined above, a search for common ground is essential. In these situations, the benefits and burdens of the following alternatives should be considered:
• Discontinuation of potentially life-prolonging treatments, including corticosteroids, insulin, dialysis, oxygen, or artificial hydration or nutrition
• Voluntary cessation of eating and drinking as an acceptable strategy for the patient, family, and treating practitioners
• Palliative sedation, even potentially to unconsciousness, if suffering is intractable and of sufficient severity (AAHPM Statement on Palliative Sedation)

Despite all potential alternatives, some patients may persist in their request specifically for PAD. The AAHPM recognizes that deep disagreement persists regarding the morality of PAD.
   Sincere, compassionate, morally conscientious individuals stand on either side of this debate. The AAHPM takes a position of "studied neutrality" on the subject of whether PAD should be legally regulated or prohibited, believing its members should instead continue to strive to find the proper response to those patients whose suffering becomes intolerable despite the best possible palliative care. Whether or not legalization occurs, AAHPM supports intense efforts to alleviate suffering and to reduce any perceived need for PAD.

For physicians practicing in regions where PAD is legal, the AAHPM advises great caution before instituting PAD, including assurance that

- The patient has received the best possible palliative care. The permissibility of PAD is dependent upon access to excellent palliative care. No patient should be indirectly coerced to hasten their death because he or she lacks the best possible medical and palliative care.
- Requests for PAD emanate from a patient with full decision-making capacity.
- All reasonable alternatives to PAD have been considered and implemented if acceptable to the patient
- The request is voluntary. Safeguards should focus in particular on protection of vulnerable groups, including the elderly, frail, poor, or physically and/or mentally handicapped. Coercive influences from family or financial pressure from payers cannot be allowed to play any role.
- The practitioner is willing to participate in PAD, never being pressured to act against his or her own conscience if asked to assist a patient in dying.

Whenever PAD is being considered by a patient with his or her physician, patients should continue to receive the best possible palliative care. Although many hospice and palliative care practitioners find it morally unacceptable to participate in PAD even where legal, neither a person requesting PAD nor the family should be deprived of any other measure of ongoing palliative care during the dying process and period of bereavement.

The most essential response to the request for PAD in the practice of palliative care is to attempt to clearly understand the request, to intensify palliative care treatments with the intent to relieve suffering, and to search with the patient for mutually acceptable approaches without violating any party's fundamental values".

Ethics committees and ethics consultations

Most hospitals in the United States have an ethics committee that should provide an invaluable resource to clinicians who are dealing with challenging ethical situations. The ethics committee should include a diverse group of health-care professionals and community representatives whose goal is to support patients and staff understand and apply ethical principles to health care.

The ethics committee performs clinical consultations at the request of clinicians and/or patients. These consultations may be performed by one individual (typically an ethics consultant with professional credentials in clinical ethics) or a team consisting of members of the committee.

Ethics consultations should be considered when there is a perceived ethical problem in the care of a patient that cannot be resolved by the parties concerned. Most so-called ethical problems are usually a breakdown in communication and can be resolved through facilitated meetings involving the consultation team.

Clinicians and patients should be encouraged to request ethics consultations without any fear of negative repercussions.

Clinical pearls

- The four principles of bioethics are autonomy, nonmaleficence, beneficence, and justice.
- Withdrawing unwanted treatment is consistent with the principles of bioethics.
- Every time we enter into a treatment contract with a patient, we are making a de facto determination of their decisional capacity.
- The physician's intent is the key to the doctrine of double effect.
- Most "ethical problems" can be resolved through better communication among the parties involved.

Further reading

Beauchamp TL, Childress JF (1979). *Principles of Biomedical Ethics*. New York: Oxford University Press.

Claessens P, Menten J, Schotsmans P, Broeckaert B (2008). Palliative sedation: a review of the research literature. *J Pain Symptom Manage* 36(3):310–333.

Gavrin JR (2007). Ethical considerations at the end of life in the intensive care unit. *Crit Care Med* 35(2 Suppl):S85–S94.

Hasselaar JG, Verhagen SC, Vissers KC (2009). When cancer symptoms cannot be controlled: the role of palliative sedation. *Curr Opin Support Palliat Care* 3(1):14–23.

Lemiengre J, de Casterlé BD, Van Craen K, Schotsmans P, Gastmans C (2007). Institutional ethics policies on medical end-of-life decisions: a literature review. *Health Policy* 83(2-3):131–143.

National Ethics Committee, Veterans Health Administration (2006–2007). The ethics of palliative sedation as a therapy of last resort. *Am J Hosp Palliat Care* 23(6):483–491.

Szalados JE (2007). Discontinuation of mechanical ventilation at end-of-life: the ethical and legal boundaries of physician conduct in termination of life support. *Crit Care Clin* 23(2):317–337.

Tillyard AR (2007). Ethics review: "living wills" and intensive care—an overview of the American experience. *Crit Care* 11(4):219.

Prognostication in palliative care

David Hui, MD

Introduction

Prognostication, an underused clinical skill, is an essential component of patient management along with diagnosis and therapeutics. Patients' predicted survival has a significant impact on many medical decisions, including the initiation of specific medications, avoidance of aggressive therapies, and palliative care and hospice referral. As patients progress over the course of their disease, knowing what to expect could provide them with a sense of control and facilitate the process of advance care planning.

Prognostication consists of two parts: foreseeing (estimating prognosis) and foretelling (discussing prognosis). *Foreseeing* requires knowledge of the natural history of disease (Fig. 25.1), an understanding of how treatment could modify survival, and an appreciation of individual patient-related factors such as comorbidities. *Foretelling* entails the delivery of prognostic information in a clear, sensitive, and compassionate manner and represents a longitudinal process of communication rather than a single discussion.

In this chapter, we discuss the science and art of prognostication, specifically related to patients with advanced cancer, congestive heart failure (CHF), chronic obstructive pulmonary disease (COPD), and dementia.

Clinical pearl

- Clinicians generally tend to overestimate prognosis. Use of prognostic tools such as the Palliative Prognostic Score for cancer patients can help improve accuracy.

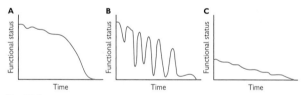

Fig. 25.1 Trajectories of advanced disease. (**A**) The trajectory for cancer patients tends to be predictable, with a rapid decline in function close to the end of life. (**B**) This is in contrast to COPD and CHF, with multiple acute exacerbations and a higher chance of sudden death. (**C**) Patients with dementia generally experience a slow and steady decline over time.

Prognostication in general palliative care and advanced-cancer patients

Much of the literature regarding prognostication is derived from patients with advanced cancer.[1] However, many of the key principles of survival predictions can be applied to other palliative care populations.

Clinician predicted survival (CPS) is formulated solely on the basis of the clinician's knowledge and experience. While this intuitive estimation correlates with survival to a certain extent, clinicians tend to be overly optimistic in their estimations and even more generous when communicating prognosis.

Clinicians who are more experienced and who have not yet established a strong relationship with the patient are more likely to be accurate with their predictions.

Prognostic factors

A number of signs and symptoms have been found to confer a poor prognosis in advanced-cancer patients:
- Performance status—ECOG performance status, Karnofsky Performance Status (KPS), Palliative Performance Scale (PPS) (Table 25.1)
- Delirium
- Dyspnea
- Cachexia–anorexia–dysphagia

The following laboratory variables are also associated with a shorter survival:
- Leukocytosis
- Lymphocytopenia
- Hypoalbuminemia
- Elevated lactate dehydrogenase (LDH)
- Elevated C-reactive protein (CRP)

Prognostic models

A number of prognostic models are available for predicting survival in general palliative care and advanced-cancer patients, with the Palliative Prognostic Score (PaP Score)[2] being the most validated (Table 25.2).

A Web-based prognostic model is also available at http://web.his. uvic.ca/research/NET/tools/PrognosticTools/. It provides an estimated survival based on patient's age, gender, cancer diagnosis, and Palliative Performance Scale.

Table 25.1 Palliative Performance Scale (PPS)

PPS Level	Ambulation	Activity & Evidence of Disease	Self-Care	Intake	Conscious Level
100%	Full	Normal activity & work No evidence of disease	Full	Normal	Full
90%	Full	Normal activity & work Some evidence of disease	Full	Normal	Full
80%	Full	Normal activity with Effort Some evidence of disease	Full	Normal or reduced	Full
70%	Reduced	Unable Normal Job/Work Significant disease	Full	Normal or reduced	Full
60%	Reduced	Unable hobby/house work Significant disease	Occasional assistance necessary	Normal or reduced	Full or Confusion
50%	Mainly Sit/Lie	Unable to do any work Extensive disease	Considerable assistance required	Normal or reduced	Full or Confusion
40%	Mainly in Bed	Unable to do most activity Extensive disease	Mainly assistance	Normal or reduced	Full or Drowsy +/− Confusion
30%	Totally Bed Bound	Unable to do any activity Extensive disease	Total Care	Normal or reduced	Full or Drowsy +/− Confusion
20%	Totally Bed Bound	Unable to do any activity Extensive disease	Total Care	Minimal to sips	Full or Drowsy +/− Confusion
10%	Totally Bed Bound	Unable to do any activity Extensive disease	Total Care	Mouth care only	Drowsy or Coma +/− Confusion
0%	Death	—	—	—	—

Copyright © 2001 Victoria Hospice Society
Median survival periods for PPS of 60–70%, 30–50%, and 10–20% are 108 days, 41 days, and 6 days, respectively.
Reprinted with permission © Victoria Hospice Society, BC, Canada (2001) www.victoriahospice.org

Table 25.2 Palliative Prognostic Score (PaP)

Scoring	
Clinician prediction of survival (weeks)	
>12	0
11–12	2
7–10	2.5
5–6	4.5
3–4	6
1–2	8.5
Dyspnea	1
Anorexia	1.5
Karnofsky performance status 10–40	2.5
Total WBC count	
8501–11000 cells/mm^3	0.5
>11000 cells/mm^3	1.5
Lymphocyte percentage	
12–19.9%	1
0–11.9%	2.5

Interpretation of PaP Score*

Total score	Advanced-cancer patients (out/inpatients)	Advanced-cancer patients (inpatients only)	Cancer and non-cancer patients (consult service)
0–5.5	87%	97%	66%
	76 days	17 weeks	60 days
5.6–11	52%	59%	55%
	32 days	7 weeks	34 days
11.1–17.5	17%	25%	5%
	14 days	≤1 week	8 days

* The percentage on the top row represents 30-day survival, while the number below it represents median survival.

Prognostication in patients with heart failure

Predicting survival in patients with CHF is more challenging than for cancer patients because of the relatively unpredictable disease trajectory, with a 25–50% chance of sudden death.[3]

Prognostic factors

Functional capacity indicated by New York Heart Association (NYHA) Class is the most important indicator of prognosis:
- Class II (dyspnea with normal activity)—1-year survival: 90–95%
- Class III (dyspnea with mild activity)—1-year survival: 85–90%
- Class IV (dyspnea at rest)—1-year survival: 30–40%

Other clinical prognostic factors include the following:
- Decreased left ventricular ejection fraction
- Ventricular arrhythmia
- Hospitalization for cardiac reasons
- Cachexia
- Comorbidities such as diabetes, COPD, cirrhosis, cerebrovascular disease, cancer, and HIV

Laboratory variables associated with poor prognosis are as follows:
- Anemia
- Hyponatremia
- High creatinine (>1.4 mg/dL) or urea (above upper normal limit)

Prognostic models

For hospitalized patients with acutely decompensated heart failure, a 3-risk factor model based on admission characteristics provides the probability of in-hospital mortality (Table 25.3).

For longer-term prognostication, the Seattle Heart Failure Model (http://www.SeattleHeartFailureModel.org) includes 24 variables related to demographics, medications, laboratory data, and devices and provides an estimate of 1-, 2- and 3-year survival with or without interventions.

Table 25.3 Prognostic model for inpatient mortality in heart failure

Urea (≥43 mg/dL)	Systolic blood pressure (<115 mmHg)	Creatinine (≥2.75 mg/dL)	In-hospital mortality predictions
(−)	(−)		2.1%
(−)	(+)		5.5%
(+)	(−)		6.4%
(+)	(+)	(−)	12.4%
(+)	(+)	(+)	21.9%

Prognostication in patients with COPD

The disease course of COPD is similar to that for CHF, with a gradual deterioration of organ function and increasing frequency of exacerbations over time.[4]

Clinical prognostic factors

Forced expiratory volume in 1 second (FEV_1) is the most important indicator of prognosis. Specifically, FEV_1 <35% is associated with a 2-year survival of 75% and 4-year survival of 45%. Other factors associated with decreased survival include old age, weight loss, and poor functional status.

Clinical prognostic factors for in-hospital mortality are as follows:

- $PaCO_2$ level >50 mmH_2O
- Prolonged (>72 hour) or recurrent mechanical ventilation
- Comorbidities
- Hypoalbuminemia
- Anemia

Prognostic models

The BODE Index is a prognostic model developed and validated for COPD patients (Table 25.4).

For critically ill COPD patients requiring admission to the intensive care unit, the APACHE IV score is a reliable tool for prediction of in-hospital mortality (www.icumedicus.com/icu_scores/apacheIV.php).

Table 25.4 BODE Index

Scoring	
Body mass index (BMI)	
0 = >21	0
1= ≤21	1
Obstruction (post-bronchodilator FEV₁)	
≥65% predicted	0
50–64%	1
36–49%	2
≤35%	3
Distance walked in 6 minutes	
≥350 m	0
250–349 m	1
150–249 m	2
≤149 m	3
Exercise MMRC dyspnea	
1	0
2	1
3	2
4	3

Interpretation of BODE Score*

Total score	1-year mortality	2-year mortality	52-mo. mortality
0–2	2%	6%	19%
3–4	2%	8%	32%
5–6	2%	14%	40%
7–10	5%	31%	80%

* Hazard ratio for death from any cause per one-point increase in BODE score is 1.34.

Reprinted with permission from Celli BR, Cote CG, Marin JM, et al. (2004). The body-mass index, airflow obstruction, dyspnea, and exercise capacity index. *N Engl J Med* 350(10):1005–1012. Copyright © 2004 Massachusetts Medical Society. All rights reserved.

Prognostication in patients with dementia

Dementia is a neurocognitive syndrome with persistent intellectual and functional decline.[5] The different stages of dementia are shown in Table 25.5.

Prognostic factors

A number of signs and symptoms are associated with poor prognosis in patients with dementia:

- Older age
- Male sex
- CNS—altered level of consciousness
- Respiratory—dyspnea, supplemental oxygen
- GI—dysphagia, aspiration, anorexia, weight loss, bowel incontinence
- Comorbidities—diabetes, CHF, COPD, cancer
- Recent hospitalization

Prognostic models

The Mortality Risk Index (MRI) is a 12-factor prognostic model developed in nursing home residents with advanced dementia and has been validated for this purpose (Table 25.6).

Table 25.5 Functional assessment staging[6]

Stages	Functional level
1	No difficulty either subjectively or objectively
2	Complains of forgetting location of objects. Subjective work difficulties
3*	Decreased job functioning evident to co-workers. Difficulty in traveling to new locations. Decreased organizational capacity
4*	Decreased ability to perform complex tasks, e.g., planning dinner for guests, handling personal finances (such as forgetting to pay bills), difficulty marketing, etc.
5*	Requires assistance in choosing proper clothing to wear for the day, season, or occasion, e.g., patient may wear the same clothing repeatedly unless supervised
6*	A) Improperly putting on clothes without assistance or cueing (e.g., may put street clothes on over night clothes, or put shoes on wrong feet, or have difficulty buttoning clothing) occasionally or more frequently over the past weeks
	B) Unable to bathe properly (e.g., difficulty adjusting the bath-water temperature) occasionally or more frequently in the past weeks
	C) Inability to handle mechanics of toileting (e.g., forgets to flush the toilet, does not wipe properly or properly dispose of toilet tissue) occasionally or more frequently over the past weeks
	D) Urinary incontinence (occasionally or more frequently over the past weeks)
	E) Fecal incontinence (occasionally or more frequently over the past weeks)
7	A) Ability to speak limited to approximately a half a dozen intelligible words or fewer, in the course of an average day or in the course of an intensive interview
	B) Speech ability is limited to the use of a single intelligible word in an average day or in the course of an intensive interview (the person may repeat the word over and over)
	C) Ambulatory ability is lost (cannot walk without personal assistance)
	D) Cannot sit up without assistance (e.g., the individual will fall over if there are not lateral rests [arms] on the chair)
	E) Loss of ability to smile
	F) Loss of ability to hold head up independently

*Scored primarily on the basis of information obtained from knowledgeable informant.

Table 25.6 Mortality Risk Index (MRI)

Score Sheet to Estimate 6-Month Prognosis in Nursing Home Residents With Advanced Dementia

Risk Factor From Minimum Date Set	Points	Score
Activites of Daily Living Scale =28*	1.9	—
Male Sex	1.9	—
Cancer	1.7	—
Congestive Heart Failure	1.6	—
Oxygen Therapy Needed in Prior 14 Days	1.6	—
Shortness of Breath	1.5	—
<25% of Food Eaten at Most Meals	1.5	—
Unstable Medical Condition	1.5	—
Bowel Incontinence	1.5	—
Bedfast	1.5	—
Age >83 y	1.4	—
Not Awake Most of the Day	1.4	—
Total Risk Score, Rounded to Nearest integer Possible Range, 0-19		☐

* The Activities of Daily Living Scale is obtained by summing the resident's self-performance ratings on the Minimum Date Set for the following 7 functional activities: bed mobility, dressing, toileting, transfer, eating, grooming, and locomotion. In the Minimum Date Set, functional ability is rated on 5-point scale for each activity (0, independent; 1, supervision; 2, limited assistance; 3, extensive assistance; and 4, total dependence). A total score of 28 represents complete functional dependence.

If Total Risk Score is ...	Risk Estimate of Death Within 6 Months, %
0	8.9
1 or 2	10.8
1 or 2	23.2
3, 4, or 5	40.4
6, 7, or 8	57.0
9, 10, or 11	70.0
≥ 12	

Adapted with permission from Mitchell et al. (2004). *JAMA* 291(22):2734–2740. Copyright © (2009). American Medical Association. All rights reserved.

Communicating prognosis

Even with the most sophisticated prognostic model, it is important to recognize that there will always be uncertainty in survival predictions given the inherent nature of death, mediated by acute complications such as infections and thromboembolism. Thus, it is imperative for clinicians to not only polish the science of prognostication but also further the art of communication, gently guiding patients and families through times of uncertainty.

Instead of avoiding bad news, most patients prefer to receive honest, realistic, and accurate information regarding their prognosis. At the same time, they want to have control over what, when, and how much information is given.

Physicians tend to underestimate patients' need for information yet at the same time overestimate patients' appreciation of their prognosis.[7] Thus, it is important for clinicians to find out about patients' preferences in communication prior to prognostic disclosure, to frequently assess patients' understanding, and provide ample opportunities for questions.

With disease progression, patients tend to want more discussions around their psychosocial needs rather than biomedical issues. In fact, patients generally want less information as they get closer to the end of life, whereas caregivers tend to need more. Thus, separate discussions with patients and caregivers may be useful for some situations.

Discussing prognosis can be a challenging task, trying to strike a balance between honesty, hope, and empathy. Rather than destroying hope, prognostic information should be framed in such a way to sustain existing goals and/or to create new ones.

While each patient–physician interaction should be individualized, Table 25.7 lists a number of communication strategies that may be helpful for clinicians when sharing prognosis.

Clinical pearl

- Patients generally want to know how long they have to live. The art of prognostication is in delivering the appropriate amount of information at the right time, the proper setting, and in a manner tailored to the patient's level of comprehension and emotional state.

Table 25.7 General strategies for discussing prognosis[8]

Key element	Comments
Context	Ensure a quiet, comfortable, and safe environment.
	Sit down and speak to the patient at eye level.
	Ask the patient if he or she wants to be accompanied by family or friends during the discussion.
How much does the patient know?	Explore the patient's understanding of his or her illness and expectations.
How would learning about prognosis help the patient?	A clear understanding of the patient's reasons to explore prognosis can help clinicians to shape their discussion that addresses the patient's goals and to provide a personalized management plan.
Deliver information	Emphasize the uncertainties in prognostication.
	Discuss prognosis in terms of days, weeks, and months, rather than providing specific numbers or median survivals. Information should be related such that it is measured to the perceptions of the patient's intellectual comprehension and emotional resilience.
Empathic response	Simple remarks such as "This is a difficult time for you" can be helpful. Be prepared to acknowledge and grieve losses.
Empowering	Take this opportunity to help patients define achievable goals and remain hopeful. Initiate discussions about important advance care planning issues such as philosophy of care, living will, and code status.
Provide follow-up and support resources	Reassure patients regarding non-abandonment and symptom control.
	Introduce other members of the interprofessional team, such as the chaplain and social worker, who will be able to provide further counseling.

References

1. Glare PA, Sinclair CT (2008). Palliative medicine review: prognostication. *J Palliat Med* 11(1):84–103.
2. Maltoni M, Nanni O, Pirovano M, Scarpi E, Indelli M, Martini C, Monti M, Arnoldi E, Piva L, Ravaioli A, Cruciani G, Labianca R, Amadori D (1999). Successful validation of the palliative prognostic score in terminally ill cancer patients. Italian Multicenter Study Group on Palliative Care. *J Pain Symptom Manage* 17(4):240–247.
3. Reisfield GM, Wilson GR (2007). Prognostication in heart failure. *J Palliat Med* 10(1):245–246.
4. Childers JW, Arnold RM, Curtis JR (2007). Prognosis in end-stage chronic obstructive pulmonary disease. *J Palliat Med* 10(3):806–807.

5. Tsai S, Arnold RM (2007). Prognostication in dementia. *J Palliat Med* 10(3):807–808.
6. Reisberg B (1998). Functional assessment staging (FAST). *Psychopharmacol Bull.* 24(4):653–659.
7. Parker SM, Clayton JM, Hancock K, Walder S, Butow PN, Carrick S, Currow D, Ghersi D, Glare P, Hagerty R, Tattersall MH (2007). A systematic review of prog-nostic/end-of-life communica-tion with adults in the advanced stages of a life-limiting illness: patient/caregiver preferences for the content, style, and timing of informa-tion. *J Pain Symptom Manage* 34(1):81–93.
8. Back AL, Anderson WG, Bunch L, Marr LA, Wallace JA, Yang HB, Arnold RM (2008). Communication about cancer near the end of life. *Cancer* 113(7 Suppl):1897–1910.

Frequent pharmacological interactions in palliative care

Mary Lynn Mcpherson, PharmD, BCPS, CDE

Introduction

Medications are indispensable in managing symptoms associated with advanced illness. Patients with an advanced illness such as cancer take an average of five medications (range 0–13), which increases the risk for experiencing an adverse drug event or a drug interaction.[1,2] The risk for experiencing an adverse drug-related outcome is increased by patient fragility, comorbid conditions, and increased age.

Palliative care practitioners frequently add medications to the patient's regimen to control symptoms as the disease progresses, but we also take away medications as the patient declines and therapeutic goals change. It is imperative that palliative care practitioners understand the clinical effects of both adding and taking away medications from a patient's medication regimen.

A *drug interaction* is defined as "a measurable modification (in magnitude or duration) of the action of one drug by prior or concomitant administration of another substance (including prescription and nonprescription drugs, food, or alcohol).[3] This includes drug–drug (prescription or nonprescription), drug–food, drug–herbal, drug–lab, drug–disease, and drug–chemical interactions.

In this chapter we will focus on interactions between drugs (known as drug–drug interactions). Drug–drug interactions primarily fall into two categories: pharmacodynamic and pharmacokinetic.

Pharmacodynamic drug interactions

Pharmacodynamics describes the study of the action and effects of medications on physiological function. Therefore, drug interactions that are said to be pharmacodynamic in nature result in either an additive, synergistic, or antagonistic pharmacologic effect.

Pharmacodynamic drug interactions can produce either the intended pharmacological effect of a medication or the adverse effect. An example of an antagonistic pharmacodynamic drug interaction would be using dexamethasone and glyburide in the same drug regimen. Dexamethasone increases blood glucose, while glyburide is used to decrease blood glucose. Frequently, we use this type of "interaction" to our advantage; one example is using a stimulant laxative to increase peristalsis to combat opioid-induced slowed peristalsis.

Additive pharmacodynamic drug interactions can also have a beneficial effect, such as using more than one medication to achieve better blood pressure–lowering effects or to achieve better analgesia.

Conversely, there are several examples of common adverse additive or synergistic pharmacodynamic drug interactions seen in palliative care practice. Some examples include the following.

Central nervous system (CNS) depression

Patients receiving one or more CNS depressant medications may experience sedation, agitation, and/or confusion and may progress to respiratory depression.

Examples include opioids, benzodiazepines, non-benzodiazepine sedative–hypnotic agents, barbiturates, alcohol, antipsychotic agents, antidepressants, antihistamines (especially the first-generation agents such as diphenhydramine), antiemetics, anticonvulsants, and illicit drugs.

Less obvious causative agents include medications such as cimetidine, anticholinergic agents, and drugs that reduce glomerular filtration, such as nonsteroidal anti-inflammatory drugs and angiotension-converting-enzyme inhibitors.

Anticholinergic (antimuscarinic) adverse effects

These commonly include constipation, urinary retention, blurred vision, dry mouth, and cognitive impairment. Medications that may cause anticholinergic effects include the antidepressants, antipsychotics, antihistamines, atropine, scopolamine, and hyoscyamine, among others.

Constipation

Constipation may be related to anticholinergic drug use as well as use of a variety of other medications such as opioids, iron and calcium supplements, and many medications for chronic disease states (e.g., antihypertensives and diuretics).

QTc prolongation

Palliative care practitioners think of methadone as one medication associated with long QT syndrome and the associated life-threatening arrhythmia, torsades de pointes. This is just one medication that may cause this effect.

Common examples include antiarrhythmic agents (such as quinidine, procainamide, dofetilide, sotalol, and amiodarone), antihistamines, antibiotics, gastrointestinal prokinetic agents, and antipsychotic agents. For a more complete listing of medications that can prolong the QTc, refer to the Web site www.torsades.org.[4]

Serotonin syndrome

This is a potentially life-threatening condition caused by excess serotonergic stimulation of the CNS.[5] Clinical findings range from mild symptoms to life-threatening toxicity and include akathisia, tremor, altered mental status, clonus, muscular hypertonicity, and hyperthermia.

Drugs known to cause serotonin syndrome include the antidepressants, valproic acid, analgesics (meperidine, fentanyl, tramadol, pentazocine, methadone), antiemetics (ondansetron, granisetron, metoclopramide), sumatriptan, sibutramine, linezolid, ritonavir, dextromethorphan, some drugs of abuse, some dietary supplements (e.g., tryptophan, St. John's worst, ginseng) and lithium.[5]

Agents affecting seizure

Some medications can lower the seizure threshold, including meperidine, tramadol, phenothiazines (such as chlorpromazine and haloperidol), tricyclic antidepressants, venlafaxine, propofol, and bupropion. Abrupt discontinuation of antiepileptic agents and benzodiazepines can also increase the risk for seizures.

Pharmacokinetic drug interactions

Pharmacokinetics describes the process of what the body does to a drug after administration: absorption, distribution, metabolism, and excretion. While there is little consistent information available regarding pharmacokinetic changes associated with terminal illness, some predictable changes have been shown with aging.

Examples of these changes and their impact on drug therapy are as follows.[6]

Absorption
- Decrease gastrointestinal acidity (decreased absorption of some drugs)
- Decreased surface area of small bowel (may reduce absorption of some sustained release drug products)

Distribution
- Increase in adipose tissue (may increase half-life of lipid-soluble drugs)
- Decrease in lean body mass (may increase serum concentration of water-soluble drugs)
- Reduced serum albumin (increased free fraction of highly albumin-bound drugs)

Metabolism
- Reduced phase I metabolism (prolonged half-life of drugs metabolized by this route)
- Phase II metabolism largely unchanged

Elimination
- Reduced glomerular filtration ratio (prolonged half-life of drugs that are renally excreted)
- Reduced renal plasma flow

In addition to age-related changes affecting the pharmacokinetics of drug therapy, pharmacogenetic variability may influence drug metabolism, and drug interactions may affect all four phases of pharmacokinetics (absorption, distribution, metabolism, excretion).

A discussion and examples of the impact on each phase follow, with an emphasis on the role of drug-metabolizing enzymes in the liver and other organ sites.

Absorption

After administration, most medications must be absorbed into the systemic circulation to be effective (obviously, some medications are intended for a local or topical effect at the site of application). Drugs given by the intravenous (IV) route of administration are not subject to variables that may adversely affect absorption because the drug is placed into the systemic circulation.

Similarly, medications given by the intramuscular (IM) and subcutaneous (SC) routes generally have a high degree of absorption. Oral medication administration is subject to variability in gastric emptying, absorption via passive diffusion, and presystemic elimination.

Examples of drug interactions subject to these variables are as follows:

- Antacids, anticholinergic drugs, and opioids may slow gastric emptying; this may slow the onset of action of coadministered medications.
- Some medications may be inactivated in the acid environment of the stomach, such as penicillin G and levodopa. Delayed gastric emptying may decrease bioavailability of these agents.
- Metoclopramide enhances gastric emptying and may cause an earlier and higher peak concentration of some drugs.
- Some medications require an acidic environment for absorption (such as griseofulvin, itraconazole, ketoconazole azole, gabapentin); enhanced gastric emptying may reduce absorption of these medications. Acid suppression by proton pump inhibitors, histamine-2-receptor antagonists, or antacids may also reduce the absorption of these medications.
- Sucralfate, aluminum- and magnesium-containing antacids, calcium, iron or zinc may reduce the absorption of quinolone antibiotics (e.g., levofloxacin and ciprofloxacin), tetracycline, minocycline, and azithromycin

Distribution

Medications such as phenytoin, diazepam, warfarin, and others are highly bound to serum protein such as albumin or alpha-1-acid glycoprotein (AAG).

When combined, some drugs can "bump" other drugs off proteins in the plasma, increasing the free fraction of drug (which is the portion of drug that causes the pharmacological and potentially toxic effect). These drug interactions are rarely clinically significant because this effect is transient and a compensatory increase in drug elimination.

Metabolism

Variables that can affect the metabolism of medications include rates of metabolism, diet, age, race, genetics, disease states, and drug dosage. For example, some patient populations may be deficient in the CYP2D6 enzyme, the enzyme responsible for the metabolism of codeine to morphine. Most pharmacokinetic drug interactions are due to altered drug metabolism via the cytochrome P450 (CYP450) enzyme system.

Drug metabolism occurs primarily in the liver, but also in the intestinal mucosa and other parts of the body. Generally speaking, drug metabolism converts an active, nonpolar drug to one or more polar metabolites (that may or may not be pharmacologically active). These polar metabolites are generally cleared by the kidneys.

The CYP system consists of more than 20 families of isoenzymes; the enzymes most important in drug metabolism are CYP1A2, 2C9, 2C19, 2D6, and 3A4.

The CYP3A4 group accounts for about 40–60% of all hepatic CYP isoenzymes and is most frequently implicated in drug–drug interactions. Many medications commonly used in palliative care are metabolized by the 3A4 enzyme such as dexamethasone, prednisone, midazolam, triazolam, alprazolam, methadone, fentanyl, and haloperidol.[7]

When we consider drug interactions involved in drug metabolism, the drug or substance being acted upon is known as a *substrate*. Some medications act as *enzyme inhibitors*, inhibiting the activity of one or more specific enzymes. Enzyme-inhibiting drugs reduce the metabolism of the substrate drug, resulting in an increased serum concentration.

For example, when fluconazole, a potent 3A4 inhibitor, is added to an established methadone regimen (methadone is the substrate in this case), the metabolism of methadone is inhibited, increasing the serum methadone concentration and potentially resulting in sedation or respiratory depression.

Conversely, some medications act as *enzyme inducers*, increasing the activity of one or more enzymes. When an enzyme inducer is introduced, metabolism of the substrate drug is enhanced, resulting in a lower serum concentration, possibly causing a loss of effectiveness.

Using methadone as an example again, if phenytoin is added to an established methadone regimen, the methadone will be metabolized to a greater extent with a likely loss of analgesia.

Common symptoms experienced by patients with advanced illness include pain, constipation, diarrhea, anorexia, cachexia, nausea, vomiting, dyspnea, confusion, anxiety, depression, insomnia, and fatigue. The International Association for Hospice and Palliative Care (IAHPC) collaborated with other organizations to develop a list of "essential" palliative care drugs.[8]

Table 26.1 is a listing of selected moderately severe and severe drug interactions associated with the medications on this list. Practitioners are encouraged to consult a more comprehensive description of these drug interactions as needed for patient care activities.[8]

Table 26.1 Drug interactions associated with selected palliative care drugs

Interacting medication	Interaction effect	Probable mechanism	Severity*	Clinical management
Antidepressants				
Amitriptyline				
Carbamazepine	Decreased amitriptyline effectiveness	Increased amitriptyline metabolism	Moderate	Monitor for clinical efficacy of the amitriptyline and for signs of carbamazepine toxicity
Duloxetine	Increased amitriptyline serum concentration	Duloxetine-induced inhibition of CYP2D6 metabolism of amitriptyline	Moderate	Use caution with combination; monitor amitriptyline serum concentration
Fluconazole	Increased risk of amitriptyline toxicity	Inhibition of amitriptyline metabolism by CYP enzymes	Major	Use caution with combination
Fluoxetine	Increased amitriptyline toxicity	Decreased amitriptyline metabolism	Major	Concurrent use is not recommended
Phenytoin	Increased risk of phenytoin toxicity	Inhibition of phenytoin metabolism	Moderate	Monitor serum levels of both drugs
Sertraline	Increased amitriptyline serum level	Inhibition of amitriptyline metabolism	Major	Use caution with concurrent administration
St. John's wort	Decreased effect of amitriptyline	Induction of metabolizing enzymes	Moderate	Avoid concurrent use

Drug	Interacting drug	Effect	Mechanism	Severity	Management
	Valproic acid	Increased serum concentrations of amitriptyline	Decreased amitriptyline plasma clearance	Moderate	Monitor serum level of amitriptyline
	Warfarin	Increased risk of bleeding	Reduced warfarin metabolism and increased absorption	Moderate	Monitor INR closely
Citalopram	Bupropion	Increased plasma level of citalopram	Inhibition of citalopram metabolism by buproprion	Moderate	Use combination with caution and monitor for excessive citalopram adverse effects (CNS)
	Desipramine	Increased desipramine serum concentration	Inhibition of desipramine metabolism	Moderate	Use combination with caution and monitor patient response
	Fluconazole	Increased risk of serotonin syndrome	Inhibition of CYP2C19-mediated citalopram metabolism by fluconazole	Major	Use combination with caution and monitor patient for signs and symptoms of serotonin syndrome or other adverse effects from citalopram
	Imipramine	Increase in bioavailability and half-life of desipramine, major metabolite of imipramine	Inhibition of desipramine metabolism, the major metabolite of imipramine	Moderate	Use combination with caution and adjust dosing as clinically indicated

Table 26.1 (Contd.)

	Interacting medication	Interaction effect	Probable mechanism	Severity*	Clinical management
Gastrointestinal agents					
Loperamide	Gemfibrozil		Inhibition of CYP2C8-mediated loperamide metabolism	Moderate	Use with caution, especially with high loperamide doses. Monitor for loperamide adverse effects, including nausea, vomiting, dry mouth, dizziness, or drowsiness
	St. John's wort	Delirium with symptoms of confusion, agitation, and disorientation	Unknown	Moderate	Use with caution, monitor for signs of altered mental status
	Valerian	Delirium with symptoms of confusion, agitation, and disorientation	Unknown	Moderate	
Mineral oil enema	Docusate	Inflammation of intestinal mucosa, liver, spleen, and lymph nodes	Enhanced mineral oil absorption (shown with mineral oil liquid paraffin)	Moderate	Avoid concurrent oral administration of docusate salts and mineral oil
Senna	Digoxin	Increased risk of digoxin toxicity	Senna may cause potassium loss with excessive or prolonged use	Moderate	Avoid concurrent use, or monitor potassium serum concentration

Droperidol	Increased risk of cardiotoxicity (QT prolongation, torsdes de pointes, cardiac arrest)	Senna may cause potassium and magnesium loss with excessive or prolonged use; may precipitate QT prolongation	Major	Droperidol should be used with extreme caution with laxatives
Anticonvulsants				
Gabapentin	Aluminum, dihydroxyalumin, and magnesium salts	Reduces gabapentin bioavailability by 20%	Decreased gabapentin bioavailability	Moderate — Avoid antacid use within 2 hours of taking gabapentin
Opioids				
Fentanyl	Carbamazepine	Decreased plasma fentanyl concentrations	Induction of CYP enzymes, increasing clearance of fentanyl	Moderate — Monitor response to fentanyl and increase dose as appropriate
	Clarithryomycin	Increased fentanyl toxicity (CNS and respiratory depression)	Inhibition of CYP3A4-mediated fentanyl metabolism	Major — Monitor patient and reduce fentanyl dose
	Diltiazem	Severe hypotension and increased risk of fentanyl toxicity (respiratory depression)	Inhibition of CYP3A4-mediated fentanyl metabolism	Major — Monitor blood pressure and reduce/adjust fentanyl dose as appropriate
	Erythromycin	Increased fentanyl toxicity (CNS and respiratory depression)	Inhibition of CYP3A4-mediated fentanyl metabolism	Major — Monitor patient and reduce fentanyl dose
	Fluconazole	Increased fentanyl toxicity	Inhibition of CYP3A4-mediated fentanyl metabolism	Major — Monitor patient and reduce fentanyl dose

Table 26.1 (Contd.)

	Interacting medication	Interaction effect	Probable mechanism	Severity*	Clinical management
	Ketoconazole	Increased fentanyl toxicity	Inhibition of CYP3A4-mediated fentanyl metabolism	Major	Monitor patient and reduce fentanyl dose
	Phenytoin	Decreased fentanyl serum concentrations	Induction of fentanyl metabolism by phenytoin	Moderate	Adjust fentanyl dose as appropriate
Methadone	Erythromycin	Increased serum methadone concentrations	Inhibition of CYP3A4-mediated methadone metabolism	Moderate	Use caution with combination; consider lowering methadone dose
	Fluconazole	Increased plasma methadone levels	Inhibition of CYP3A4-mediated methadone metabolism	Moderate	Monitor therapy closely; consider lowering methadone dose empirically
	Ketoconazole	Increased plasma methadone levels	Inhibition of CYP3A4-mediated methadone metabolism	Moderate	Monitor therapy closely; consider lowering methadone dose empirically
	Phenobarbital	Decreased methadone effectiveness	Induction of CYP3A4-mediated methadone metabolism	Moderate	Combination may result in lower methadone serum concentration; increase dose as required
Morphine	Cimetidine	Increased morphine toxicity	Unclear, possibly decreased metabolism	Major	Use caution with combination, start with lower dose of morphine and titrate as appropriate

Tramadol	Carbamazepine	Decreased tramadol efficacy	Induction of CYP3A4 metabolism of tramadol by carbamazepine	Major	Concurrent administration is not recommended
	Erythromycin	Increased tramadol serum level	Inhibition of CYP3A4 metabolism of tramadol by erythromycin	Moderate	Monitor patient for signs and symptoms of tramadol overdose
	Ketoconazole	Increased tramadol serum level	Inhibition of CYP3A4 metabolism of tramadol by ketoconazole	Moderate	Monitor patient for signs and symptoms of tramadol overdose
	St. John's Wort	Decreased tramadol serum level	Induction of CYP3A4 metabolism of tramadol by St. John's Wort	Moderate	Monitor for tramadol efficacy
Nonopioid analgesics					
Acetaminophen	Carbamazepine	Increased risk of acetaminophen toxicity	Carbamazepine may induce metabolism of acetaminophen resulting in increased level of hepatotoxic metabolites	Moderate	At usual therapeutic oral doses of acetaminophen and carbamazepine, no special monitoring is required
	Phenytoin	Decreased acetaminophen effectiveness and increased risk of hepatotoxicity	Phenytoin increases metabolism of acetaminophen by more than 40% and decreases acetaminophen half-life by about 25%. Increases production of toxic acetaminophen metabolites.	Moderate	Avoid large or chronic doses of acetaminophen. Monitor patient for signs or symptoms of hepatotoxicity

Table 26.1 (Contd.)

	Interacting medication	Interaction effect	Probable mechanism	Severity*	Clinical management
	Warfarin	Increased risk of bleeding due to increased hypoprothrombinemic effect of warfarin. Two to 4 g/day of acetaminophen increases INR within 1–2 weeks	Acetaminophen may inhibit metabolism of warfarin or acetaminophen may interfere with formation of clotting factors	Moderate	Limit intake of acetaminophen. Monitor INR for several weeks when acetaminophen is added or discontinued in patients taking warfarin.
Ibuprofen	Desipramine	Increased risk of desipramine toxicity	Inhibition of desipramine metabolism by ibuprofen	Moderate	Monitor desipramine concentration and monitor for adverse effects
	Lithium	Increased risk of lithium toxicity	Decreased lithium clearance	Moderate	Monitor for signs of lithium toxicity; lithium dosage reduction may be necessary
	Phenytoin	Increased risk of phenytoin toxicity	Increased free phenytoin serum concentration and/ or altered metabolism of either phenytoin or ibuprofen	Moderate	Monitor patients receiving this combination for signs of phenytoin toxicity and monitor serum levels (free and total phenytoin)

Corticosteroids

Drug	Interacting drug	Effect	Mechanism	Severity	Management
Dexamethasone	Carbamazepine	Decreased dexamethasone effectiveness	Increased dexamethasone metabolism	Moderate	Monitor response to dexamethasone and increase dose as clinically indicated
	Phenobarbital	Decreased dexamethasone effectiveness	Induction of hepatic metabolism	Moderate	Monitor response to dexamethasone and increase dose as clinically indicated
	Phenytoin	Decreased dexamethasone effectiveness	Increased dexamethasone metabolism	Moderate	Monitor therapeutic response to dexamethasone and increase dose as clinically indicated

Benzodiazepines

Drug	Interacting drug	Effect	Mechanism	Severity	Management
Diazepam	Erythromycin	Increased benzodiazepine toxicity	Decreased hepatic metabolism	Moderate	Monitor patient for excessive benzodiazepine effects and adjust therapy as appropriate
	St. John's wort	Reduced diazepam effectiveness	St. John's wort inhibits CYP3A4 enzyme activity	Moderate	Monitor for altered therapeutic and adverse effects of diazepam

Table 26.1 (Contd.)

	Interacting medication	Interaction effect	Probable mechanism	Severity*	Clinical management
Lorazepam	St. John's wort	Reduced lorazepam effectiveness	St. John's wort inhibits CYP3A4 enzyme activity	Moderate	Monitor for altered therapeutic and adverse effects of lorazepam.
	Valproic acid	Increased lorazepam concentration	Decreased lorazepam metabolism	Moderate	Reduce lorazepam dose by 50% and monitor for increased adverse effects
Midazolam	Carbamazepine	Decreased efficacy of midazolam	Induction of CYP3A enzymes by carbamazepines	Moderate	Larger doses of midazolam may be required to achieve desired response
	Clarithromycin	Increased midazolam toxicity	Inhibition of CYP3A4-mediated midazolam metabolism	Moderate	Monitor patient and reduce midazolam dose empirically
	Erythromycin	Increased midazolam sedation	Inhibition of CYP3A4-mediated midazolam metabolism	Moderate	Monitor patient and reduce midazolam dose empirically
	Fluconazole	Increased midazolam serum concentration and toxicity	Inhibition of CYP3A4-mediated midazolam metabolism	Moderate	Monitor patient and reduce dose of midazolam
	Ketoconazole	Increased midazolam serum concentration and toxicity	Inhibition of CYP3A4-mediated metabolism of midazolam	Major	Combination not recommended

Phenytoin	Decreased efficacy of midazolam	Induction of CYP3A4-mediated metabolism of midazolam	Moderate	Larger doses of midazolam may be required
St. John's wort	Reduced midazolam effectiveness	Inhibition of CYP3A4-mediated metabolism of midazolam	Moderate	Monitor response and increase midazolam dose as required
Non-benzodiazepine sedatives/hypnotics				
Trazodone				
Amiodarone	Amiodarone and trazodone are both metabolized by CYP3A4, and amiodarone inhibits this enzyme. Combination increases risk of QT interval prolongation and torsade de pointes	Unknown	Major	Use caution if these drugs are used in combination and monitor cardiac function
Carbamazepine	Decreased trazodone plasma concentration	Induction of CYP3A4 metabolism	Moderate	Monitor trazodone serum concentration and response; adjust therapy as needed
Clarithromycin	Increase in trazodone plasma levels	Inhibition of CYP3A4 metabolism	Moderate	Use lower dose of trazodone in patients receiving clarithromycin and monitor for adverse effects

Table 26.1 (Contd.)

	Interacting medication	Interaction effect	Probable mechanism	Severity*	Clinical management
	Digoxin	Increased serum digoxin concentration and possible toxicity	Unknown	Moderate	Monitor serum digoxin concentration with combination
	Fluoxetine	Increased trazodone toxicity and/or serotonin syndrome	Decreased trazodone clearance	Major	Monitor for trazodone toxicity and adjust dose as necessary
	Itraconazole, ketoconazole	Increased trazodone serum concentrations	Inhibition of CYP3A4-mediated trazodone metabolism	Moderate	Use a lower dose of trazodone and monitor adverse effects
	Phenytoin	Increased phenytoin serum concentrations and increased risk of toxicity	Unknown, possibly due to competitive inhibition of phenytoin metabolism, protein binding, or excretion	Moderate	Monitor serum phenytoin concentration
	Ritonavir	Increased trazodone plasma level and increased risk of adverse effects	Inhibition of CYP3A-mediated trazodone metabolism by ritonavir	Moderate	Monitor patient for increased sedative effects and hypotension. May require trazodone dosage reduction
Zolpidem	Ketoconazole	Increased zolpidem plasma level and increased risk of adverse effects	Impaired metabolism of zolpidem	Moderate	If used together, monitor for decreased concentration and increased somnolence

Dopamine antagonists

Haloperidol	Bupropion	Increased plasma levels of haloperidol	Inhibition of CPY2D6-mediated haloperidol metabolism	Moderate	Use combination with caution, and start with lower dose of haloperidol
	Carbamazepine	Decreased haloperidol effectiveness	Increased CYP 2D6 and 3A4-mediated haloperidol metabolism	Moderate	Monitor effectiveness of haloperidol and increase dosage as appropriate

Antihistamines/anticholinergics

Diphenhydramine	Metoprolol	Increased metoprolol plasma concentrations with prolonged negative chronotropic and inotropic effects of metoprolol, especially in poor CYP2D6 metabolizers	Diphenhydration inhibits CYP2D6 enzyme, which reduces metoprolol metabolism	Moderate	Use combination with caution; monitor for increased metoprolol adverse effects

Elimination

There are few pharmacokinetic interactions caused by alterations in drug elimination because most drugs have multiple mechanisms of elimination (e.g., biliary, renal).[8]

Probenecid has been shown to affect drug secretion in the kidney, prolonging elimination of methotrexate and penicillin and other beta-lactam antibiotics.

Drug–disease interaction is more likely to cause drug toxicity, specifically renal and/or hepatic impairment.

Conclusion

Medications are commonly used to palliate symptoms associated with advanced illness. Practitioners must be vigilant in monitoring this frail patient population for drug-induced illness, including those caused by drug–drug interactions.

References

1. Davis M, Homsi J (2001). The importance of cytochrome P450 monooxygenase CYP2D6 in palliative medicine. *Support Care Cancer* 9:442–451.
2. Curtis E, Walsh T (1993). Prescribing practices of a palliative care service. *J Pain Symptom Manage* 8:312–316.
3. Wright J (1992). Drug interactions. In: Melmon K, Morrelli H, Hoffman B, Nierenberg D (Eds.), *Melmon and Morrelli's Clinical Pharmacology: Basic Principles in Therapeutics*. New York: McGraw-Hill, p. 1012.
4. Arizona Cert: Center for Education and Research on Therapeutics. QT drug lists by risk group. Retrieved October 25, 2009, from www.torsades.org
5. Boyer E, Shannon M (2005). The serotonin syndrome. *N Engl J Med* 352:1112–1120.
6. Mihelic R (2005). Pharmacology of palliative medicine. *Semin Oncol Nurs* 21:29–35.
7. Haddad A, Davis M, Lagman R (2007). The pharmacological importance of cytochrome CYP3A4 in the palliation of symptoms: review and recommendations for avoiding adverse drug interactions. *Support Care Cancer* 15:251–257.
8. Micromedex Healthcare Series [Internet database] (2009). Thomson Reuters (Healthcare) Inc. Retrieved November 10, 2009, from http://www.micromedex.com/

Pediatric palliative care

Donna Zhukovsky, MD
Rhonda Robert, PhD

What is pediatric palliative care and whom does it involve?

Definition of pediatric palliative care

Pediatric palliative care (PPC) is a family-centered approach to care for children and their families living with life-threatening illness. The goal of PPC is to manage pain and other physical symptoms while addressing the psychological, social, and spiritual problems of the child and the child's family.

As defined by the World Health Organization,[1] effective palliative care for children

- Involves giving active total care of the child's body, mind, and spirit as well as support to the family
- Begins when illness is diagnosed and continues regardless of whether or not a child receives treatment directed at the disease
- Requires that the health-care provider evaluate and alleviate the child's physical, psychological, and social distress
- Requires a broad multidisciplinary approach that includes the family and effectively uses available community resources
- Can be provided in tertiary-care facilities, community health centers, and the child's home

Who are the affected children?

Typically, people think of children diagnosed with cancer and other life-limiting illnesses as the exclusive recipients of PPC. However, their siblings are also important beneficiaries, as are the child's community of friends, peers, and classmates and children of adult cancer patients, an expanding group due to childbirth into later years.

Affected children are often overlooked by health-care professionals and receive less attention from their parents than the ill child in part because of care-giving needs and the emotional distress associated with parenting a seriously ill child.

Clinical pearl

- Pediatric palliative care is not limited to child and adolescent patients. All children whose lives are affected by serious medical illness in a loved one are potential beneficiaries: pediatric patients, their siblings, peers, parents, and family caregivers, as well as children and grandchildren of adult patients.

Differences from palliative care for adults

While the overall approach to palliative care for children is similar to that provided for adults, there are several differences that influence the provision of care (Table 27.1).[2]

Child's developmental stage

In addition to physiological and pharmacokinetic differences that influence pharmacotherapy, developmental factors that impact communication, as well as the understanding of illness and death, distinguish care of the child

Table 27.1 Pediatric palliative care: differences from care of adult patients

- Child's developmental stage
- Family life cycle stage
- Disease spectrum
- Illness trajectories

from that of adults. Health-care providers must be familiar with these differences in order to provide effective and compassionate care.

Family life cycle

Parents or adult siblings function as proxy reporters and decision-makers. When children are very young or ill, these proxies may be the only source of input. Assuming these new roles and responsibilities is emotionally taxing on parents and siblings, and they need additional emotional support.

For older children who are healthy enough to provide self-report and participate in decision-making, both parents and patients often participate in reporting and decision-making. Differences in parent and patient wishes may result in ethical dilemmas.

Disease spectrum

Death is an uncommon phenomenon in children, with 53,000 deaths per year in the United States. Approximately one-half of deaths occur during the first year of life, with congenital defects, prematurity, and sudden infant death syndrome representing the most common causes.

From ages 1 to 19, the overwhelming causes of death result from traumatic accidents and injuries, raising the need for acute palliative care for bereaved families that may have no or very little time to adjust to the threat of premature mortality.

Of medical causes, cancer is the most common at 2200 annually in the United States, followed by cardiac diseases, congenital anomalies, and multiple other uncommon diseases. The relative rarity of pediatric death and limited availability of disease-specific expertise often requires medical care in locations distant from the family's home.

Illness trajectories

The spectrum of illness trajectories that accompany life-limiting illness is different from those associated with adult causes of mortality, some without the predictable decline that is common to adults[3]:

- Potentially curable conditions, such as cancer (over 70% of children with cancer are cured)
- Progressive conditions for which intensive therapy prolongs and enhances life, such as cystic fibrosis
- Progressive conditions for which curative or disease-altering therapy is not available, such as a variety of neurodegenerative conditions
- Nonprogressive conditions for which death before adulthood is likely from complications, such as prolonged seizures or respiratory failure with cerebral palsy

Role of family-centered care

Family-centered care, integral to the definition of palliative care in general, plays an especially strong role in caring for children living with life-limiting illness and their families. In pediatrics, family-centered care recognizes that parents are the true experts regarding their own children and that they are the primary source of information, strength, and support for each child.

To provide for a true partnership, health-care professionals must step back from their customary roles as experts to realize that families are experts in their own right and must be involved at all levels of health-care delivery, including development and execution of treatment plans.

Symptom assessment and management

Symptom epidemiology

Available data, while limited, suggest that children living with life-limiting illnesses experience a high symptom burden. The data are best described in cancer patients.

Almost two-thirds of children with non-CNS tumors have symptoms at diagnosis, which typically resolve with initiation of treatment. However, multiple symptoms are common throughout the course, with inpatients and those receiving chemotherapy reporting more symptoms than outpatients.[4,5]

Unrelieved symptoms are also prevalent at the end of life, with pain, fatigue, dyspnea, and anorexia being the most common. In addition to the cancer, symptoms may occur as a result of the treatment or procedures or from non-cancer etiologies.

Causes of treatment and procedure-related pain are noted in Tables 27.2 and 27.3. These can often be anticipated and prevented. In non-cancer illnesses, symptoms vary depending on the diagnosis, but often reflect respiratory, neurological, or feeding problems.

Paradigm for symptom assessment and management

As for adults, optimal management of pain and other disease-associated symptoms is predicated on an understanding of the multidimensional nature of the symptom experience. Contributing to symptom expression are medical factors, including underlying pathophysiological mechanisms and comorbid medical conditions, as well as psychological, social, and spiritual factors.

Table 27.2 Treatment-related pain in children with cancer

Chemotherapy	Surgery
• Myalgias	• Postoperative
• Mucositis	• Phantom limb
• Extravasation	• (preoperative analgesia)
• Neuropathy	**Radiation**
• GVHD (allogeneic BMT)	• Mucositis
	• Dermatitis

BMT, bone marrow transplantation; GVHD, graft-versus-host disease.

Table 27.3 Procedure-related pain in children with cancer

- Needles
- Bone marrow
- Aspiration and biopsy
- Central line removal
- Diagnostic procedures

Symptom assessment includes a systematic symptom survey, a symptom-specific history, oncological history, including disease-directed therapies, general medical history, spiritual review, and psychosocial and family history that includes screening for substance abuse. When available, validated age- and developmentally appropriate symptom screening batteries such as the pediatric versions of the Memorial Symptom Assessment Scale[4,5] and symptom-specific scales should routinely be incorporated into the clinical history.

Optimal management is contingent upon ongoing assessment of the symptom experience, physical examination, and indicated diagnostic testing, as expert assessment is the basis for a working diagnosis and treatment plan in keeping with the goals of care.

Pain assessment tools

Types of assessment tools include behavioral, numeric rating, categorical, and visual analog scales. For pain, behavioral observation scales are the primary assessment method for neonates, infants, and children under 4 years of age and those with developmental disabilities.

Children ages 3 to 8 years are usually able to use faces scales with a series of photographs or drawings depicting varying degrees of distress. Children aged 8 years and older can generally also use verbal rating scales (no pain, mild, moderate, severe) and horizontal versions of adult visual analog scales, for example, measuring pain against a horizontal ruler.[6]

Examples of age-appropriate pain assessment scales are noted in Box 27.1.

Assessment of psychological distress

Assessment of psychological distress should be an early and ongoing component of care for persons with a life-threatening illness. Learning of and living with the illness are both initially and intermittently distressing and often relate to losses.

Box 27.1 Pain assessment: examples of age and developmentally appropriate scales

Children <4 years or with developmental disabilities
- Behavioral observation scales
- FLACCS (Face, Legs, Activity, Cry, Consolability)
- Children's Hospital of Eastern Ontario Pain Scale (CHEOPS)
- Gustave Roussy pain scale

Children 3–7 years
- Faces scales (e.g., Oucher, revised Bieri, Baker–Wong)
- Color analog scale (e.g., pain thermometer)
- Poker chip tool
- Body maps

Children ≥8 years
- Verbal rating scales
- Numeric rating scales
- Visual analog scales (horizontal)

Acutely, losses may include disruption of daily life and loss of physical well-being. Progressive losses may include deaths of friends at the same treatment center and health decline from advanced disease or treatment side effects. Examples of anticipated losses include independence from caregiver or career options.

With most life-threatening or life-limiting illnesses, persons are at risk for symptoms of depression and anxiety, including traumatic stress. A source for reviewing the symptoms of possible diagnoses is *the Diagnostic and Statistical Manual of Mental Disorders (DSM)*, published by the American Psychiatric Association. Portions of the DSM are available online at www.psyweb.com.

Given that depression, anxiety, and traumatic stress need to be evaluated, assessing sleep quality is a nonthreatening way to begin screening for these conditions. Sleep has behavioral qualities and concrete descriptors, is usually not stigmatizing to discuss, and involves personal disclosure. Easily disrupted by emotional distress, sleep patterns provide some transparency regarding a person's emotional state.

A possible questioning sequence may be "How have you been sleeping? How long do you take to fall asleep? Once you are asleep, do you awaken? If so, what causes you to awaken? What is on your mind when you awaken? How are you feeling when you awaken?"

Questions about feeling states such as worry and sadness are a natural progression. When assessing concerns, normalizing the experience is important before asking questions: "Many people have new worries and concerns when they are feeling sick. Some people have never been to a hospital before, and others have never spent a night away from home before. I would like to know how you feel."

The fear thermometer is a single-item numeric rating scale that can be used to simplify assessment of worry.[7,8] Similar to a pain thermometer, it is a type of tool with which many children are already familiar.

Online screening tools and resources developed for assessing depression and anxiety are available from the International Psycho-oncology Society (www.ipos-society.org), the American Psychosocial Oncology Society (www.apos-society.org), and the National Child Traumatic Stress Network (www.NCTSNet.org).

Clinical pearl

• Asking about sleep is a nonthreatening way to begin screening for depression and anxiety.

Synthesis of symptom diagnosis and management plan

Once a working diagnosis is established, treatment is directed at modifying the underlying causes as well as palliation of the symptom itself. Symptom-directed therapy (i.e., analgesics for pain) is often an integral component of the treatment plan while awaiting the benefit of disease-directed therapy or when primary therapy is ineffective.

Psychological, social, and spiritual concerns often exacerbate the symptom and necessitate corresponding interventions for optimal symptom management and to avoid unnecessary drug toxicity.

Modalities of symptom control

Modalities of symptom control, reviewed elsewhere in this book, are numerous and include disease-specific, pharmacological, anesthetic, surgical, psychiatric, psychological, spiritual, and integrative-medicine interventions.

Optimal management is often multimodal and best configured with the interdisciplinary input of team members working closely together. Understanding the impact of illness and associated symptoms on the child is essential. If barriers are present, psychosocial staff, including a child-life specialist when available, can foster communication about these issues.

Principles of pharmacotherapy

Pharmacotherapy is a mainstay of treatment for most children. There is a paucity of studies conducted in children, thus use is largely based on clinical experience. Principles of management are noted in Box 27.2.

Indications for most medications and medication side effects are similar to those for adults in most cases.

Given the variation in starting doses and dose range due to developmental issues (see Developmental issues in drug use, below), specific dose recommendations are beyond the scope of this text.

Developmental issues in drug use

Factors that influence drug management include ratio of body compartments, differences in plasma protein binding, development of hepatic enzyme systems for drug metabolism, extent of renal filtration and excretion of drugs and their metabolites, metabolic rate, oxygen consumption, and degree of maturation of respiratory function.[6]

For individuals not experienced in working with premature infants or children of different developmental stages, close coordination with pediatricians and pediatric pharmacists is essential to providing safe and expert pharmacotherapy, and use of pediatric-specific resources is advised.

Box 27.2 Principles of pharmacotherapy for symptom management

- Start one drug at a time and allow an adequate trial to assess benefit and side effects.
- Choose the appropriate route of administration.
- Use the oral route whenever possible.
- Avoid the intramuscular route.
- Provide regularly scheduled medication for continuous pain.
- Use PRN or "breakthrough" doses for prevention of predictable incident pain and treatment of pain exacerbations.
- Anticipate and manage side effects, e.g., bowel management with narcotics.

Communication issues in pediatric palliative care

Communication: the principle determinant of high-quality care

The literature consistently demonstrates that parents value direct, clear and caring communication about what to expect and that this is a primary determinant of quality pediatric palliative care.[8] Involvement of the child, when considered age- and culturally appropriate by the parents, is key to satisfaction with care.

Furthermore, most children adjust best to death, be it their own, their sibling's, or their parent's, when provided with a safe and permissive environment in which they are allowed to openly ask questions, voice concerns, and participate in care.

Clinical pearl

- Parents value direct, clear, and caring communication about what to expect; this is a primary determinant of quality of care.
- Involvement of the child in discussions about the illness and care plans, when considered age- and culturally appropriate by the parents, is key to parents' satisfaction with care.

Formats for medical conversations

The format of medical conversations may be 1) patient only; 2) patient and parent simultaneously; 3) parent first, followed by parent and patient simultaneously; or 4) parent only. Problems commonly arise when negotiation of the format does not occur, for example:

- Patient: "The worst part was waiting in the lobby when my parents and doctor were talking about me."
- Parent: "The doctor just said the diagnosis. I was not prepared. I was so upset. I wished I had been able to support my child."

The medical-conversation formats used in these examples are reasonable but not suited to the participants' needs. Once the conversations have taken place, fit of the conversation should be reassessed: What about the format worked? What did not work? What modifications should be made?

As participants gain treatment experience, the format may need to be changed. Optimally initiated at the beginning of the patient–professional caregiver relationship, these conversations should continue throughout the course of care and provide the opportunity for the medical professional to learn what is important to both the parent and child.

Empathic listening

Communication requires both an empathic listening component and a treatment leadership component. Most often, the empathic listening component is omitted and communication is limited to biomedical information.

The patient needs permission and invitation to be heard; the medical professional can extend this invitation by asking open-ended questions.

Open-ended questions are an invitation for the recipient to reflect, feel, and self-disclose.

Mack and Wolfe offer suggestions for best practice in this area, including how to initiate medical conversations, introduce the possibility of death, elicit care goals, introduce palliation, talk about expectations, and address children directly.[9]

Transitioning between or participating in simultaneous curative and palliative care services

Communicating during transitions in care can be challenging. Language may become vague, euphemistic, autocratic, and/or complex biomedical speak, resulting in confusing communications.

Clear language, support, and commitment from the medical team along with active engagement with the family in decision-making is the ideal; for example: "It is time to rethink our goals and plans. We had each hoped that the treatment would cure the disease, but we now know the disease is worsening. Our goal is to help you in the best way possible. Do you have ideas regarding what is best for you? Would examples of goals, options, or plans help us start the conversation?"

Core concepts to complete understanding of death

Core concepts to a mature understanding of illness and death develop during childhood.[10] The first concept to develop is the *irreversibility* of death. Dead people do not come back to life the way that cartoon characters do.

Finality signifies that all body functions cease. When the concept of finality has not yet been grasped, children will ask how the deceased will eat or breath, once buried. Failure to address these developmentally appropriate concerns can lead to misperceptions, which can be traumatic if not corrected.

Universality implies that death happens to all living things and that, one day, death will happen to the child.

Causality is the understanding that death occurs for a proximate reason independent of oneself. Younger children commonly blame themselves for the death, rather than a cause independent of themselves. This misattribution of cause and effect is labeled "magical thinking."

Young children may believe that they have "wished" somebody dead; their misbehavior caused the death; or that death is contagious. Given the likelihood that these beliefs will occur, it is important to identify and rectify misattributions.

Age-specific recommendations regarding care of children exposed to life-threatening illness and death

Pre-school-age children understand physical discomfort. Parents' presence and soothing of the child are the focal parenting tasks. Pre-school-age children live in the present. They do not have "issues" to resolve or need "closure" before death.

Young school-age children need help with magical thinking, as discussed above. A sample script is as follows: "The (name of illness) is stronger, and the medicines are not able to help as much as they had. You worked hard and followed the prescriptions. We are very proud of you. You did not cause the (illness), nor did you do anything to make it stronger. No one knows why this happened. We will do everything possible to help you and one other."

Older school-age children and adolescents have a broad range of concerns and need for information. Commonly reported concerns include the following:
- What dying feels like, including whether dying will be painful
- Separation from loved ones
- How others will fare after the child dies
- What happens to the child after death

School-age children and adolescents need permission to voice concerns. Some may need to hear examples of commonly experienced concerns, as most are apprehensive to disclose private thoughts about death. They may need a neutral party with whom to disclose concerns, wanting to protect loved ones from sadness.

Grief and bereavement in pediatric palliative care

Children may cross many milestones during the course of an illness. Normalizing life as much as possible by facilitating participation in milestones important to the child is necessary. If this is not done, treatment adherence and psychological adjustment may both deteriorate.

The child patient: disclosure of impending death

Parental grief

Parents may need to grieve the anticipated death of their child, spouse, or other beloved individual before they are able to assist their child or children in the grieving process. This timing may conflict with the health-care professional's readiness to discuss dying with the child. The health-care professional should discuss timing of disclosure with the parent.

Negotiating a balance between the parents' needs and the child's needs is the goal. In addition to reflective listening and empathic responses from the medical professional, the parent(s) may benefit from additional services to work through their grief.

Describing the role and accessibility of expert assistance and offering to facilitate the connection is ideal. If such an expert is not available within the institution, a member of the treatment team should assume the responsibility of making a community-based referral.

A national locator for licensed psychologists is provided by the National Registry of Health Service Providers at www.findapsychologist.org. State licensing boards provide online rosters of licensees by city or zip code. The key search words are "state board of examiners of (psychologists, psychiatrists, licensed professional counselors, or social workers)."

Parental role in protecting the child from harm

Parents' jobs involve protection of their child from harm; accordingly, they may want to protect their child by avoiding discussion of death. However, one cannot be protected from one's own death. Parents may need input, discussion, and suggestions as to how to help their dying child with developmentally appropriate information.

When a child does not have adequate, age-appropriate information, what the child imagines is likely worse than the truth. With information, the child can trust in others, know what to expect, and be part of the family experience. By modeling how persons are helped, regardless of circumstances, death need not be feared.

Parents may benefit from opportunities to plan and rehearse ways to discuss the possibility and likelihood of the child's dying with the treatment team or community experts.

Clinical pearl

- Giving children permission to talk about the impending death of themselves or of a loved one is important, as it demonstrates confidence in their ability to cope and allows for correction of potentially distressing misperceptions.

Psychosocial support of parents and siblings of a child with life-limiting illness

During illness

Healthy siblings need to maintain normalcy. Maintaining contact with the familiar is important. Routines such as school and peer-based activities need to continue. When parents are unable to sustain these routines, surrogate caregivers should be identified to help.

In addition, the healthy sibling needs consistent, trustworthy information regarding the ill sibling and contact with parents and the ill sibling during the course of medical care. To foster contact, sibling-oriented services are often available, e.g., sibling support groups and summer camps that include healthy and ill sibling groups.

Parents may need suggestions of how best to parent a healthy child when another child in the family is ill. National organizations, such as Candlelighters (www.candlelighters.org), provide parent support, and Supersibs (www.supersibs.org) provides sibling support and parenting information.

During bereavement

Psychosocial support and intervention subsequent to the death of a patient is also an important and often neglected aspect of care. Brief contact by phone or mail by the primary medical team members provides both the opportunity for the shared loss to be recognized and an offer to locate local bereavement resources.

Bereaved parents often do not fit into generic, community grief support groups because of the rarity of and aspects unique to a child's death.

National organizations available to facilitate identification of local bereavement resources include the following:

- *Compassionate Friends* (www.compassionatefriends.org) is a national organization for bereaved parents, with local chapters that provide parent support groups.
- *Dougy Center* (www.dougy.org) provides sibling bereavement services and an international listing of similar organizations.

Palliative care for the child whose parent is dying

A child whose parent is at the end of life can be an important beneficiary of palliative care services, either directly or through the proxy of their parent. Like parents of seriously ill children, parents affected by a terminal illness may need help in learning how to talk with a child about their own or the other parent's illness.

Assistance in talking with their children about the illness should be offered at the beginning of treatment and whenever health status changes significantly. Parents are encouraged to do the following:

- Openly discuss the illness
- Involve the treatment team expert as needed
- Use proper name of the illness
- Clarify whether or not the illness is contagious
- Dispel magical thinking regarding causality
- Bring the child to an appointment

- Encourage visitation during hospitalizations
  • Visitation is the child's choice; most children wish to visit.
  • Prepare the child before the visit; explain the parent's status, the medical equipment being used, treatment of the disease, and treatment for comfort.
- Foster discussions about dying; ensure an age-appropriate understanding of what dying means (e.g., the body stops working).
- Reassure the child regarding who and how the child will be cared for during end of life and after the parent's death.
- Inform and update school counselors and other involved adults.
- Maintain normalcy as much as possible.

Kathleen McCue provides more detailed guidance in her book *How to Help Children through a Parent's Serious Illness* (1994), published by St. Martin's Press, New York.

Grieving children: how do they differ from adults?

Whenever possible, children should be offered the opportunity to be present with the ill individual and to participate in death rituals such as funerals to the extent that they would like. Explanations of what to expect and provision of an adult dedicated to that child in the event that the child's needs change is integral to a successful bereavement outcome.

Unlike most adults, children do not exhibit intense emotional and behavioral expressions of grief in a continuous fashion. For example, a typical developmental response for a school-age child might be to exhibit intense signs of grief, followed by a request to play at the neighbor's house. While grief may not be continuous, it can last longer than grief of adults, with the need to repeat the work of mourning at developmental and chronological milestones.

The bereavement process itself is affected by many factors, including closeness of relationship with the deceased, family functioning, and family style of communication. For most families, the process is a successful one.

Pediatric palliative care: what do parents need?

There is a consistent theme:
- Good pain and symptom control
- Direct, sensitive, and clear communication, as influenced by culture
- Collaborative, caring relationships (child, family, and health-care team)
- Parent and child (when age appropriate) involvement in decision-making, including at the end of life
- Health-care professional availability (24/7)
- Continued relationships with health-care professionals in bereavement

References

1. World Health Organization (2002). *National Cancer Control Programmes: Policies and Managerial Guidelines*, 2nd ed. Geneva: World Health Organization.
2. Field JM, Behrman RE (Eds.) (2003). *When Children Die: Improving Palliative and End-of-Life Care for Children and Their Families*. Washington, DC: National Academies Press, pp. 41–71.
3. Hynson JL, Sawyer SM (2001). Paediatric palliative care: distinctive needs and emerging issues. *J Paediatr Child Health* 37:323–325.
4. Collins JJ, Byrnes ME, Dunkel IJ, Lapin J, Nadel T, Thaler HT, Polyak T, Rapkin B, Portenoy RK (2000). The measurement of symptoms in children with cancer. *J Pain Symptom Manage* 19:363–377.
5. Collins JJ, Devine TD, Dick GS, Johnson EA, Kilham HA, Pinkerton CR, Stevens MM, Thaler HT, Portenoy RK (2002). The measurement of symptoms in young children with cancer: the validation of the Memorial Symptom Assessment Scale in children aged 7–12. *J Pain Symptom Manage* 23:10–16.
6. Berde CB, Sethna NF (2002). Analgesics for the treatment of pain in children. *N Engl J Med* 347(14):1094–1103.
7. Silverman W, Kurtines W (1996). *Anxiety and Phobic Disorders: A Pragmatic Approach*. New York: Plenum Press.
8. Walk RD (1956). Self-ratings of fear in a fear-invoking situation. *J Abnorm Social Psychol* 52:171–178.
9. Mack J, Wolfe J (2006). Early integration of pediatric palliative care: for some children, palliative care starts at diagnosis. *Curr Opin Pediatr* 18:10–14.
10. Himelstein BP, Hilden JM, Boldt AM, Weissman D (2004). Pediatric palliative care. *N Engl J Med* 350:1752–1762.

Palliation in the care of older adults

Christine S. Ritchie, MD, MSPH

Aging with chronic disease

In the year 2000, the average American life expectancy was 76 years. Those who survive to age 65 can anticipate living another 17 to 19 years, and Americans who live to age 85 are likely to survive to age 92.[1]

Also in 2000, 66% of Medicare beneficiaries aged 65–74 reported two or more chronic health conditions, and 21% reported fair or poor health. Among respondents age 85 and older, 80% reported more than two chronic conditions and 36% described fair or poor health.[2]

Given that older adults are surviving into advanced age with chronic disease, the majority of hospice diagnoses are now non-cancer related, e.g., congestive heart failure (CHF), chronic obstructive pulmonary failure (COPD), or dementia.

Palliative care providers need to become familiar with managing the symptoms of chronic disease as well as prognosticating in the setting of variable chronic disease courses.

Palliative care needs in older adults

The symptom burdens of chronic disease can exceed terminal illness burdens but are frequently underrecognized and undertreated, e.g., COPD-related dyspnea and anxiety in the setting of lung cancer.[3]

Functional and mobility decline complicate symptom management and care planning for frail elders—e.g., ambulatory function and the ability to get to the bathroom while using diuretics or laxatives, or fall-risk management for frail elders on psychoactive medication who live in multi-story housing.

Psychosocial and caregiver support can be tenuous because of spousal loss, social isolation, and geographically dispersed extended families.

Generational and cultural factors may affect a patient's comfort level with caregiving dependence on others. This can be very challenging for patients who embrace a Western concept of autonomy and independence but are no longer able to function independently because of illness and physical decline.

Settings of care for palliative care and hospice

Palliative care services are provided in multiple settings (Table 28.1):
- Inpatient
- Outpatient
- Long-term care facilities

Outpatient palliative care is covered by Medicare Part B or by private insurance, making it compatible with hospice benefits.

Medicare Part A does not pay for rehabilitation services and hospice simultaneously. Medicare Part A covers hospice services but not custodial care at a long-term care facility.

The goals of skilled nursing rehabilitation and hospice are often at odds in the final weeks of a patient's life.

Table 28.1 Settings of palliative care and hospice for older adults

Benefit	Goals	Location	Services	Services excluded	Eligibility	Payer
Skilled nursing rehabilitation	Rehabilitation of physical deconditioning to achieve optimal health and functional autonomy	Long-term care facilities	Physical therapy, occupational therapy, speech therapy, and skilled nursing care. Room and board, medications, and medical supplies are covered	Prohibits simultaneous enrollment in hospice	Meet skill needs in 3 therapy areas, or have at least one skillable nursing care need, e.g., wound care, IV antibiotics, tube-feeding, catheter care	Medicare Part A or private insurance (if under 65 years of age)
Hospice	Provides palliation of symptoms, spiritual and psychosocial support at the end of life	Can provide services at long-term care facilities, residential hospices, inpatient hospices, and at home	Nursing care, medications, supplies, durable medical equipment, pastoral care, social work, personal aid and attendance, bereavement support	Does not pay for room and board in long-term care facilities. Cannot receive Medicare-reimbursed rehabilitation services simultaneously while on hospice	Physician-documented life-limiting illness with a prognosis of 6 months or less	Medicare Part A or private insurance

Barriers to hospice for older adults

- Absence of caregiver support at home, especially for widowed, older females
- Inability of patient or family to pay for custodial care at a long-term care facility
- Patient fears of medical abandonment once on hospice

Goals of care discussions

Ageism bias occurs when health-care providers withhold more aggressive treatments or interventions because of consideration of age alone rather than functional and cognitive abilities or anticipated survival. People desire prolonged life at all ages. We cannot assume that people of advanced age will necessarily choose against life-prolonging therapy.

Quality of life, even in the cognitively impaired, is best assessed by the patient, not by proxies or health-care providers.[4,5] A person's functional capacity and quality of life influence the decision to endure procedures or treatments.[6]

Prognostication becomes difficult as the population lives longer with chronic diseases that have variable survival courses, e.g., CHF, COPD, and Alzheimer's disease.

Patients and families may feel strongly about the continued use of medications for chronic conditions unrelated to terminal illness, e.g., cholesterol medication. The health-care provider needs to balance the need for rapport-building and trust with the goal of reducing unnecessary polypharmacy.

Despite the tendency to approach dementia as if it were a single entity, it is important to recognize that different types of dementia present with different symptoms, clinical courses, and prognoses. Lewy body, vascular, and Alzheimer's dementia all have different clinical presentations and prognoses, necessitating nuanced, disease-specific care planning.

Clinical pearl

- Age alone should not dictate treatment choices, rather functional status, expected survival, and patient preferences should be the determining factors.

Biology of aging and pharmacokinetics

Decreased renal function, liver size, and hepatic blood flow occur with aging, leading to reduced drug metabolism.

Hydrophilic drugs have a lower volume of distribution due to decreased total body water in geriatric patients, leading to an increased risk of toxicity. Such drugs include ethanol, lithium, and digoxin.

Lipophilic drugs, e.g. benzodiazepines, barbiturates, trazodone, take longer to reach steady state and eliminate because of increased fat stores.

Decreased albumin levels cause increased unbound drug fractions, risking greater drug toxicity, e.g., with phenytoin, valproate, benzodiazepines, and warfarin.

Drugs using hepatic phase I pathways (diazepam, propoxyphene, miperidine, tricyclic antidepressants, carisoprodol) produce active metabolites that result in prolonged clinical effects and toxicity. Drugs using phase II pathways (lorazepam) result in inactive metabolites and are preferred in geriatric care.

Given age-related changes in drug metabolism and excretion, psychoactive medications (opioids, sedatives, tricyclic antidepressants) can cause central nervous system toxicity and delirium in older adults.

The general guideline when starting a medication in an older adult is to "start low and go slow," with frequent reassessments for side effects and efficacy.

Clinical pearl

- Psychoactive medications commonly used in palliative care increase risk for delirium in older adults.

Symptom management in geriatric populations

The side effects from drugs and polypharmacy in older adults often make symptom management more challenging.

Infection

Prolonged or recurrent antibiotic use can cause side effects (nausea, decreased appetite, diarrhea, infectious colitis, yeast infections) and drug resistance.

However, antibiotic use at the end of life may decrease symptom burden and therefore improve quality of life, even when it does not prolong survival.[7]

Pressure ulcers

Despite excellent skin care and pressure relief, pressure ulcers (PU) can be difficult to avoid at the end of life. Pressures ulcers tend to heal poorly in malnourished, frail older adults, particularly those with mobility limitations and incontinence.

Pressure ulcers are easier to prevent than to heal. Prevention measures include pressure-relieving mattresses, frequent turning, and good perineal hygiene.

Diverting colostomies may be appropriate in incontinent individuals with chronic sacral PU, provided there is reasonable life expectancy.

In patients who are actively dying, the goal is to effectively manage symptoms. Metronidazole gel and frequent dressing changes help odor control and drainage. Patients should be premedicated as needed for incident pain from dressing changes.

Kennedy terminal ulcers, usually a reddish-black area located over the sacrum, can appear suddenly during the last days to week of life, prognosticating short survival. It is hypothesized that they occur from progressive multiorgan failure involving the skin.

Pain

Many providers erroneously assume that older adults don't experience pain as intensely as younger patient populations.

Pain from a terminal illness may be complicated by pain from chronic underlying conditions, such as osteoarthritis, which are frequently unrecognized and undertreated. Pain assessment in cognitively impaired adults requires observation for pain behaviors (grimacing, crying, withdrawing, behavioral and sleep disturbances, diminished appetite).

Avoid use of medications such as NSAIDs (risk of GI upset, GI bleeding, and renal damage), opioids with toxic metabolites (miperidine, propoxyphene), and tricyclic antidepressants for neuropathic pain.

Exercise caution with sustained-release opioid preparations in patients with renal impairment because of the risk of increased neurotoxicity. In such circumstances, it is safer to use cleaner-metabolizing, short-acting opioids, such as oxycodone.

Nausea and vomiting
- Metoclopramide can cause extrapyramidal side effects.
- Promethazine and benzodiazepines increase the risk of falls and can cause delirium.
- Steroids can precipitate delirium.
- Ondansetron worsens constipation.

Constipation
Many geriatric patients chronically use laxatives, do not drink adequate fluids, or have fluid restrictions placed for cardiac or renal conditions.

Elderly patients should avoid fiber and bulking agents in opioid-induced constipation because of prolonged gut transit time resulting in increased water reabsorption and risk for obstruction.

Anticholinergic medications (bladder antispasmodics, antihistamines, tricyclic antidepressants) and calcium channel blockers all worsen constipation.

Diarrhea
Consider medication-induced causes (recent antibiotic use, chemotherapy) or infectious causes (*Clostridium difficile* colitis) of diarrhea.

Rule out infection before empirically using an antidiarrheal agent in patients who have recently taken antibiotics or who live in an institutional facility.

Cough
Some medications, such as calcium channel blockers and angiotensin-converting enzyme (ACE) inhibitors, can induce chronic cough weeks to months after initiation of the medication.

Gastric reflux can cause coughing and should be considered in patients who are tube fed.

Oral complaints
Poor dentition, ill-fitting dentures from weight loss, oral candidasis, and oral ulcerations can cause discomfort, resulting in decreased oral intake.

Depression and anxiety
Depression is often underrecognized in older adults as they may not acknowledge "feeling depressed" because of perceived social stigmas associated with depression. The Geriatric Depression Scale (GDS) is a good clinical tool for capturing unrecognized depressive behaviors.

Stimulants, such as methylphenidate, can quickly improve depressive symptoms in advanced terminal illness. Caution is advised for long-term treatment with stimulants in the setting of severe underlying coronary artery disease, CHF, or history of stroke.

SSRIs, such as citalopram and sertraline, are generally well tolerated in older adults. They can, however, contribute to hyponatremia, particularly in patients who suffer hyponatremia from volume overload conditions.

Incontinence
Fecal and urinary incontinence are common in older adults with mobility, cognitive, and neurogenic impairments. Incontinence is an important cause of institutionalization.

Bladder antispasmodics can cause delirium, severe bladder retention, constipation, and dry mouth, requiring close monitoring for tolerance.

Long-term indwelling Foley catheters promote recurrent urinary tract infection and antibiotic resistance.

Long-term use of rectal tubes is not advised.

Mobility and sensory impairment

Both mobility and sensory impairment increase the risk of falls, particularly if psychoactive medications are being used.

Decreased proprioception and hand coordination make self-care and medication administration difficult, e.g. glucose monitoring, shot administration, and opening pill bottles. Such impairments challenge patients and caregivers, contributing to the decision to institutionalize.

Insomnia

Insomnia results from sleep-cycle changes, medication use (some antidepressants, chemotherapy, steroids, sedatives/somniferents), day and nighttime inversion in dementia, occult alcohol use, and poor sleep hygiene.

Tricyclic antidepressants should not be used for insomnia because of anticholinergic side effects causing delirium and falls.

Use caution when prescribing benzodiazepines and zolpidem because of the risk of delirium and falls. In geriatric populations, lorazepam is preferred over diazepam, clonazepam, and alprazolam.

Low-dose trazodone is usually recommended as a safe first choice. Low-dose mirtazapine can improve both insomnia and appetite stimulation in patients suffering from anorexia.

Nutrition

Taste and smell diminish as we age, lowering appetite. In dementia, dietary modification using salty, sweet, and sour flavors can improve appetite, as can temperature adjustment (hot instead of cold dishes).

Modified consistencies, such as pureed foods, and tube-feeding are often less appealing to patients even though they may be safer in the setting of dysphagia.

Value judgments weighing quality of life vs. swallowing safety need to be assessed by the care team, patient, and family.

Cognitive impairment and delirium

Regardless of whether cognitive impairment is mild or severe, patients are at increased risk for suffering delirium. Delirium in cognitively impaired individuals may last as long as weeks to months following the precipitating event(s).

Delirium is often multifactorial, resulting from the underlying terminal illness, drugs, infection, dehydration, or change in environmental circumstances, e.g., hospitalization.

In addition to treating the underlying causes, short-term use of haloperidol for behavioral disturbances is helpful.

If antipsychotic use is anticipated to last for months, atypical neuroleptics (quetiapine, risperdal, olanzapine) usually result in fewer extrapyramidal side effects. However, the practitioner must weigh the increased risk of cerebrovascular events and mortality in patients with dementia who take these medications for extended periods of time.[8]

Quetiapine is usually the antipsychotic of choice in the setting of Parkinsonism.

Ethical and social issues

Artificial hydration and nutrition

There is no clear evidence that tube-feeding of institutionalized patients with dementia does or does not prolong survival. Since different types of dementia have different clinical presentations and survival courses, we cannot assume that tube-feeding uniformly provides the same survival benefits.[9]

Proxy and decision making

Patients with mild to moderate cognitive impairment are able to express preferences for treatments and interventions, even when they cannot provide formal consent. A common dilemma is when a patient's prior living will or advance directive does not coincide with expressed preferences once the person is cognitively impaired.

While this predicament involves value judgments, it is important for patient proxies and health-care providers to be sensitive to the patient's preferences, since cooperation is necessary for successful treatment and care planning.

Financial interdependence

It is not uncommon for spouses and family members to resist institutionalization of a loved one if they are still dependent on the patient for housing or financial support.

Medicaid protects spouses against losing their homes in the setting of a Medicaid spend-down. But it does not extend the same benefit to adult children or other family members living in the patient's home. This dilemma is ethically challenging if the health-care provider feels that the patient is not getting adequate care or supervision at home and needs institutionalization.

Existential suffering

Many older adults endure the loss of a spouse, face marginal care-giving support, and shoulder economic worries due to constrained income. Autonomy may be tenuous at best, only to become logistically and functionally compromised after the diagnosis of a life-limiting illness.

The way in which older adults face these challenges is often framed through cultural and religious lenses. These concerns lead to fears of institutionalization and abandonment for many elders. Such fears can compromise the fluid communication of needs between patients and health-care providers, underscoring the importance of a "whole-patient assessment" of needs.

Proper use of the interdisciplinary team model, through social work assistance, pastoral care, and psychology support services, can improve resource access and help patients cope with anxiety and stress.

Care of the caregiver

Compared to younger patients, older patients are frequently more dependent in activities of daily living (bathing, dressing, toileting, eating, transferring) and instrumental activities of daily living (banking, shopping, cleaning). This dependency is very physically and emotionally challenging for caregivers of all ages.

Older, frail spouses or siblings often care for their loved ones at home, jeopardizing caregiver well-being. This makes the patient vulnerable to institutionalization if the caregiver falls ill or dies.

Working-age caregivers frequently forego employment to provide informal care for a loved one, resulting in economic losses for the caregiver. In 2006 in the United States, the economic cost of informal caregiving was estimated at $350 billion in lost wages.[10] Social work services can help families identify and maximize available resources to help reduce caregiving strain.

When institutionalization does occur, it can produce feelings of guilt in caregivers of all ages.

When an older spouse, sibling, or adult child cares for a patient during a protracted illness, the caregiver is at risk for complicated grief and depression after the care-giving role is lost, particularly in families with enmeshed emotional dynamics. The risk for complicated grief should be explored by the interdisciplinary team prior to the patient's death. Team members should probe for suicidal ideation.

Palliative psychology support services and contact with caregiver support groups can help surviving family members cope with loss.

Clinical pearl

• Caregivers are at higher risk for depression, mortality, and complicated grief when their care recipient dies.

References

1. Life expectancy in the United States. Data from *National Vital Statistics Report* 2002; 51(3):2.
2. Terrell S, Berkman ND, Kuo M, Anderson W, Bonito A (2002). Analysis of Medicare Beneficiary Knowledge Data Using the Medicare Current Beneficiary Survey (MCBS) http:// aspe.hhs.gov (Accessed Dec. 2010).
3. Elkington H, White P, Addington-Hall J, Higgs R, Edmonds P (2005) The healthcare needs of chronic obstructive pulmonary disease patients in the last year of life. *Palliat Med* 19(6):485–491.
4. Hoe J, Katona C, Orrrell M, Livingston G (2007) Quality of life in dementia: care recipient and caregiver perceptions of quality of life in dementia: the LASER-AD study. *Int J Geriatr Psychiatry* 22(10):1031–1036.
5. Berlowitz DR, Du W, Kazis L, Lewis S (1995) Health-related quality of life of nursing home residents: differences in patient and provider perceptions. *J Am Geriatr Soc* 43 (7):799–802.
6. McCarthy EP, Pencina MJ, Kelly-Hayes M, et al. (2008) Advance care planning and health care preferences of community-dwelling elders: the Framingham Heart Study. *J Gerontol A Biol Sci Med Sci* 63(9):951–959.
7. Van der Steen JT, Ooms ME, van der Wal G, Ribbe MW (2002) Pneumonia: the demented patient's best friend? Discomfort after starting or withholding antibiotic treatment. *J Am Geriatr Soc* 57(10):1681–1688.
8. Schneider LS, Dagerman KS, Insel P (2005) Risk of death with atypical antipsychotic drug treatment for dementia: meta-analysis of randomized placebo-controlled tirals. *JAMA* 294(15):1934–1943.
9. Casarett D, Kapo J, Caplan A (2005) Appropriate use of artificial nutrition and hydration— fundamental principles and recommendations. *N Engl J Med* 353(24):2607–2612.

10. Gibson MJ, Houser A. Valuing the invaluable: a new look at the economic value of family caregiving. *Issue Brief (Public Policy Inst (Am Assoc Retired Pers))* 2007 Jun;(IB82):1–12.

Further reading

Brown JA, Von Roenn JH (2004). Symptom management in the older adult. *Clin Geriatr Med.* 20(4):621–640.

Duncan JG, Forbes-Thompson S, Bott MJ (2008). Unmet symptom management needs of nursing home residents with cancer. *Cancer Nurs.* 31(4):265–273.

Evers MM, Meier DE, Morrison RS (2002). Assessing differences in care needs and service utilization in geriatric palliative care patients. *J Pain Symptom Manage* 23(5):424–432.

Meier D, Monias A (2004). Palliative medicine and care of the elderly. In Doyle D, Hanks G, Cherny N, Calman KC (Eds.), *Oxford Textbook of Palliative Medicine*, 3rd ed. Oxford, UK: Oxford University Press, pp. 935–944.

Schwartz CE, Wheeler HB, Hammes B, et al. (2002) Early intervention in planning end-of-life care with ambulatory geriatric patients: results of a pilot trial. *Arch Intern Med* 162(14):1611–1618.

Wijnia JW, Corstiaensen IJ (2008). A poor prognosis: guide or misleading? *Am J Hosp Palliat Care* 25(1):5–8.

Palliative care in end-stage heart failure

Sandra P. Gomez, MD, FAAHPM,
Jaime S. Gomez, MD, FACC, FSCAI

Introduction

The syndrome of heart failure is one of the most common constellation findings encountered in medicine today. It accounts for at least 20% of medical admissions to all hospitals for patients older than 65 years of age. It is, of course, quite prevalent in terminally ill patients not only as a primary diagnosis but also as a complication of other disease processes. It is important to recognize this syndrome and some of its most common causes in order to be an effective palliative care team.

The definition of heart failure can be summed up into a few key concepts: 1) the inability of the heart to deal with the metabolic demands of the body, and 2) the constellation of symptoms associated with this phenomena. In essence, this syndrome has different stages that can roughly be divided into acute decompensation and chronic disease.

The *acute* syndrome of heart failure, better know as congestive heart failure (CHF), is not a specific disease but rather a collection of symptoms, physical findings, and classic laboratory findings that help the clinician develop a differential diagnosis of more specific disease entities.

Very much like a fever, which can help the clinician narrow the differential diagnosis, it is best to think of the phenomena of CHF as a symptom or problem rather than a specific disease process. In contrast, the patient with *chronic* heart failure has some, but certainly not all, of the many characteristic findings of congestive heart failure.

One of the most challenging aspects is diagnosis, as many other diseases can mimic the syndrome.

Epidemiology

Cardiac disease was listed as the most common cause of death in the United States in 2005. With life expectancy hitting a record high in 2006 and Centers for Disease Prevention and Control (CDC) data showing the average life expectancy of white males to be 76 years, black males 70 years, white females 81 years, and black females 76.9 years, it is likely that most of us will develop some sort of cardiac issues before our death.

The physical and psychological symptom burden in patients dying from heart failure is similar to that in those dying from terminal cancer. Table 29.1 illustrates some of the common symptomatology suffered by patients with heart failure.

Fatigue, difficulty ambulating, and edema are other common symptoms that can at times be alleviated with maximal medical management, which should be continued until the burden of administration outweighs the benefits.

Table 29.1 Common symptoms experienced by patients with heart failure and common interventions

Symptom	Affected	Intervention
Pain	78%	Identify etiology, if possible Consider opioids for angina
Dyspnea	61%	Optimize medication Treat reversible causes—effusions, dysrhythmias, COPD
Depression	59%	Screen for hypoactive delirium, screen for chemical coping, CAGE* Consider SSRI, use psychostimulants with caution**
Insomnia	45%	Screen for delirium Screen for depression Treat reversible causes, i.e., pain or dyspnea
Anorexia	43%	Screen for treatable causes—depression, delirium, constipation
Anxiety	30%	Screen for delirium, depression, spiritual, or emotional suffering Consider SSRI
Constipation	37%	Monitor fluid balance Appropriate bowel program when using opioids

* CAGE, Cut back, Annoyed, Guilt, Eye opener.

** The drugs of choice are still the SSRIs because they preserve ejection fraction, lack hypotensive and dysrhythmogenic effects, and have few drug interactions. There are no data documenting the safety of psychostimulants in heart failure, thus they should be initiated with caution.

Medical management

Medical management of CHF has been refined over the past 10 years. The efforts at medical management are to improve the symptoms suffered by those with the disease. In palliative care, all efforts should be made to ensure that patients are receiving evidence-based medical management.

Systolic dysfunction vs. diastolic dysfunction

The causes of heart failure are many, and an exhaustive list is beyond the scope of this chapter. The palliative care team should be aware of the most common types of heart failure.

Roughly, patients should be divided into two groups: those with systolic dysfunction and those with diastolic dysfunction, sometimes referred to a congestive heart failure with normal left ventricular systolic function. The 2D echocardiogram is the most reliable and widely available diagnostic test used for this purpose. Most patients will have this information available before a palliative medicine consult is called.

Patients with predominantly diastolic heart failure are typically less complicated to treat. Most of these patients will have hypertensive heart disease. Treatment for these patients is usually directed at blood pressure management with a variety of agents (i.e., beta-blockers, ACE inhibitors, angiotensin II receptor blockers [ARBs], calcium channel blockers, hydralazine, nitroglycerin [NTG], etc.). However, diuretics are also frequently employed in the management of this syndrome.

In the patient whose pain is being managed, careful review of medications must be done to identify medications that may antagonize the effects of diuretics or affect renal function (e.g., NSAIDs).

Patients with systolic dysfunction usually present a more difficult task to the clinician. While the mainstay of treatment is with similar agents, as with the previous syndrome, symptoms can be significantly more refractory to treatment. These patients tend to have multiorgan failure by the time they are referred to palliative care, so special care must be taken with the use of certain drugs that may exacerbate end-organ damage.

Changing oral diuretics to the intravenous or subcutaneous route can produce symptom relief within minutes. Furosemide is the mainstay of treatment and usually is used in incremental doses until symptoms subside or improve. Significant renal toxicity can result from aggressive use of these agents.

Because of this risk of renal toxicity and, ultimately, failure, patients on opioids, particularly morphine, should be opioid rotated to an agent that is not primarily cleared by the kidneys.

Intravenous inotrope therapy

Agents such as dobutamine, milrinone, and dopamine have a substantial record of use but lack data on their use in the home setting. While these agents may help to improve symptoms, the data show an increased risk of death. Intravenous inotrope therapy may help hospitalized inotrope-dependent heart failure patients be transferred to die at home.

The cost of these agents may be prohibitive to some hospices because of the capitated reimbursement system. They may be more feasible in the home health setting with the addition of hospice once the infusions are stopped.

Device therapies

Cardiac pacemakers in advanced heart failure and at end of life

Patients with congestive heart failure have been known to benefit from biventricular pacemakers for palliating and improving symptoms. This section will focus not on the selection of patients for a pacemaker but rather on the pacer's function at the time of death, indications for deactivation, and other end-of-life issues.

Each year about 600,000 new pacemakers are implanted, and the majority are implanted in patients over the age of 60.

Do pacemakers prolong the dying process?

No. Pacemakers do not prolong the dying process, as they are not resuscitative devices. When the patient is in the active stages of dying, the myocardium is usually too sick to respond to the pacemaker-generated signals.

When is pacer deactivation indicated?

Most patients are not pacer dependent, particularly during the active stages of dying when the most common rhythm is tachycardia. When a pacemaker's role is not meeting the goals of care, a family meeting to discuss expectations on its role should take place with the patient, family, primary medical team, and interdisciplinary team.

Routine deactivation is not recommended, as this can lead to bradycardia, which can produce worsening symptoms of heart failure such as dyspnea and fatigue. Family education should focus on what the pacemaker does *not* do, which is to prolong the dying stage and thus prolong suffering.

If an interdisciplinary discussion leads to the decision to deactivate the pacer, the cardiology team and pacemaker service should be informed of the decision. A patient's right to request withdrawal of life-sustaining medical interventions, including pacemakers, is legal and ethical.

During this time, advance directives and code status should be discussed with the patient and family and documented.

Implantable cardioverter defibrillator (ICD) at the end of life

The purpose of an ICD is to monitor cardiac rhythm and deliver electric cardioversion when ventricular tachycardias are detected. It has been shown that ICD therapy significantly prolongs life in patients at increased risk for sudden death from depressed left ventricular function. However, whether this increased longevity is accompanied by deterioration in the quality of life is unclear.

ICDs can also deliver pacing therapy aimed at increasing heart rate when slow rhythms are detected. The pacing and shocking capabilities of an ICD can be independently turned off.

ICDs and quality of life

In a randomized trial, ICD therapy or amiodarone was compared with state-of-the-art medical therapy alone in 2521 patients who had stable heart failure with depressed left ventricular function. Quality of life was retrospectively measured at baseline and at 3, 12, and 30 months after the ICD was implanted. No clinically or statistically significant differences in physical functioning between the study groups were observed.

Psychological well-being in the ICD group, as compared with medical therapy alone, was significantly improved at 3 months ($P = 0.01$) and at 12 months ($P = 0.003$) but not at 30 months. Additional quality-of-life measures were improved in the ICD group at 3 months, 12 months, or both, but there was no significant difference at 30 months. ICD shocks in the month preceding a scheduled assessment were associated with a decreased quality of life.

The use of amiodarone had no significant effects on the primary quality-of-life outcomes.

Turning off an ICD

Indications

When a patient or family requests the deactivation of an ICD, this is acceptable both legally and ethically. This is done when an ICD is inconsistent with the patient's goals of care, when an antiarrhythmic medication is withdrawn and there is concern of impending arrhythmias, when death is imminent, and/or when the patient and family are concerned about the inconsistencies of having a functioning ICD and a DNR or AND (allow for natural death) directive.

Family and patient discussion

The physician primarily responsible for the ICD and the device company that has been monitoring the ICD should be informed of the patient's decision to deactivate the ICD. This can provide a level of comfort and closure for the patient and family and involve the ICD's primary medical team in the decision-making and goals of care.

At this point it is important to discuss expectations once the ICD is deactivated and to answer any related questions or concerns. With an actively dying patient, families often expect that the patient will expire immediately after the ICD is deactivated. Families should be educated on what to expect; most patients do not expire soon after deactivation. Rather, the disease must continue to follow its normal course.

Deactivation

The cardiologist or electrophysiologist and device company are contacted and arrangements are made for deactivation. Advance directives should be discussed and documented and the patient and family must understand that the goal of deactivation is to allow for natural death.

If a patient and family expect heroics at the time of death, the goals of care must be discussed to clarify the purpose of deactivation of the ICD. It is important to note that most device manufacturers will not send representatives to a patient's home for the purpose of deactivating the device. These issues are best handled before the patient is discharged from the hospital.

Left ventricular assist devices (LVADs)

Many types of LVADs have been developed to assist patients with advanced heart disease. Most devices consist of an axial flow pump that provides a significant amount of blood flow to the body in the setting of severe systolic left ventricular heart failure.

The original intent of these devices was to provide a bridge to transplant; however, with the advent of smaller, easier-to-insert devices, they are now used for a variety of purposes, from destination therapy to ultra-high-risk percutaneous revascularization.

The lack of heart donors and the prolonged survival of heart failure patients have led to applications of LVADs that were not previously expected. Patients previously too sick to undergo revascularization can now be treated effectively with the aid of these devices.

The palliative care team must collaborate closely with the cardiovascular team and be aware of this very dynamic area of medicine.

Mortality after LVAD implantation

Data from 2006 show that 1-year survival after LVAD implantation was 56%. The in-hospital mortality after LVAD surgery was 27%. Main causes of death included sepsis, right heart failure, and multiorgan failure. The most important determinants of in-hospital mortality were poor nutrition, hematological abnormalities, markers of end-organ or right ventricular dysfunction, and lack of inotropic support.

The appropriate selection of candidates and timing of LVAD implantation are critical for improved outcomes of destination therapy.

Quality of life after LVAD implantation

The overall quality of life of patients with LVAD implantation as a destination therapy can be adversely affected in some cases by serious infections, neurological complications, and device malfunction. LVADs alter end-of-life trajectories, and caregivers of recipients may experience significant caregiver burden and financial strain.

Thus, appropriate informed consent is vital.

Ethical challenges with LVADs as destination therapy

Because LVADs can prolong the survival of average recipients over that with optimal medical management of chronic end-stage heart failure, which affects quality of life and increases caregiver burden, it is vital that recipients and their caregivers receive adequate informed consent.

Early use of a palliative care approach is recommended when use of an LVAD as a destination therapy is being considered, as this approach will help make the process a well-informed one.

Recommendations regarding a palliative care approach to LVAD use include but are not limited to the following:

- Participation of a multidisciplinary care team, including palliative care specialists
- A concise plan of care for anticipated device-related complications
- Careful surveillance, counseling, and community support for caregivers, to minimize caregiver burden
- Advance-care planning for anticipated end-of-life trajectories and timing of device deactivation when it no longer benefits or supports the patient's goals of care
- A plan to address the long-term financial burden on patients, families, and caregivers
- Appropriate spiritual and emotional support for recipients as their devices alter end-of-life trajectories

Prognostication

Providing accurate prognostic data for 6- to 12-month morality in heart failure is nearly impossible. Many factors are involved, including the unpredictability of disease trajectory, high risk of sudden death, disparities in the application of evidence-based guidelines, and other issues.

Based on data from the SUPPORT study, Framingham study, and IMPROVEMENT, 1-year mortality estimates are as follows:
- Class II (mild symptoms)   5–10% mortality
- Class III (moderate symptoms) 10–15% mortality
- Class IV (severe symptoms)   30–40% mortality

Other factors associated with a limited prognosis are listed in Table 29.2.

Appropriate referrals to hospice

Given the difficulty in prognosticating the last 6 months of life in heart failure patients, hospice referrals are usually made very late in the course of the illness. The 1996 National Hospice and Palliative Care Organization (NHPCO) criteria are not predictors of a 6- to 12-month mortality. These criteria can, however, serve as guidelines to aid clinicians in identifying the decline of a patient and help hospice staff focus their documentation when recertifying a patient for hospice benefits.

A clinician should simply ask the question, "Would I be surprised if this patient died in the next 6 months?" If the answer is no, the patient would be best served by being referred to hospice. This decision should also involve the cardiovascular specialist because of the complexity of therapies and prognostic trajectories.

NHPCO criteria include the following:
1. Symptoms of recurrent heart failure at rest NYHA class IV
2. Optimal medical management
3. Ejection fraction of <20%
4. Treatment-resistant ventricular or supraventricular arrhythmias
5. History of cardiac arrest in any setting

Table 29.2 Factors associated with a limited prognosis in heart failure

Factor	Effect on prognosis
Recent cardiac hospitalization	Triples 1-year mortality
SBP <100 mmHG and/or pulse >100 bpm	Each doubles 1-year mortality
Hospitalized heart failure patient with acute decompensation	*In-hospital mortality rates*
BUN >43 mg/dL	2% for 0/3 risk factors
Creatinine >2.75 mg/dL	20% for 3/3 risk factors
SBP <115 mmHg	
Anemia	Each 1 g/dL reduction associated with a 16% increase in mortality

6. History of unexplained syncope
7. Cardiogenic brain embolism
8. Concomitant HIV disease

Further reading

Verma A, Solomon SD (2007). Optimizing care of heart failure after acute MI with an aldosterone receptor antagonist. *Curr Heart Fail Rep* 4(4): 183–189.

Mark DB, Anstrom KJ, Su JL, et al. (2008). Quality of life with defibrillator therapy or amiodarone in heart failure. *N Engl J Med* 359(10): 999–1008.

MacIver J, Rao V, Delgado DH (2008). Choices: a study of preferences for end-of-life treatments in patients with advanced heart failure. *J Heart Lung Transplant* 27(9):1002–1007.

Powell LH, Calvin JE Jr, Mendes de Leon CF, et al. (2008). The Heart Failure Adherence and Retention Trial (HART): design and rationale. *Am Heart J* 156(3):452–460.

Holst M, Strömberg A, Lindholm M, Willenheimer R (2008). Description of self-reported fluid intake and its effects on body weight, symptoms, quality of life and physical capacity in patients with stable chronic heart failure. *J Clin Nurs* 17(17):2318–2326.

Rizzieri AG, Verheidje JL, Rady MY, McGregor JL (2008). Ethical challenges with the left ventricular assist device as a destination therapy. *Philos Ethics Humanit Med* 3:20.

Lietz K, Long JW, Kfoury AD, et al. (2007). Outcomes of left ventricular assist device implantation as destination therapy in the post-REMATCH era: implications for patient selection. *Circulation* 116(5):497–505.

Bieniarz MC, Delgado R (2007). The financial burden of destination left ventricular assist device therapy: who and when? *Curr Cardiol Rep* 9(3):194–199.

Harrington MD, Luebke DL, Lewis WR, Aulisio MP, Johnson NJ (2004). Cardiac pacemakers at end of life. Fast Facts and Concepts #111. Retrieved December 28, 2010, from http://www.eperc.mcw.edu/fastfact/ff_111.htm

Harrington MD, Luebke DL, Lewis WR, Aulisio MP, Johnson NJ (2004). Fast Facts #112, Implantable cardioverter defibrillator (ICD) at end of life. Fast Facts and Concepts #112. Retrieved December 28, 2010, from http://www.eperc.mcw.edu/fastfact/ff_112.htm

Reisfield GM, Wilson GR (2005). Fast Facts #143, Prognostication in heart failure. Fast Facts and Concepts #143. Retrieved December 28, 2010, from http://www.eperc.mcw.edu/fastfact/ff_143.htm

Reisfield GM, Wilson GR (2005). Fast Facts # 144, Palliative care issues in heart failure. Fast Facts and Concepts #144. Retrieved December 28, 2010, from http://www.eperc.mcw.edu/fastfact/ff_144.htm

Palliative care in end-stage liver disease

Valentina Medici, MD
Lorenzo Rossaro, MD, FACP
Frederick J. Meyers, MD, MACP

Definition and prevalence

End-stage liver disease (ESLD) is the final result of various pathophysiological disturbances that underlie chronic liver diseases (Table 30.1), including chronic viral hepatitis ([hepatitis B virus [HBV], hepatitis C virus [HCV]), alcohol abuse, and nonalcoholic steatohepatitis.

Cirrhosis is the common histological finding in all of these chronic processes. It can be described as a diffuse process of advanced fibrosis and conversion of the normal liver architecture into abnormal regenerative nodules of hepatocytes.

Portal hypertension is the most common manifestation of ESLD, and as a direct consequence of the increased portal pressure, esophageal and gastric varices, ascites, and peripheral edema develop. Other common complications of ESLD are hepatic encephalopathy, coagulopathy, renal failure, malnutrition, and hepatocellular carcinoma.

Prevalence and mortality

About 5.5 million people (2% of the U.S. population) are affected by cirrhosis, with approximately 26,000 deaths each year, making this condition one of the leading cause of terminal illness among people between 25 and 65 years old.[1]

Twenty thousand patients with advanced ESLD are waiting for liver transplantation in the Unites States. But with the scarcity of donors (about 5000 yearly), most ESLD patients will have no chance of receiving a graft and will need medical management (Table 30.2).

ESLD is characterized by significant physical and emotional suffering. This erosion of quality of life represents a significant challenge to patients with ESLD and their families. These patients should receive intensive palliative care, to a degree that increases as the disease progresses, and should include timely hospice referral.

Table 30.1 Etiologies of chronic liver disease

Chronic hepatitis related to infectious agents	• HCV
	• HBV/HDV
	• HIV-associated hepatobiliary disease
	• Protozoan amoebiasis
	• Malaria
	• Toxoplasmosis
Toxic injury-related liver diseases	• Alcohol
	• Nonalcoholic fatty liver disease and nonalcoholic steatohepatitis
	• Drug-induced liver diseases
Immune system-related diseases	• Autoimmune hepatitis
	• Primary biliary cirrhosis
	• Primary sclerosis cholangitis
Genetic diseases	• Hemochromatosis
	• Wilson disease
	• α_1-Antitrypsin deficiency
Other	• Amyloidosis
	• Budd–Chiari syndrome

Table 30.2 Management of the most common signs and symptoms of end-stage liver disease

Sign/symptom	Treatment	Dose	Note
Ascites	Sodium restriction (2 g/daily)		Increase the diuretics dose once a week, checking electrolytes levels.
	Spironolactone	50–400 mg daily	
	Fursomide	20–150 mg daily	TIPS frequently induces encephalopathy.
	Paracentesis		
	TIPS	if >4 liters with IV albumin	
Spontaneous bacterial peritonitis (SBP)	Cefotaxime	2 g every 8 hours	After SBP resolution with IV antibiotics, prophylactic therapy with norfloxacin 400 mg daily for an indefinite time is recommended. Oral treatment can be considered in inpatients without vomiting, shock, encephalopathy ≥ grade 2, with creatinine <3 mg/dL.
	Albumin	1.5 g/kg of body weight at diagnosis followed by 1 g/kg of body weight on day 3	
	Ofloxacin	400 mg twice daily	
Hyponatriemia	Recommend water restriction when Na⁺ ≤120 mmol/L		Volume expansion with colloid or saline might be recommended. Avoid increasing serum sodium by 12 mmol/L per 24 hours.
Hyperkalemia	Stop spironolactone; start kayexalate		In case of severe hyperkalemia
Hepatic encephalopathy	Lactulose	Titrated to 3–4 bowel movements daily	Protein restriction is recommended only at the onset of severe hepatic encephalopathy.
	Neomycin	4–12 g daily	
	Rifaximin	400 mg three times daily	

Table 30.2 (contd.)

Sign/symptom	Treatment	Dose	Note
Esophageal varices	Beta-blockers:		Beta-blockers can induce fatigue and dizziness. Relative contraindications are peripheral vasculopathy and insulin-dependent diabetes with recurrent hypoglycemia. Nadolol might be associated with less side effects.
	Propranolol	20 mg twice daily	
	Nadolol	40 mg daily	
	Endoscopic variceal ligation		
	TIPS		
Pruritus	Cholestyramine	4 g 3–4 times daily	
	Ursodiol	15–30 mg/kg daily	
	Rifampin	150–300 mg twice daily	
Hepatorenal syndrome	Octreotide	100–200 mg SC three times daily	
	Midodrine	7.5–12.5 mg orally three times daily	
	Albumin 20%	20–40 g IV daily	Maximum of 2 months
	Ornipressin	2–6 IU/h IV 3 days	3 days
	Albumin 20%	20–60 g daily	
	Terlipressin	0.5–2 mg IV every 4 hours	
	Albumin 20%		Maximum of 15 days
	20–40 g IV daily		

TIPS, transjugular intrahepatic portosystemic shunt.

Complications of end-stage liver disease

Ascites

Ascites, or fluid collection in the peritoneal cavity, is the most common complication of ESLD. It is characterized by abdominal distension and often pain and dyspnea. The diagnosis is based on the physical examination or by abdominal ultrasound.

Primary management includes sodium restriction (maximum 2 g/day) and diuretic therapy, with the combination of spironolactone and furosemide achieving the best control of fluid retention and least electrolytes imbalances.

When diuretics are not sufficient, repeated paracentesis may be effective and safe, provided that it is associated with intravenous albumin infusion, 8 g/L removed, during or just after the end of any large volume paracentesis (>4 L).

The control of refractory ascites may also be accomplished using the transjugular intrahepaic portosystemic shunt (TIPS), which is superior to repeated paracentesis in controlling ascites but is complicated by worsening hepatic encephalopathy.[2]

Nevertheless, ascites often becomes refractory to medical management and can be a focus of care at the end of life.

Spontaneous bacterial peritonitis (SBP)

SBP, or ascitic fluid infection, possibly secondary to bacterial translocation from the intestinal lumen, is a common complication of ascites. The diagnosis is made when there is a positive ascitic fluid bacterial culture and/or an elevated ascitic fluid absolute PMN count (i.e., $\geq$250 cells/mm^3) without an evident intra-abdominal source of infection.

IV cefotaxime or a similar third-generation cephalosporin is the first-line treatment for suspected SBP. Normally, the results of the ascitic fluid culture are not required to start the antibiotic treatment. The concomitant administration of intravenous albumin can prevent the development of hepatorenal syndrome and reduce mortality.[2]

Oral ofloxacin has been reported to be as effective as intravenous cefotaxime in patients without vomiting, shock, grade II (or higher) hepatic encephalopathy, or serum creatinine >3 mg/dL.[3]

Electrolytes imbalances

The activation of the renin–angiotensin–aldosteron system is responsible of hyponatremia and hyperkalemia. Most patients with ESLD tolerate relatively well low sodium levels, provided that hyponatremia develops gradually.

The best treatment when the sodium level is below 120 mmol/L is water restriction and temporary cessation of diuretics.

Hepatic encephalopathy

Hepatic encephalopathy, characterized by several neuropsychiatric disturbances from insomnia and tremor to stupor and coma, is very frequent in ESLD.

The preferred treatment is a cathartic, nonabsorbable disaccharide, typically lactulose, which will acidify the luminal contents that promote the formation of ammonia, with consequent increased excretion with the stool. With lactulose intolerance or reduced efficacy, nonabsorbable antibiotics can be used (i.e., neomycin and rifaximin).

Dietary protein restriction is not indicated, except during the onset of severe encephalopathy. It worsens the risk of malnutrition.[4]

Esophageal varices

Various degrees of esophageal varices are a frequent finding in ESLD, being present in about 50% of patients with cirrhosis. Their rupture results in variceal hemorrhage, which is the most lethal complication of portal hypertension.

Variceal hemorrhage occurs at a yearly rate of 5%–15%. The most important predictor of hemorrhage is the size of varices, which is determined by the esophagogastroduodenoscopy (EGD).

Pharmacological therapy consists of nonselective beta-blockers (propranolol and nadolol) and endoscopic therapy, based on variceal banding ligation or sclerotherapy.[5] The combination of pharmacological and endoscopic therapy decreases short-term mortality, but only liver transplant can offer long-term survival.

Pruritus

Pruritus in ESLD is multifactorial. It is more frequently associated with cholestasis, but the use of opioids has also been associated with pruritus. The most common but relatively ineffective treatment is oral antihistamines, which have a nonspecific sedating effect.

Cholestyramine is also used for its effect in preventing bile acid uptake in the terminal ileum, however it can interfere with the absorption of other medications. Other options in patients with ESLD are ursodiol and rifampin.

Hepatorenal syndrome (HRS)

The HRS is the most feared complication of ESLD and is defined as a clinical condition of renal failure that is associated with advanced hepatic failure and portal hypertension. It is characterized by impaired renal function and marked abnormalities in the arterial circulation and in the activity of the endogenous vasoactive systems. The major criteria for the diagnosis of the HRS are as follows:

1. Low glomerular filtration rate (serum creatinine >1.5 mg/dL)
2. Absence of shock, ongoing bacterial infection, current treatment with nephrotoxic drugs, gastrointestinal fluid losses, renal fluid losses >500 g/day
3. Proteinuria <500 mg/dL
4. No ultrasonographic sign of primary renal disease

In the palliative care setting, the administration of agonists of vasopressin receptors (ornipressin and terlipressin) may improve renal function. Octreotide and midodrine (an alpha-adrenergic agonist) has been used with promising results,[6,7] but no controlled randomized trials have ever shown increased survival.

Hepatocellular carcinoma (HCC)

HCC occurs at an estimate rate of 1–6% per year in patients with ESLD. Potentially curative treatments for HCC include surgical resection, radi-ofrequency ablation (RFA), percutaneous ethanol injection (PEI), and liver transplantation (Table 30.3).[8]

The most commonly used criteria for liver transplantation for HCC are the Milan Criteria (Table 30.4).

Palliative treatments for HCC include transarterial chemoemboliza-tion (TACE), which offers palliative benefits for patients with large and/or multifocal HCC without vascular invasion or extrahepatic metastasis, with 1- and 2-year survival rates of 82% and 63%, respectively.[8] This technique is based on the induction of embolization, which causes ischemic tumor necrosis, combined with selective intra-arterial chemotherapy with doxo-rubicin, mitomycin, or cisplatin and a contrast agent, lipiodol.

In the spectrum of the palliative options, promising results have been reported for the use of sorafenib, a small molecular inhibitor of several protein kinases.

Table 30.3 Therapeutic options for hepatocellular carcinoma (HCC) management and their indications

Surgical resection	Best option for patients without cirrhosis. Solitary HCC of the liver, without vascular invasion, no evidence of portal hypertension, and well-preserved hepatic function.
Radiofrequency ablation (RFA)	Best outcomes are in patients with a single tumor <4 cm in diameter. For cirrhotic patients, some clinicians restrict RFA to those with Child–Pugh class A or B.
Percutaneous ethanol injection (PEI)	PEI is often considered for patients with small HCCs who are not candidates for resection because of their poor functional hepatic reserve.
Transarterial chemoembolization (TACE)	Most often used for large unresectable HCCs that are not amenable to other treatments such as resection or RFA; sometimes it is used as a bridging therapy prior to transplant to downstage the tumor.
Liver transplantation	Best option for unresectable patients who meet the Milan criteria (Table 30.4)

Table 30.4 Milan staging criteria for hepatocellular carcinoma

Single tumor	Multiple tumors	
Single tumor maximum diameter	Maximum number	Largest tumor size
≤5 cm	3	≤3 cm

A large multicenter, randomized, placebo-controlled phase III trial studied the efficacy of sorafenib vs. placebo in 602 patients with advanced HCC who had had no prior systemic therapy. The median overall survival was 10.7 vs. 7.9 months ($p = 0.00058$) (sorafenib vs. placebo). The time to symptom progression was significantly longer for sorafenib than for placebo (5.5 vs. 2.8 months; $p = 0.000007$), and the disease control rate was higher in the sorafenib than in the placebo group (43% vs. 32%).[9]

Malnutrition

Weight loss and muscle wasting are very frequent in ESLD and are related to increased metabolic needs as well as reduced caloric intake. Contributing factors are protein loss associated with paracentesis, early satiety and gastroesophageal reflux related to abdominal distention, and gastroparesis.

Timely hospice referral for ESLD patients

Patients with ESLD have significant physical and emotional suffering and are thus excellent candidates for hospice care. Timely referral to hospice service should result in median length of stay on hospice of more than 2 months. While some patients and families may resist acceptance of hospice, most do not. Physician delay in referral is the most common cause of delayed or non-referral.

Hospice provides 24-hour on-call, regular nurse and social worker home visits; provision of needs related to the terminal illness, including medications, durable medical equipment, and volunteer and pastoral services; and bereavement services.

Hospice is associated with the highest rates of patient family satisfaction in most medical systems and not only reduces the cost of care but can also prolong survival. Pre-hospice DNR is not required for admission to hospice for most programs.

A reliable tool to guide hospice referral is the Model of End Stage Liver Disease (MELD) score, which is calculated on the base of three laboratory values: PT-INR, creatinine, and bilirubin, and can be easily calculated using several Web sites (i.e., http://www.unos.org/resources/meldpeldcalculator.asp).[10]

We reported a negative correlation between MELD score and length of hospice stay. That is, as the MELD score increases, the average survival decreases.

The MELD score is a very useful guide to support a clinician recommendation to families for hospice care, achieving one of the national benchmark goals of increasing hospice care duration beyond the current median of 2–3 weeks.[11] A higher MELD score should augment physician judgment regarding hospice referral. We recommend that referral to hospice be introduced when the MELD score reaches 17–20.

The MELD score has been used to guide prioritization for liver transplantation. How does one decide between liver transplantation and hospice in patients with increasing MELD scores?

Hospice care can be an important tool in the liver transplant setting. Patients on the liver transplant list suffer all of the chronic conditions that require close monitoring and continuous support when frequent hospitalizations are not indicated. Conversely, when potential candidates for liver transplantation are not considered for this option because of worsening medical condition and the occurrence of absolute contraindications to the procedure, they can be referred to hospice service.

The potential use of hospice service as a means of integration between palliative care and liver transplantation is described in Figure 30.1.

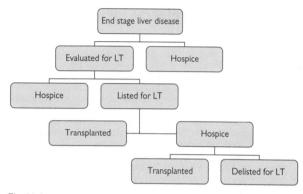

Fig. 30.1 Integration model between hospice care and liver transplant (LT).

Clinical pearls

- Encephalopatic patients should not be protein restricted.
- Na$^+$ restriction is the cornerstone of management of ascites and peripheral edema in ESLD.
- Patients with a previous episode of spontaneous bacterial peritonitis should receive long-term prophylaxis with daily norfloxacin or trimethoprim/sulfamethoxazole.

References

1. Hoyert DL, Kung HC, Smith BL (2005). Deaths: preliminary data for 2003. *Natl Vital Stat Rep* 53:1–48.
2. Runyon BA (2004). Management of adult patients with ascites due to cirrhosis. *Hepatology* 39:841–856.
3. Navasa M, Follo A, Llovet JM, Clemente G, Vargas V, Rimola A, Marco F, Guarner C, Forné M, Planas R, Bañares R, Castells L, Jimenez De Anta MT, Arroyo V, Rodés J (1996). Randomized, comparative study of oral ofloxacin versus intravenous cefotaxime in spontaneous bacterial peritonitis. *Gastroenterology* 111:1011–1017.
4. Blei AT, Córdoba J (2001). Practice Parameters Committee of the American College of Gastroenterology. Hepatic encephalopathy. *Am J Gastroenterol* 96:1968–1976.
5. Garcia-Tsao G, Sanyal AJ, Grace ND, Carey W. (2007) Prevention and management of gastro-esophageal varices and variceal hemorrhage in cirrhosis. *Hepatology* 46:922–938.
6. Kashani A, Landaverde C, Medici V, Rossaro L (2008). Fluid retention in cirrhosis: pathophysiology and management. *QJM* 101:71–85.
7. Angeli P, Volpin R, Gerunda G, Craighero R, Roner P, Merenda R, Amodio P, Sticca A, Caregaro L, Maffei-Faccioli A, Gatta A (1999). Reversal of type 1 hepatorenal syndrome with the administration of midodrine and octreotide. *Hepatology* 29:1690–1697.
8. El-Serag H, Marrearo JA, Rudolph L, Reddy KR (2008). Diagnosis and treatment of hepatocellular carcinoma. *Gastroenterology* 134:1752–1763.
9. Llovet J (2007). Sorafenib improves survival in advanced hepatocellur carcinoma (HCC): results of the phase III randomized placebo-controlled trial (SHARP trial). *J Clin Oncol* 25(18S, June 2 Suppl):LBA1.
10. Kamath PS, Kim WR (2007). Advanced Liver Disease Study Group. The Model for End-stage Liver Disease (MELD). *Hepatology* 45:797–805.
11. Medici V, Rossaro L, Wegelin JA, Kamboj A, Nakai J, Fisher K, Meyers FJ (2008). The utility of the Model for End-stage Liver Disease score: a reliable guide for liver transplant candidacy and, for select patients, simultaneous hospice referral. *Liver Transpl* 14:1100–1106.

Renal palliative care

David Hui, MD, MSc, FRCPC
Sara Davison, MD, MSc, FRCPC

Introduction

Chronic kidney disease (CKD) is defined as either kidney damage or glomerular filtration rate (GFR) <60 mL/min/1.73 m^2 for ≥3 months and may develop as a result of chronic disorders such as diabetes, hypertension, and polycystic kidney disease or from renal injuries such as glomerulonephropathy, tubular necrosis, and interstitial nephritis.

The National Kidney Foundation classifies CKD into five stages (Table 31.1). Stage 5 is also known as end-stage renal disease (ESRD), in which patients require renal replacement therapy in the form of either dialysis or a kidney transplant.

As renal function declines, patients with CKD typically experience significant morbidity and mortality. Given that the annual mortality rate for dialysis patient approaches 25%,[1] early integration of palliative care into renal care is essential. Specifically, palliative care can help to optimize symptom control, facilitate advance care planning, and ease transitions at the end of life.[2,3]

In this chapter, the prognosis, decision-making around the initiation and withdrawal of dialysis, and symptom management for patients with ESRD are discussed.

Clinical pearl

- Patients with stage 5 chronic kidney disease have poor prognosis, with a median survival of 2–3 years. Early involvement of palliative care for symptom control and transition of care is essential.

Table 31.1 National Kidney Foundation classification of CKD

Stage	GFR (mL/min/1.73m^2)*
1	>90, proteinuria
2	60–89
3	30–59
4	15–29
5	<15

*GFR is estimated (eGFR) from serum creatinine (Cr) using the Modification of Diet in Renal Disease Study (MDRD) equation based on age, gender, and race. GFR can also be estimated by creatinine clearance (CrCl) using the Cockroft Gault formula:

CrCl = (140 − age) × (weight in kg)/(72 × serum creatinine in mg/dL) × 0.85 if woman

Reprinted with permission from the National Kidney Foundation.

Prognosis of patients with ESRD

The life expectancy of patients on dialysis is approximately 25% of age-matched individuals without renal disease (Table 31.2).

Factors associated with poor prognosis include the following:

- Advanced age
- Poor nutritional status
- Low serum albumin <3.5 g/dL is associated with 50% 1-year mortality
- Low functional status
- Comorbidity—modified Charlson Comorbidity Index >8 is associated with a 50% 1-year mortality

The ability to accurately estimate prognosis is of great importance to patients, families, and clinicians. As patients progress over the course of their disease, knowing what to expect can give them with a sense of control and facilitate the process of advance care planning.

Patients' projected survival is a key consideration in many medical decisions, such as initiating and withdrawing dialysis, and referral to palliative care and hospice. Chapter 25 provides a general approach to discussing prognosis.

Table 31.2 Unadjusted survival probabilities (%) for patients with incident ESRD[1]

Age	1 year	2 years	3 years	5 years	10 years
40–49	89.6	81.6	73.5	61.9	37.7
50–59	86.2	75.9	65.4	49.5	21.8
60–64	83.0	69.6	58.3	38.1	12.3
65–69	79.1	63.1	50.8	30.7	6.4
70–79	71.2	53.5	39.0	20.2	2.7
80+	60.5	40.8	25.7	9.6	0.9

Incident cohorts include only those patients who survive the first 90 days.

Source: U.S. Renal Data System (2008). USRDS 2008 Annual Report: Atlas of End-Stage Renal Disease in the United States. Bethesda, MD: National Institutes of Health, National Institute of Diabetes and Digestive and Kidney Diseases.

Decision-making regarding dialysis

As patients progress toward ESRD, discussions regarding dialysis should be initiated with the nephrology team. Decision-making for initiation and withdrawal of dialysis is a complicated process, with clinical, psychosocial, ethical, and legal implications.[3]

While dialysis is generally associated with survival and quality-of-life benefits, in a minority of patients (i.e., those with poor prognostic factors), survival benefit may be minimal and dialysis may worsen quality of life. Hemodialysis requires visits to the dialysis unit 3 times per week, whereas peritoneal dialysis necessities multiple exchanges every day.

Patients on dialysis tend to experience multiple, complex symptoms as a result of CKD, comorbidities, or the dialysis treatment itself. These, coupled with frequent clinic visits and investigations, can worsen the already compromised quality of life of patients. Furthermore, potentially life-threatening acute complications such as infections and cardiovascular incidents are common.

Even with dialysis, patients eventually succumb to their disease (as seen in Table 31.2). Thus, patients should be educated on the risks and benefits of dialysis prior to committing to this aggressive intervention.

For patients with acute life-threatening illnesses who develop acute renal failure (with or without pre-existing renal disease), the mortality rate is 50–75%. Dialysis should be decided on a case-by-case basis.

Initiating dialysis

General indications for initiating dialysis in CKD patients include the following:
- Creatinine clearance <15 mL/min/1.73 m^2 in combination with uremic symptoms
- Uremic symptoms: anorexia, nausea, fatigue, restless legs/muscle cramps, paresthesias

Acute indications are as follows:
- Uremic pericarditis or encephalopathy
- Persistent metabolic acidosis, hyperkalemia, or fluid overload despite optimal medical treatment
- Intoxications (ASA, lithium, methanol, digoxin)

It is important to recognize that medical factors represent only a portion of the complex decision-making process regarding dialysis (see Table 31.3). The Renal Physician Association and American Society of Nephrology developed a clinical practice guideline on the initiation of and withdrawal from dialysis[4] and recommends a shared decision-making process between the nephrologists and patient, taking into account the patient's overall prognosis and goals of care.

In patients for whom dialysis affords no tangible benefits and may negatively affect their quality of life, conservative management with palliative care is appropriate. Criteria for withholding dialysis include patient or surrogate wishes, profound neurological impairment, the presence of a nonrenal terminal condition, or a medical condition that precludes the technical process of dialysis.

Table 31.3 Decision-making in initiating dialysis

Prognosis	Patient's interest in dialysis	Recommendations
Good (years)	Yes	Initiate dialysis
Good (years)	No	Dialysis is strongly recommended, although patient holds the right to refuse treatment
Poor (months)	Yes	Consider time-limited dialysis trial of 1 to 3 months to determine benefit, or no dialysis if obvious harm without benefit
Poor (months)	No	No dialysis

Time-limited trials of dialysis may be reasonable when faced with uncertainty about the potential benefits of dialysis.

Withdrawal of dialysis

Once dialysis is initiated, the dialysis team works closely with patients for regular assessments to evaluate the utility of dialysis. It is now a widely accepted practice in most countries to stop dialysis when it is no longer achieving a meaningful goal for the patient.

Approximately 25% of deaths of dialysis patients are preceded by a decision to discontinue dialysis. Failure to thrive, associated with decreased functional status and cachexia, is the most common reason to stop dialysis for patients dying at home. Medical complications are the most common reasons for hospitalized patients.[1]

The palliative care team should work closely with the renal replacement team to provide longitudinal counseling, optimal symptom control, and end-of-life preparations. Once dialysis is stopped, patients have an average survival of 8–10 days.

Hospice is underused by ESRD patients. It is important to note that dialysis patients in the United States are eligible to receive hospice while receiving dialysis if they have a non-ESRD diagnosis that affords them a prognosis of less than 6 months.

In some cases, this may be a "failure to thrive" diagnosis. If a dialysis patient withdraws from dialysis, they are immediately eligible to receive hospice care. Thus, the decision to continue dialysis should not defer hospice referral in the appropriate patient.

Clinical pearl

- The decision to initiate and withhold dialysis should be highly individualized, taking into account patient preference, risks, and benefits, after extensive counseling.

Symptom management for CKD

Patients with ESRD may experience significant symptoms from progressive renal disease, from comorbidities (e.g., diabetes, peripheral vascular disease), or from the dialysis procedure itself:

- Constitutional—fatigue, generalized weakness
- Neurological—decreased memory and concentration, slow and slurred speech, myotonic jerks, seizures, altered smell and taste, peripheral neuropathy, sleep disturbances, restless leg syndrome
- Gastrointestinal—anorexia, nausea and vomiting, gastritis
- Hematological—anemia, platelet dysfunction and bleeding
- Musculoskeletal—bone disorders, arthropathy, muscle cramps
- Dermatological—pruritus, uremic frost, sallow
- Sexual—amenorrhea, sexual dysfunction, infertility

In this section, discussion is focused on pain, fatigue, pruritus, anorexia and sleep disturbances.[5,6] Management of other common symptoms in ESRD patients can be found in Chapter 16 of this Handbook.

Pain

Approximately 50% of dialysis patients experience chronic pain. Common causes include the following:

- Infections—osteomyelitis, cellulitis
- Procedures—dialysis catheter insertion, surgeries
- Peripheral neuropathy—diabetic neuropathy, uremic neuropathy
- Peripheral vascular disease—diabetes, hypertension
- Musculoskeletal—renal osteodystrophy, osteoarthritis, osteoporosis

Calcific uremic arteriolopathy (CUA)

CUA, or "calciphylaxis," a relatively rare but serious disorder seen almost exclusively in ESRD patients, is characterized by tissue ischemia due to metastatic calcification of subcutaneous tissue and small arteries.

Patients develop painful violaceous mottling of the skin that can progress to extremely painful ulcers and eschar formation. Even with aggressive therapy, 60–90% of patients with CUA die from sepsis. This condition may be related to secondary hyperparathyroidism, elevated serum calcium/phosphate levels, and the use of calcitriol.

No definitive treatment regimens are available. However, hyperbaric oxygen may cure the cutaneous ulcers of CUA, and most reports recommend normalization of serum calcium, phosphorous, and parathyroid levels. This often includes cessation of calcitriol and may require surgical parathyroidectomy. Treatment may also include sodium thiosulfate.

Nephrogenic systemic fibrosis (NSF)

NSF is a recently recognized disorder in CKD patients that causes substantial pain and disability characterized by an acute onset of hardening of the skin of the extremities and trunk, nodules with hyperpigmentation, and flexion contractures. Patients typically describe pain and pruritus at the site of the fibrosis. This disorder may be related to gadolinium-containing contrast agents for magnetic resonance imaging.

There is no consistently effective treatment, although physical therapy, steroids, thalidomide, methotrexate, and UVA light therapy have all been tried. Principles of pain management can be found in Chapter X. Optimal use of analgesics in patients with CKD requires a good understanding of the pharmacokinetics of various medications.

Acetaminophen

Acetaminophen is metabolized by the liver and does not require dose adjustment in ESRD. It is considered the non-narcotic of choice for mild to moderate pain in patients with CKD.

A typical dose is 325–650 mg PO q6h PRN.

Nonsteroidal anti-inflammatory drugs (NSAIDs)

NSAIDs may increase the risk of gastrointestinal bleeding in patients with ESRD because of their effects on platelet function, and they have potential cardiovascular risks and may cause loss of residual renal function. For these reasons, NSAIDs should be used for precise indications (e.g., gout) and for a limited time only in patients with ESRD.

Opioids

Methadone and fentanyl are opioids of choice for patients with ESRD.

- Methadone may be safely used in CKD patients, as it is excreted in the stool in ESRD patients. A reasonable starting dose is 5 mg PO bid. Methadone does not appear to be dialyzable and thus does not require supplement post-dialysis.
- Fentanyl is generally considered safe for patients with ESRD. However, up to 10–25% of fentanyl is excreted in urine unchanged, thus dose reduction may be required with ESRD.
- Hydromorphone and oxycodone—the active metabolites of these drugs are primarily renally excreted. Exercise caution when using these opioids in CKD patients, particularly at high doses, with long-term use or if GFR <30 mL/min. The general principle is to start low (~25% dose if CrCl 10–50 mL/min, and 50% dose if CrCl <10 mL/min), titrate slowly, and monitor patients closely for opioid toxicity.
- Morphine—because of reports of toxicity in ESRD it is not recommended for chronic pain management. If monitored carefully, it may still be an appropriate opioid for acute pain management.
- Meperidine is not recommended in CKD patients, as it is associated with significant neurotoxicity and anticholinergic effects.

Gabapentin and pregabalin

These are first-line drugs for management of neuropathic pain, although the maximum dose should be limited to 300 mg/day (given post-hemodialysis).

Tricyclic antidepressants (TCAs)

TCAs are effective in the management of neuropathic pain, but they are poorly tolerated in patients with ESRD because of anticholinergic, histaminergic, and adrenergic side effects resulting in symptoms such as dry mouth, orthostatic hypotension, and somnolence. For these reasons, TCAs are considered second-line therapy for neuropathic pain in ESRD.

If TCAs are to be used, they should be initiated at lower doses, given in divided daily doses, and titrated slowly.

Fatigue

Fatigue is one of the most common symptoms in CKD patients, affecting approximately 80% of patients on dialysis. Causes include rapid osmotic shifts during hemodialysis, dialysis-related hypotension, blood dialysis membrane interaction, carnitine deficiency, electrolytes imbalance, sleep disturbances, malnutrition, anemia, medications, and depression.

Management of fatigue should be focused on treatment of any reversible causes, such as anemia and depression, along with optimization of dialysis with a Kt/V >1.2. The target hemoglobin should be between 10– and 12 g/dL. A higher target (13.5 g/dL) has been shown to be associated with more complications and may result in increased mortality, without improvement in quality of life.

Patients should also be encouraged to exercise regularly, if possible.

Pruritus

Pruritus is one of the most frustrating and challenging conditions for CKD patients and is experienced by up to 60% of ESRD patients. The pathophysiology is not well understood, but may be related to accumulation of calcium-phosphate and/or toxins in the skin, low-grade hypersensitivity reactions to dialysis products, and xerosis.

The key to management of pruritus is to make sure that the patient is receiving an adequate dose of dialysis and is adherent to dietary phosphate restriction and phosphate-binding therapy. For pruritus that occurs during dialysis, switching the dialysis membrane may sometimes help.

Symptomatic management of uremic pruritus includes emollients (ammonium lactate cream), capsaicin 0.025% cream, antihistamines, gabapentin, UVB light therapy, and naltrexone.

Anorexia

Anorexia is common in patients with ESRD and is frequently associated with malnutrition and cachexia. Many factors may contribute to anorexia, including inadequate dialysis, nausea, taste alterations, xerostomia, gastroparesis, pain, constipation, and depression.

In addition to ensuring that an adequate dialysis dose is delivered, a number of strategies may be useful to improve appetite, including antiemetics for nausea; zinc 220 mg PO daily for taste change; artificial saliva every 1–2 hours or pilocarpine 5–10 mg PO tid for dry mouth; metoclopramide 10 mg PO q4h for early satiety; and megestrol acetate 100–400 mg PO daily and dronabinol 2.5–5 mg bid for appetite stimulation.

Further discussions on anorexia–cachexia can be found in Chapter 6.

Sleep disturbances

Patients with CKD commonly report sleeping disturbances, including insomnia, periodic leg movement disorders, restless leg syndrome, and sleep apnea. Insomnia is present in 50–90% of patients and may be related to pain, pruritus, medications, and emotional distress.

Restless leg syndrome occurs in 20–40% of patients and may be associated with uremic neuropathy (inadequate dialysis), iron deficiency, and hypoparathyroidism. It is characterized by a restless sensation that is brought on by rest, particularly at night, and relieved with movements. Treatment options for restless leg syndrome include dopamine agonists (pergolide, pramipexole or ropinirole), gabapentin, clonazepam, and oxycodone if precipitated by pain.

Clinical pearl

• Patients with ESRD often experience a multitude of symptoms related to progressive renal disease, comorbidities, dialysis, and psychosocial issues. Frequent assessments, early intervention, and involvement of the interprofessional team are key to poviding care for these patients.

References

1. The 2008 United States Renal Data System (USRDS) Annual Data Report. Bethesda, MD: National Institutes of Health, National Institute of Diabetes and Digestive and Kidney Diseases. Retrieved January 4, 2009, from http://www.usrds.org/adr.htm
2. Chambers EJ, Germain M, Brown E (Eds.) (2004). *Supportive Care of the Renal Patient*. New York: Oxford University Press.
3. Cohen LM, Moss AH, Weisbord SD, Germain MJ (2006). Renal palliative care. *J Palliat Med* 9:977–992.
4. Moss AH; Renal Physicians Association; American Society of Nephrology Working Group (2000). A new clinical practice guideline on initiation and withdrawal of dialysis that makes explicit the role of palliative medicine. *J Palliat Med* 3:253–260.
5. Moss AH, Holley JL, Davison SN, Dart RA, Germain MJ, Cohen L, Swartz RD (2004). Palliative care. *Am J Kidney Dis* 43:172–173.
6. Davison SN (2003). Pain in hemodialysis patients: prevalence, etiology, severity, and management. *Am J Kidney Dis* 42(6): 1239–1247.

Palliative care in patients with AIDS

Kirsten Wentlandt
Camilla Zimmermann, FRCPC, MD, MSc

Introduction

The human immunodeficiency virus (HIV) is a retrovirus that causes acquired immune deficiency syndrome (AIDS), a syndrome once considered rapidly fatal. Since the introduction of antiretroviral drugs, HIV has become a manageable chronic illness: over 33 million people across the globe are living with HIV, of whom 1.93 million are North Americans.[1]

Effective prevention strategies, earlier diagnosis, and the use of antiretroviral therapy (ART) have all improved survival rates. Despite this, there remain approximately 22,000 AIDS deaths per year in the United States alone.[1]

The purpose of this chapter is to review how clinicians can improve patient care by combining recent disease-specific therapies with palliative care practices.

Clinical course and WHO staging

HIV is transmitted by sexual contact, exposure to contaminated blood products and bodily fluids, or perinatal transmission from mother to child. The acute phase of HIV infection is characterized by a febrile illness, much like a typical flu.

This is followed by an asymptomatic second phase lasting 4–5 years, and then a more chronic symptomatic phase in which patients develop persistent lyphadenopathy and AIDS-defining malignancies.

The final stage is clinical AIDS, defined as a CD4 count <200/µL or occurrence of AIDS-defining conditions.

The World Health Organization (WHO) has developed a clinical staging paradigm for HIV/AIDS, which enables a clinician to stage patients on the basis of clinical features, rather than laboratory values (Table 32.1).

The impact of antiretrovirals on survival has made it difficult to use traditional prognostic indicators. For many patients, mortality results not from end-stage HIV disease but from other comorbidities, such as hepatitis C or B (cirrhosis and liver failure) or HIV-related malignancies.

Overall, the clinical course of HIV/AIDS is fluctuating, with considerable variation among patients, and is marked by a number of opportunistic infections requiring treatment. Specific guidelines have been developed to prevent opportunistic infections, including tuberculosis, *Pneumocystis carinii*, toxoplasmosis, *Mycobacterium avium* complex, and varicella (Table 32.2).

AIDS is defined as a CD4 count <200/µL or occurrence of AIDS-defining conditions.

Table 32.1 Revised WHO clinical staging of HIV/AIDS for adults and adolescents

Primary HIV infection
- Asymptomatic
- Acute retroviral syndrome

Clinical stage 1
- Asymptomatic
- Persistent generalized lymphadenopathy

Clinical stage 2
- Moderate unexplained weight loss
- Recurrent respiratory tract infections
- Herpes zoster
- Angular cheilitis
- Recurrent oral ulcerations
- Papular pruritic eruptions
- Seborrhoeic dermatitis
- Fungal nail infections of fingers

Clinical stage 3
- Severe weight loss (>10% of presumed or measured body weight)
- Unexplained chronic diarrhea for longer than 1 month
- Unexplained persistent fever (intermittent or constant for longer than 1 month)
- Oral candidiasis
- Oral hairy leukoplakia
- Pulmonary tuberculosis (TB) diagnosed in last 2 years
- Severe presumed bacterial infections (e.g., pneumonia, empyema, pyomyositis, bone or joint infection, meningitis, bacteremia)
- Acute necrotizing ulcerative stomatitis, gingivitis, or periodontitis
- Unexplained anemia (<8 g/dL) for >1 month
- Neutropenia (<500/mm^3) >1 month
- Thrombocytopenia (<50,000/mm^3) >1 month

Clinical stage 4
- HIV wasting syndrome
- Pneumocystis pneumonia
- Recurrent severe or radiological bacterial pneumonia
- Chronic herpes simplex infection (>1 month's duration)
- Esophageal candidiasis
- Extrapulmonary TB
- Kaposi's sarcoma
- Central nervous system toxoplasmosis
- HIV encephalopathy

Diagnostic testing is needed to confirm
- Extrapulmonary cryptococcosis
- Disseminated non-tuberculous mycobacteria

Diagnostic testing is necessary to confirm the following:
- Progressive multifocal leukoencephalopathy
- Candida of trachea, bronchi, or lungs
- Cryptosporidiosis or isosporiasis
- Visceral herpes simplex infection
- Cytomegalovirus (CMV) infection
- Any disseminated mycosis
- Recurrent non-typhoidal salmonella
- Lymphoma (cerebral or B-cell non-Hodgkin)
- Invasive cervical carcinoma
- Visceral leishmaniasis

Reprinted with permission from World Health Organization (2005). Interim WHO Clinical Staging of HIV/AIDS and HIV/AIDS Case Definitions for Surveillance: African Region.

Table 32.2 Opportunistic infection prevention and prophylaxis

	Indications for prophylaxis	Prophylaxis
P. carinii pneumonia	CD4 <200	Trimethoprim 160 mg/ sulfamethoxazole 800 mg PO od
Toxoplasmosis	CD4 <100	Trimethoprim 160 mg/ sulfamethoxazole 800 mg PO od
M. avium complex	CD4 <50	Clarithromycin 500 mg PO bid or Azithromycin 1200 mg every week
Tuberculosis	PPD + High-risk exposure	Izoniazid 300 mg PO od + Pyridoxine 50 mg PO od for 6–12 months
Varicella	Exposure with no history	Varicella immune globulin (VZIG) 625 units IM <96 hours post-exposure

From World Health Organization (2007), HIV/AIDS Treatment and Care. Copenhagen: WHO Regional Office for Europe.

Antiretroviral therapy

Antiretroviral therapy (ART) has had a profound effect on the clinical course of HIV/AIDS. Since the introduction of zidovudine in the 1980s, several new classes of HIV medications have been developed that have differing mechanisms of action and are used together to produce durable suppression of HIV. The combinations of these drugs were initially known as highly active antiretroviral therapy (HAART) and are now commonly termed ART.

The introduction of ART has dramatically changed the clinical features of HIV/AIDS. As a result of suppressing the virus, ART is associated with symptom improvement (e.g., reducing weight loss, fatigue, and dementia) and a decrease in opportunistic infections. There has also been a decrease in AIDS-defining malignancies, including Kaposi's sarcoma and cerebral lymphoma.

Unfortunately, ART is plagued by substantial side effects. These result mainly from mitochondrial toxicity, hypersensitivity reactions, and lipodystrophy, which commonly produce anorexia, diarrhea, nausea, vomiting, and pain. Side effects heavily contribute to nonadherence to ART but can be minimized by proper symptom management and palliative care.

There are many potential drug interactions when using ART. Most are related to the liver's cytochrome P-450 system, and many involve medications central to palliative care and pain management (e.g., benzodiazepines, opioids, anticonvulsants, and antidepressants).

Table 32.3 shows a list of potential drug interactions with medications commonly used in palliative care. Methadone levels are decreased by several non-nucleocide reverse transcriptase inhibitors (i.e., nevirapine and efavirenz), requiring dosage adjustments. In some cases, medications may be contraindicated; for instance, midazolam is contraindicated with use of most protease inhibitors.

A useful online resource on HIV drug interactions has been designed by the University of Liverpool and can be found at http://www.hiv-druginteractions.org/.

Potential interactions with antiretroviral therapy should be checked before prescribing medications for symptoms.

Table 32.3 Possible HIV and palliative care drug interactions

HIV medications	Palliative care medication
Protease inhibitor interactions	
Atazanavir, darunavir, fosamprenavir, indinavir, lopinavir, nelfinavir, ritonavir, saquinavir, tipranavir	**Analgesics:** codeine, fentanyl, methadone, morphine, tramadol
	Anticonvulsants: carbamazepine, clonazepam, phenobarbital, phenytoin
	Antidepressants: all classes
	Antipsychotics: chlorpromazine, clozapine, haloperidol, olanzapine, quetiapine
	Anxiolytics: diazepam, flurazepam, zolpidem Contraindicated: midazolam, triazolam
	Gastrointestinal agents contraindicated: cisapride
	Steroids: dexamethasone, prednisone
Non-nucleoside reverse transcriptase inhibitor interactions	
Group 1 Delavirdine, efavrenz, etravirine, nevirapine *Group 2* Abacavir, didanosine, emtricitabine, lamivudine, stavudine, tenofovir, zidovudine	**Analgesics:** codeine, fentanyl, methadone, morphine, tramadol
	Anticonvulsants: carbamazepine, clonazepam, phenobarbital, phenytoin (contraindicated with use of delavirdine and etravirine)
	Antidepressants: bupropirn, citalopram, mirtazapine, sertraline, trazodone, venlafaxine
	Antipsychotics: olanzapine, quetiapine
	Anxiolytics: diazepam, flurazepam, midazolam, triazolam, zolpidem
	Gastrointestinal agents: cisapride
	Steroids: dexamethasone, prednisone
	Analgesics: possible interactions with abacavir and zidovudine with all opioids
Entry and integrase inhibitor interactions	
Maraviroc, raltegravir	**Analgesics:** codeine
	Anticonvulsants: carbamazepine, phenobarbital, phenytoin
	Antidepressants: venlafaxine
	Gastrointestinal agents: antacids, cimetidine, famotidine, omeprazole, pantoprazole, ranitidine

For more details on HIV drug interactions, see the Web site http://www.hiv-druginteractions.org/

HIV-related cancer

Approximately 25% of patients with HIV/AIDS will develop cancer. Kaposi's sarcoma and cerebral non-Hodgkin's lymphoma occur more frequently as the disease progresses and are thought to be directly related to immunosuppression by HIV. Consequently, the introduction of ART has greatly reduced the incidence of these malignancies.

Several other cancers occur with a higher frequency in the HIV population. There is a greater incidence of human papilloma virus (HPV)-associated anal and cervical cancers, but this is likely related to the sexual transmission of both HIV and HPV.[2]

Other non-AIDS-defining malignancies that occur in greater frequency in HIV/AIDS patients include multiple myeloma and cancers of the head and neck, lung, and gastrointestinal tract.

Common symptoms

Patients with HIV/AIDS present with a spectrum of symptoms and medical issues. Symptom management generally follows the same basic principles as those for the oncological population, but in some instances the best treatment may be HIV/AIDS specific. Pain is a good example of this. Pain may be directly related to HIV (e.g., neuropathy, opportunistic infection, HIV-related malignancy), associated with treatment (e.g., procedures, ART, radiotherapy), or related to chronic illness (pressure sores, constipation).

An overview of symptom causes and suggested treatment regimes (for both HIV- and non-HIV-specific causes) is given in Table 32.4.[3]

Most pain syndromes in patients with HIV are neuropathic rather than nociceptive. There is a wide range of common neuropathic syndromes in HIV/AIDS patients, the most common being distal sensory polyneuropathy (DSP). DSP involves the distal lower extremities, especially the plantar aspects of both feet.

Table 32.4 Common symptoms and possible treatments in HIV/AIDS

Symptom	Causes	HIV-related and general treatment options
Fatigue	AIDS Opportunistic infection Anemia Nonspecific	**ART** **Antibiotics** **Transfusion/ erythropoeitin** Corticosteriods, stimulants Dexamethasone 4–16 mg PO/IV od Methylphenidate 2.5–5 mg PO (max daily 60 mg) Testosterone patches
Constipation	Dehydration Malignancy Medications	**Hydration** **Radiation/chemotherapy** Change medications Activity/diet changes Lactulose 15–30 mL PO od/bid Senna 2–4 tabs PO od/bid
Diarrhea	Infections ART Malabsorption	**Antibiotics/ antifungals/ antivirals** **Discontinue** **ART or change regime** Loperamide 4 mg PO, then 2 mg PO after each loose stool (maximum dose 16 mg/day)
Dyspnea	*P carinii* pneumonia Anemia Tuberculosis Pleural effusion	**Trimethoprim 320 mg/sulfamethoxazole 1600mg PO qid** **Transfusion/ erythropoeitin** **TB treatment/antibiotics** Oxygen supplementation, bronchodilators Opioids: morphine 2.5–5 mg PO q4hr

Table 32.4 (Contd.)

Symptom	Causes	HIV-related and general treatment options
Nausea/ Vomiting	Candidiasis CMV HAART Nonspecific	**Antifungals: nystatin susp 4–6 mL qid or Fluconazole 100 mg PO bid** **Antivirals: ganciclovir, acyclovir** **Discontinue ART or change regime** Dopamine antagonists, prokinetics, proton pump inhibitors, serotonin antagonists, somatostatin analogs Haloperidol 1–5 mg PO/IM bid Ondansetron 12–24 mg PO od Dronabinol 2.5–5 mg PO bid/tid
Nociceptive pain Neuropathic pain	Opportunistic infection Malignancy Nonspecific HIVrelated ART CMV Herpes Others	**Antibiotics** **Chemotherapy/ radiation** NSAIDs: naproxsyn 250–375 mg PO q6–8h Corticosteriods: prednisone 20–80 mg PO od **Add ART** **Change ART** **Antivirals: ganciclovir, acyclovir** **Acyclovir 400–800 mg PO tid– 5 times per day** NSAIDS, opioids, cannabis, TCAs, corticosteroids Lamotrigine 25 mg PO bid (max dose 300 mg/day) Nortriptylline 10 mg PO qhs (max dose 75 mg/day) Gabapentin 300–1200 mg PO tid
Weight loss	HIV Opportunistic infection Malignancy Chronic illness	**ART** **Antibiotics** **Chemotherapy/radiation** **Dietary support/elemental and polymeric diet** **Growth hormone 0.1 mg/kg/ SC od** Testosterone patches Megestrol acetate 400–800 mg PO od Prednisone 20–80 mg PO od Dexamethasone 4–16 mg PO od Dronabinol 2.5–5 mg PO bid/tid

Boldface text indicates best evidence available..

Peripheral neuropathies can be similar to DSP and may be caused by several antiretroviral medications, including didanosine, zalcitabine, and stavudine.

Most pain syndromes in patients with HIV are neuropathic rather than nociceptive.

Another notable qualification specific to the HIV population is the increased incidence of opportunistic infections. HIV/AIDS patients are at particular risk for opportunistic infections of the central nervous system, such as cryptococcal meningitis, progressive multifocal leukoencephalopathy, and toxoplasmosis.

These can cause an array of symptoms, including spastic paraplegia or paraparesis, loss of bowel and bladder function, painful muscle spasms, and dementia. The decision process of determining how to treat specific symptoms must be consistent with goals of care and follow the wishes of the patient and family.

Symptomatic complaints in the HIV/AIDS population may be due to HIV, antiretroviral treatments, or chronic illness.

Psychosocial and spiritual issues

The psychosocial context of HIV/AIDS is complex and is critical for palliative care providers to understand. HIV can be associated with a stigma, which may lead to concerns about confidentiality and inadequate care. In addition, AIDS tends to be concentrated in vulnerable populations, including those who are of low socioeconomic status or use intravenous drugs.

Suicidal ideation is relatively common in these patients. In a recent study it was reported more frequently in patients who were not heterosexual, who described elevated symptoms of depression, and who rated HIV-related symptoms and medication side effects as more severe.[4]

Another study showed that patients who strive for spiritual growth in the context of their illness experience less negative affect, highlighting the importance of spiritual care as well as attention to symptoms.[5]

Patients with HIV/AIDS are less likely to have discussed advance directives and do-not-resuscitate (DNR) orders with their physicians than other patient populations. This tendency is increased for those who are non-white, use intravenous drugs, or are less educated.[6]

However, HIV-infected adults and adolescents have expressed a preference to initiate conversations about end-of-life care earlier in the disease process, rather than at a time of acute deterioration.[7] Earlier discussions have also led to increased communication, decreased conflict and stress, and increased consistency with patient preferences.[7]

Patients with HIV/AIDS require a flexible approach to advance care planning, with frequent review of goals of care.

Patients with HIV/AIDS may have different concerns in end-of-life decision-making than those of oncology patients or other populations, and physicians should consider disease-specific issues. These may include the concerns of same-sex partners regarding health power of attorney and survivorship.

In addition, the fluctuating, uncertain course of AIDS requires a flexible, patient, and tolerant approach to advance care planning, with frequent review of the goals of care.[8]

The future outlook for palliative care in HIV/AIDS

HIV/AIDS has evolved from a fatal illness into a complex, chronic disease, driving changes in health policy, health services, and overall resource allocation. Since the introduction of ART, financial support for these treatments has taken priority over other services provided.

As health care systems adjust to this changing milieu, palliative care will need to remain flexible to provide integrated and comprehensive care for a population with diverse needs.

Palliative care remains important for patients with HIV/AIDS across the disease continuum, not only to improve adherence to active treatment but also to further patients' quality of life, address symptom or psychosocial issues, and coordinate end-of-life planning.

References

1. Joint United Nations Programme on HIV/AIDS (2009). 2008 Report on the Global AIDS Epidemic. Geneva: Author.
2. Almonte M, Albero G, Molano M, Carcamo C, Garcia PJ, Perez G (2008). Risk factors for human papillomavirus exposure and co-factors for cervical cancer in Latin America and the Caribbean. *Vaccine* 26(Suppl 11):L16–L36.
3. Selwyn PA (2005). Palliative care for patient with human immunodeficiency virus/acquired immune deficiency syndrome. *J Palliat Med* 8(6):1248–1268.
4. Carrico AW, Johnson MO, Morin SF, Remien RH, Charlebois ED, Steward WT, et al. (2007). Correlates of suicidal ideation among HIV-positive persons. *AIDS* 21(9):1199–1203.
5. Perez JE, Chartier M, Koopman C, Vosvick M, Gore-Felton C, Spiegel D (2009). Spiritual striving, acceptance coping, and depressive symptoms among adults living with HIV/AIDS. *J Health Psychol* 14(1):88–97.
6. Wenger NS, Kanouse DE, Collins RL, Liu H, Schuster MA, Gifford AL, et al. (2001). End-of-life discussions and preferences among persons with HIV. *JAMA* 285(22):2880–2887.
7. Lyon ME, Garvie PA, McCarter R, Briggs L, He J, D'Angelo LJ (2009). Who will speak for me? Improving end-of-life decision-making for adolescents with HIV and their families. *Pediatrics* 123(2):e199–206.
8. Selwyn PA, Forstein M. (2003). Overcoming the false dichotomy of curative vs. palliative care for late-stage HIV/AIDS: "let me live the way I want to live, until I can't". *JAMA* 290(6):806–814.

Palliative care in end-stage neurological disease

Tobias Walbert , MD, PhD, MPH

Introduction

Neurological disorders are among the leading causes of morbidity and death worldwide. While stroke is third leading cause of death, after heart disease and cancer, in the United States, other neurological diseases have a more chronic course that leads to protracted disability, morbidity, and, ultimately, death.

Unfortunately, for many of these disorders, such as Parkinson's disease, amyotrophic lateral sclerosis (ALS), and multiple sclerosis (MS), there is currently no cure available. Adequate symptom management and, later on, palliative care have the potential to maintain good quality of life for patients for as long as possible and ease the burden on caregivers and patients alike.

This chapter outlines the principles of clinical symptom management for some of the most important neurological diseases.

Amyotrophic lateral sclerosis

ALS is a progressive neurodegenerative disorder that results in muscle weakness, disability, respiratory insufficiency, and eventually death. The median survival duration for patients is approximately 3 years, yet 10% will survive for >10 years.

Given its highly predictable course, palliative care and symptom management should begin in the early stages of the disease. Multidisciplinary ALS clinics involving specialized neurologists, physical therapists, occupational therapists, speech therapists, and social workers have resulted in improved quality of life and lengthened survival.

The practice guidelines for treating ALS have been most recently reviewed by the American Academy of Neurology.[1,2]

Muscle weakness

A major symptom in ALS, progressive muscle weakness, should be managed by regular exercise. Physical therapy to the point of exhaustion is considered counterproductive, however. The main focus should be on maintaining mobility and the highest possible degree of independence.

As weakness progresses, passive physiotherapy gains importance in preventing prevent contractures and stiffness. Assistive devices such as canes, ankle–foot orthoses, crutches, and walking frames should be used to maintain patients' mobility.

Dysarthria

Speech impairments affect up to three-quarters of ALS patients and frequently cause major distress for them and their caregivers. For this reason, a speech and language therapist is an important member of the care team and should be involved early after disease onset to continuously evaluate the patient for dysphagia and dysarthria.

Patients should be introduced early to alternative communication devices such as alphabet boards and computer-based systems that can be operated by hand or eye control.

Sialorrhea

Another common symptom in ALS is drooling, which is caused by a combination of facial muscle weakness and a reduced ability to swallow. Sialorrhea has been linked to aspiration pneumonia.

Treatment with anticholinergic agents is generally tried first, but only treatment with botulinum toxin has been shown to be effective in a controlled trial in ALS and parkinsonism.[3]

Pharmacological treatment may include the following:

- Atropine 0.4 mg PO q4h
- Glycopyrrolate 1–2 mg PO twice to three times daily, or 0.1–0.2 mg SC/IM q4–8h
- Botulinum toxin type B, 2500 units into bilateral parotid and submandibular glands
- Transdermal hyoscine (scopolamine) 1–2 patches every 3 days
- Amitriptyline 10–150 mg PO daily at bedtime. The starting dose is 10–25 mg and is increased slowly as needed.

Pseudobulbar affect (emotional lability)

Excessive laughing or crying affects 20–50% of patients with ALS. Emotional lability is caused by bilateral corticobulbar tract degeneration and is not considered to be an emotional disorder per se.

Antidepressant medications have been used in the past, but their effectiveness has not been established. The combination of dextromorphan and quinidine has been shown to decrease rates of emotional outbursts and improve quality of life.[4]

The following treatments are used to ameliorate pseudobulbar affect:
- Dextromorphan/quinidine (30 mg/30 mg) PO twice daily
- Amitriptyline 10–150 mg PO daily at bedtime. The starting dose is 10–25 mg PO and is increased slowly as needed.
- Fluvoxamine 100–200 mg PO daily

Muscle spasticity

Increased muscle tone may be useful to help patients maintain antigravity power as weakness due to ALS progresses. However, spasticity may cause painful spasms. The muscle relaxants baclofen and tizanidine are roughly equivalent in efficacy in reducing muscle spasms and have similar rates of adverse events.

Baclofen can be associated with motor weakness. The side effect of tizanidine of dry mouth might actually help manage sialorrhea (see above).

There is less evidence to support the use of dantrolene to manage spasticity than that for baclofen or tizanidine.[1]
- Baclofen starting at 5–10 mg twice daily to three times daily and increased slowly to doses up to 120 mg/day as needed. Baclofen pumps are usually not considered.
- Tizanidine 2–4 mg PO twice daily up to a total dose of 24 mg daily

Muscle cramps

Muscle spasms or cramps due to ALS can be associated with severe pain and discomfort. The American Academy of Neurology recently evaluated the use of pharmacological agents for muscle cramps in a practice guideline.[5]

Quinine sulfate is considered the most effective treatment option but should not be used routinely because of the potential for toxicity (cardiac arrhythmias, thrombocytopenia, severe hypersensitivity reactions, and potentially serious drug interactions).

Vitamin E, gabapentin, and magnesium have been used frequently but failed to demonstrate efficacy in small clinical trials, whereas the following pharmacological agents have been shown to be beneficial:
- Quinine sulfate 325 mg twice a day
- Calcium channel blocker (such as diltiazem) 30 mg PO daily at night
- Naftidrofuryl, 300 mg PO twice daily; this drug is not available in the United States

Pain

Neuropathic pain is not a characteristic feature of ALS. However, many patients suffer from pain secondary to muscle spasms, cramps, and contractures as well as musculoskeletal pain caused by reduced mobility.

Frequent changes in position are essential to prevent the skin from breaking down. Physical therapy might help to avoid joint stiffness. Other management options include the use of nonopioid analgesics, opioid analgesics, or anti-inflammatory drugs.

Psychosocial symptoms

Most patients with ALS describe depressive symptoms, and approximately 10% are estimated to develop major depression. Both patients and caregivers should be offered counseling, and pharmacological treatment should be considered.

There are no data to suggest that one antidepressant class is more efficacious than another in ALS. However, tricyclic antidepressants (TCAs) such as amitryptiline have side effects that can help alleviate other symptoms of ALS, including drooling, pseudobulbar affect, and insomnia.

Several antidepressant options are available:

- Amitriptyline 10–25 mg by mouth at bedtime, with slow titration to 100 or 150 mg as needed and tolerated
- Sertraline 50–200 mg by mouth daily
- Paroxetine 20 mg daily to 40 mg by mouth daily

Insomnia

Sleep difficulties are mostly secondary to other problems associated with ALS. Causes of insomnia include anxiety, depression, dysphagia, dyspnea, and the inability to change posture, which can result in discomfort and pain. Thus, identification and treatment of the underlying causes is crucial to treating the insomnia.

Sedatives may be helpful; fear of respiratory depression is generally not justified.

Dysphagia

Difficulty swallowing is one of the most common symptoms of ALS, and patients should be screened for symptoms in the office setting at least once every 3 months.[2] Adjusting the consistency of the diet and teaching specific swallowing techniques are helpful in preventing aspiration in the early stages of the disease.

Choking due to food intake or weight loss of 10% or more of body weight should trigger a conversation about the placement of a percutaneous endoscopic gastrostomy (PEG) tube. For optimal safety and efficacy, PEG should be offered when the patient's vital capacity is above 50% of predicted. Studies have shown that PEG tube placement prolongs survival, but there are insufficient data on its impact on quality of life.

Dyspnea

At the onset of respiratory symptoms indicating hypoventilation or when a patient's forced vital capacity (FVC) drops below 50%, the patient should be counseled about noninvasive mechanical ventilation as well as the terminal phase of the disease. Deciding whether and when to initiate noninvasive ventilation is critical because of the risk of sudden death or ventilator dependence.

Besides assessment of vital capacity, nocturnal oximetry and polysomnography are helpful in detecting nocturnal hypoventilation. Patient survival is extended most when ventilation is initiated before vital capacity drops below 50%.

If patients decline noninvasive ventilation or do not tolerate it, options such as invasive ventilation or hospice referral should be discussed at this point.

Terminal phase

As ALS progresses, the goal of patient care should focus on effective and compassionate care rather than maximizing function. Patients who are not ventilated mechanically usually transition from sleep into coma due to increasing hypercapnia.

The following treatment is available if the patient develops dyspnea or becomes restless:

- Morphine 2.5–5 mg PO, SC, or IV every 4 hours as needed for dyspnea
- Lorazepam sublingual (start with 1–2.5 mg) or midazolam PO or SC (start with 1–2 mg) for anxiety

Palliative care in the stroke patient

Stroke is the third leading cause of death in the United States, making the need for hospice care for many victims essential.[6] The severity of the stroke, and thus the need for rehabilitative or palliative care, depends on its location within the brain and the severity of the damage to the brain tissue.

A stroke takes time to manifest its full effect, and some early symptoms might be transitory. The physician might consider a referral to hospice if the patient remains comatose or has a severely reduced level of consciousness (obtundation) with abnormal muscle contraction (myoclonus) for 3 days or longer.

Patients who survive 4 weeks and regain significant function during that time are more likely to need active rehabilitation than palliative care. Although there is almost no literature evaluating the palliative needs of patients with acute stroke, the following problems have been identified.

Dysphagia

Approximately one in three patients presents with swallowing problems immediately after the onset of a stroke. Limited oral intake is linked to malnutrition, poor outcome, and increased mortality. In turn, poor nutritional status may lead to skin breakdown, muscle weakness, and decreased ability to participate in rehabilitation programs.

If swallowing problems continue, nasogastric (NG) or PEG tube placement should be discussed with the patient and the family. Dysphagic stroke patients who receive feeding via a nasogastric tube rather than a PEG tube have better functional outcomes but do not live significantly longer.[7]

The question of whether a patient with a poor prognosis and extensive brain damage should receive artificial nutrition is a very important one and should be discussed openly with the patient's family or power of attorney.

Reduced communication

A stroke patient's ability to communicate might be hindered by aphasias, dysarthrias, or neuropsychological deficits such as agnosia, apraxia, neglect, and reduced visuospatial orientation. Stroke patients with aphasia were found to receive less pain medications than patients without aphasia.[8] Speech pathologists might be able to improve communication and implement coping strategies.

Incontinence and bowel management

Approximately one-third of stroke patients have symptoms of urinary incontinence at the point of discharge, and 20% of these patients are coping with fecal incontinence at the same time.

Incontinence is linked to higher morbidity and mortality in stroke patients. The use of indwelling catheters is associated with higher rates of infection and should be restricted as much as possible. Fecal incontinence can lead to decubitus ulcers and skin damage. Limited mobility and reduced oral intake increase the risk for constipation.

Pain

Pain in stroke patients may be directly related to the intracranial damage or to the results of plegia, such as contractures, pressure sores, or arthralgias caused by immobility.

Especially difficult to treat is the shoulder-hand syndrome. In this complex regional pain syndrome, the paretic upper arm frequently appears painful, edematous, with altered heat and tactile sensations, and has a slightly dystrophic skin. Early mobilization has been shown to prevent shoulder-hand syndrome, which otherwise affects up to 30% with hemiplegia.

Treatment options include nonpharmacological and pharmacological approaches such as psychotherapy, regional anesthesia, neuromodulation, and sympathectomy. Short courses of oral steroids have been shown to be effective in treatment and prevention of the syndrome.

Approximately 10% of patients suffer from central post-stroke pain, which is a neuropathic pain syndrome characterized by unilateral pain and dysesthesia associated with impaired sensation. The pain is thought to be due to a lesion in the thalamus and is typically resistant to opioids.

Amitriptyline is the most effective tricyclic antidepressant for central pain, but lamotrigen can be used instead. When tricyclic medications and lamotrigen are contraindicated or poorly tolerated, gabapentin or pregabalin are reasonable choices.[9]

Palliative care in demyelinating disease (multiple sclerosis)

Multiple sclerosis (MS) is the most frequent inflammatory demyelinating disorder of the central nervous system. While its exact cause is unknown, the clinical picture reflects the pathological mechanism of inflammation, demyelination, and axon degeneration.

Although new immunomodulatory therapy is able to slow disease progression, symptom management and palliative care remain important in the later stages of the disease.

The severity of MS can be divided into benign and malignant courses. *Benign MS* refers to disease in which the patient remains fully functional in all neurological systems 15 years after the disease onset. In *malignant MS*, patients display rapid disease progression leading to significant neurological disability or death in a relatively short time. However, death due to MS is rare and is most likely to occur as a result of secondary complications such as aspiration pneumonia or pulmonary embolus.

Particularly after the onset of the chronic progressive phase of the disease, symptom management with the goal of improving or maintaining function and quality of life is paramount.[10]

Muscle spasticity

Between 40% and 85% of patients with MS experience spasticity, which is associated with pain, bowel dysfunction, and bladder dysfunction.

The mainstay of therapy is regular physical therapy to maintain strength and movement and to decrease spasticity. Physical therapy should be used in combination with drug therapy.

Available medications are only partially effective and can cause adverse effects such as sedation, weakness, and cognitive problems. Therefore, antispastic medication should be started at low doses and slowly titrated against the clinical effect.

- Baclofen: 5–25 mg 3–4x daily PO (an intrathecal pump should be considered in severe cases)
- Tizanidine: 2–39 mg daily PO (titrated over 2–4 weeks; takes approximately 1 week to reach its full effect)
- Gabapentin: 600–900 mg three times daily PO
- Dantrolene: 25–200 mg twice daily PO

Fatigue

Fatigue has been reported for most patients with MS and is associated with high levels of disability. Underlying depression causing fatigue should be ruled out first.

Because fatigue can be greatly worsened by heat, cooling of the body or the extremities may alleviate the symptom. Stimulants appear to have only limited and short-term efficacy. A small study comparing aspirin to placebo showed some success.[10]

Medical options include the following:

- Modafinil 200–400 mg daily PO

- Amantadine 100 mg twice daily PO (second dose taken in the afternoon to avoid insomnia)
- Methylphenidate 10–60 mg/day taken bid or tid
- Aspirin 1300 mg daily PO

Bladder dysfunction

Bladder dysfunction develops in almost all MS patients, and bladder hyper-reflexia affects approximately 60% of patients. The latter condition results in a sense of urgency, urge incontinence, and frequent micturition.

Assessment of the urinary system is important to improve these systems and to prevent urinary tract infections and skin breakdown secondary to urinary incontinence.

Behavioral intervention in the early stages of MS include planning adequate fluid intake, with more intake in the morning than in the afternoon, and use of the bathroom every 2–4 hours.

Pharmacological management is described in Table 33.1.

Pain

Pain is a frequent symptom in MS, affecting 50–75% of patients. Pain can present as directly MS-related neuropathic pain or as secondary to MS symptoms, such as spasticity or paresis. Neuropathic pain often affects the lower extremities. Trigeminal neuralgia is seen in 1% of patients with MS and is clinically indistinguishable from the idiopathic form.

The initial treatment for both forms is carbamazepine (Table 33.2). Tricyclic antidepressants can be used to treat neuropathic pain, but they have to be started at low doses because their side effects might increase other symptoms in MS patients, such as fatigue.

Other medical options involve the use of anticonvulsants.

Table 33.1 Pharmacological management of bladder dysfunction in patients with MS

Indication	Medication	Dosage	Side effects
Detrusor hyperreflexia (overactive bladder)	Tolterodine (anticholinergic)	1–2 mg IR bid PO or 2–4 mg ER daily PO	Dryness, drowsiness (fewer side effects than with oxybutnin)
	Oxybutinin (anticholinergic)	2.5mg qd–tid PO (titration up to 20mg/day)	Dryness, drowsiness
Urinary frequency	Imipramine (alpha- agonist and anticholinergic activity)	10–25mg bid–tid PO	Sedation, dizziness
Nocturia	Desmopressin (antidiuretic hormone)	0.2–0.4 mcg nasal spray qhs	Hyponatremia

Table 33.2 Pharmacological pain management for patients with MS

Indication	Medication	Dosage	Side effects
Trigeminal neuralgia	Carbamazepine	100–200 mg bid, increased to 600–800 mg daily as tolerated	Drowsiness, dizziness, nausea and vomiting
Neuropathic pain	Nortriptyline, desipramine (tricyclic antidepressants)	10–25mg qhs, increased by 10–25 mg every 3–7 days as tolerated	Sedation, cognitive impairment
	Buproprion	100 mg bid, increased after 3 days to maximum of 150 mg/ dose and 450 mg/day	Dry mouth, dizziness

Psychobehavioral symptoms and depression

Progressive MS requires patients to constantly adjust to new symptoms and limitations. The lifetime rate of depression in MS patient reaches 40–50% by age 59 and is thought to be related to cerebral pathology and treatment with steroids.[11]

Initial reports linking disease-modifying therapy with interferon-beta to depression have not been confirmed in later studies.

Antidepressants should be selected on the basis of their side-effect profiles. Selective serotonin reuptake inhibitors (SSRIs) cause less fatigue, but tricyclic antidepressants might be more helpful in managing neuropathic pain or overactive bladder.

Denial and cognitive decline are frequently seen in the late stages of MS. Pathological laughing and crying is observed in 10% of patients, who might respond to amitryptiline. Cognitive deficits are detected in approximately half of patients, and 10% of patients with late-stage disease have moderate to severe dementia.

Management consists of cognitive training and teaching of compensatory strategies. Personality and cognitive changes can cause major distress for families and caregivers and require education and psychosocial intervention.

Palliative care in Parkinson's disease

Parkinson's disease (PD) is a chronic, progressive neurodegenerative disease defined by the classic triad of tremor, rigor, and akinesis. Patients are more likely to have idiopathic PD than an atypical or secondary parkinsonian syndrome when they present with unilateral onset, have resting tremors, and respond well to L-dopa.

In addition to the classic features, patients with PD may develop symptoms related to the disease itself or to the medications used to treat it.

Medical therapy involves a multispecialist team and good pharmacological knowledge to ensure maximal symptom control[12] (Table 33.3).

Psychosis and hallucination

Psychosis is frequently seen in PD and is closely associated with visual hallucinations and delusions. Hallucinations occur especially in the advanced stages of the disease and affect up to 40% of patients.

Because these symptoms are often drug induced, the first step should include the critical reassessment of potentially offending antiparkinsonian drugs. Hallucinations can be often ameliorated by a dose reduction with limited loss of the drug-related benefit.

Antiparkinsonian drugs should be reduced or stopped in reverse order of their potency and effectiveness if hallucinations are causing significant disability. A proposed order would be anticholinergic drugs followed by amantadine, catechol-O-methyl transferase (COMT) inhibitors, and finally dopamine agonists.

Antipsychotic therapy with clozapine and quetiapine has limited effect on parkinsonism and is preferred over other atypical neuroleptics, such as risperidone and olanzapine. Typical neuroleptics, such as haloperidol, should be avoided. Clozapine is effective but is underused because of its side effect of agranulocytosis.

Table 33.3 Typical non-motor symptoms and signs of Parkinson's disease

Symptom	Sign
Cognitive dysfunction	Dementia, confusion
Mood disorders	Depression, anxiety, apathy, or abulia
Autonomic dysfunction	Urinary urgency or frequency, constipation, orthostasis, erectile dysfunction
Pain and sensory disturbances	Secondary to dystonia, dyskinisia
Psychosis	Hallucinations, delirium
Sleep disturbances	Sleep interruption, PLMS, RBD
Fatigue	
Dermatological findings	Seborrhea

The patient's absolute neutrophil count must be closely monitored. Olanzapine is not effective and might even worsen patients' motor function.

Cognitive dysfunction and dementia

Cognitive dysfunction is common in PD, and severe dementia is a major cause of disability and mortality in patients with PD. As with other dementias, the treatment is symptomatic only and does not appear to modify the course of the disease or influence the prognosis.

The cholinesterase inhibitors donepezil and rivastigmine have modest benefit, but the latter especially can cause worsening of tremors.[12]

Depression

Approximately 40% of PD patients experience depression. Depressive symptoms are linked to increased motor disability and decreased quality of life. The tricyclic antidepressants amitriptyline and nortriptyline have been found to be effective in patients with PD; however, adverse events are thought to be lower with SSRIs.

Citalopram, sertraline, and controlled-release paroxetine do not appear to be effective in PD patients, according to results from small studies.

Adverse events are thought to be lower with SSRIs than with tricyclic antidepressants, but SSRIs should be avoided if a patient is also being treated with selegiline, a monoamine oxidase B inhibitor. This combination has been reported to exacerbate motor symptoms and to cause serotonin syndrome with severely disturbed mental, motor, and autonomic function.

Sleep disorders

Most patients with PD suffer from sleep disorders, most commonly sleep fragmentation. Frequent awakening throughout the night and early-morning awakening is often caused by nocturia, difficulty turning over in bed, cramps, vivid dreams or nightmares, and neck or back pain.

A specific sleep disorder associated with PD is periodic limb movement disorder (PLMS). PLMS is estimated to occur in 30–80% of patients with PD. This sleep disorder involves slow, rhythmic leg movements consisting of dorsal flexion of the feet and great toes and, occasionally, the knees and hips. PLMS responds to dopaminergic agents.

Another sleep disorder associated with PD is rapid eye movement (REM) sleep behavior disorder (RBD). Patients with RBD present with vigorous movements during REM sleep. Because of a lack of movement inhibition during REM sleep, they act out their dreams and present with vocalizations as well as kicking and punching motions of the limbs, sometimes injuring themselves or their bed partners.

Over one-third of patients that originally present with idiopathic RBD may eventually develop PD. Additional L-dopa or clonazepam are the agents of choice for treating RBD. Clonazepam (0.5 mg PO qhs, to be increased to 1–2 mg) is effective for nearly 90% of patients.

Clinical pearls

- Most chronic neurological disorders such as ALS, end-stage Parkinson's disease, and secondary progressive MS have a predictable course of progression. Start the conversation about palliative measures early and remain involved.
- The management of neurological disorders is a team effort. Reach out early and involve other providers as needed.
- The central nervous system is complex and full of interactions. Many symptoms, especially fatigue, can be caused by medication side effects. Therefore, set treatment priorities together with the patient and check the medication list—sometimes less is more.
- Use medications' side effects to the patient's advantage. Many medications influencing the central nervous system have several effects that might be useful treating more than one symptom. For example, amitryptiline might have a positive impact on the patient's mood and at the same time decrease drooling.
- Almost all patients with chronic neurological disorders have psychobehavioral symptoms or show signs of depression. Screen for these disorders frequently and treat proactively.

References

1. Miller RG, Jackson CE, Kasarskis EJ, et al. (2009). Practice parameter update: the care of the patient with amyotrophic lateral sclerosis: multidisciplinary care, symptom management, and cognitive/behavioral impairment (an evidence-based review): report of the Quality Standards Subcommittee of the American Academy of Neurology. *Neurology* 73:1227–1233.
2. Miller RG, Jackson CE, Kasarskis EJ, et al. (2009). Practice parameter update: the care of the patient with amyotrophic lateral sclerosis: drug, nutritional, and respiratory therapies (an evidence-based review): report of the Quality Standards Subcommittee of the American Academy of Neurology. *Neurology* 73:1218–1226.
3. Molloy L (2007). Treatment of sialorrhoea in patients with Parkinson's disease: best current evidence. *Curr Opin Neurol* 20:493–498.
4. Brooks BR, Thisted RA, Appel SH, et al. (2004). Treatment of pseudobulbar affect in ALS with dextromethorphan/quinidine: a randomized trial. *Neurology* 63:1364–1370.
5. Katzberg HD, Khan AH, So YT (2010). Assessment: symptomatic treatment for muscle cramps (an evidence-based review): report of the Therapeutics and Technology Assessment Subcommittee of the American Academy of Neurology. *Neurology* 74:691–696.
6. Stevens T, Payne SA, Burton C, Addington-Hall J, Jones A (2007). Palliative care in stroke: a critical review of the literature. *Palliat Med* 21:323–331.
7. Dennis M, Lewis S, Cranswick G, Forbes J (2006). FOOD: a multicentre randomised trial evaluating feeding policies in patients admitted to hospital with a recent stroke. *Health Technol Assess* 10:iii–iv, ix–x, 1–120.
8. Kehayia E, Korner-Bitensky N, Singer F, et al. (1997). Differences in pain medication use in stroke patients with aphasia and without aphasia. *Stroke* 28:1867–1870.
9. Frese A, Husstedt IW, Ringelstein EB, Evers S (2006). Pharmacologic treatment of central post-stroke pain. *Clin J Pain* 22:252–260.
10. Crayton HJ, Rossman HS (2006). Managing the symptoms of multiple sclerosis: a multimodal approach. *Clin Ther* 28:445–460.
11. Sadovnick AD, Remick RA, Allen J, et al. (1996). Depression and multiple sclerosis. *Neurology* 46:628–32.
12. Miyasaki JM, Shannon K, Voon V, et al. (2006). Practice parameter: evaluation and treatment of depression, psychosis, and dementia in Parkinson disease (an evidence-based review): report of the Quality Standards Subcommittee of the American Academy of Neurology. *Neurology* 66:996–1002.

Palliative care in end-stage chronic obstructive pulmonary disease

Ana Leech , MD
Sriram Yennurajalingam, MD

Introduction

Patients with end-stage chronic obstructive pulmonary disease (COPD) experience high symptom burden arising from severe dyspnea, fatigue, anxiety, depression, disability, and social isolation, resulting in poor quality of life. The caregiving burden for the family of a patient with end-stage COPD is significant. In this chapter, we discuss the key issues in assessing and managing end-stage COPD.

COPD, which affects 6% of the general population, is one of the leading causes of morbidity and mortality worldwide.[1] The incidence of COPD is increasing; it is estimated that COPD will become the third-leading cause of mortality and the fifth-leading cause of morbidity by 2020.[1]

Prognostic factors

Clinical evaluation

According to the National Hospice and Palliative Care Organization, patients who meet any of the following criteria may be suspected of having end-stage COPD:

1. Disabling dyspnea at rest
2. Poor or no response to bronchodilators
3. A bed-to-chair existence
4. Repeated emergency room visits or hospitalizations for respiratory infection or failure
5. Hypoxemia at rest (partial pressure of oxygen <55 mmHg)
6. Oxygen saturation <88% while receiving supplemental oxygen)
7. Hypercapnia (partial pressure of carbon dioxide >50 mmHg)
8. Cor pulmonale
9. Right heart failure secondary to pulmonary disease
10. Unintentional progressive weight loss (>10% over 6 months, serum albumin level <2.5 g/dL)
11. Resting tachycardia (heart rate > 100 beats/minute)

The BODE index is used to determine the severity of disease in COPD patients.[2] Please refer to Table 34.1 for details of the BODE index.

Mortality

In general, it is difficult to predict mortality in patients with long-standing COPD, but the higher the BODE index the higher the likelihood of death (see Table 34.2). Ultimately, patient satisfaction and quality of life are key factors to guiding decision-making.

Table 34.1 Variables and point values used for the computation of the body mass index, degree of airflow obstruction, degree of dyspnea, and exercise capacity (BODE) index

| Variable | Points on BODE index | | | |
	0	1	2	3
FEV_1 (% of predicted)	≥65	50–64	36–49	≤35
Distance walked in 6 min (m)	>350	250–349	150–249	≤149
MMRC dyspnea scale	0–1	2	3	4
BMI	>21	≤21		

Abbreviations: BMI, body mass index; FEV_1, forced expiratory volume in 1 second; MMRC, modified Medical Research Council.

Reprinted with permission from Celli BR, Cote CG, Marin JM, et al. (2004). The body-mass index, airflow obstruction, dyspnea, and exercise capacity index in chronic obstructive pulmonary disease. *N Engl J Med* 350(10):1005–1012. Copyright © 2004 Massachusetts Medical Society. All rights reserved.

Table 34.2 Interpretation of body mass index, degree of airflow obstruction, degree of dyspnea, and exercise capacity (BODE) index scores

BODE index score	1-year mortality (%)	2-year mortality (%)	3-year mortality (%)
0–2	2	6	19
3–4	2	8	32
5–6	2	14	40
7–10	5	31	80

Reprinted with permission from Celli BR, Cote CG, Marin JM, et al. (2004). The body-mass index, airflow obstruction, dyspnea, and exercise capacity index in chronic obstructive pulmonary disease. *N Engl J Med* 350(10):1005–1012. Copyright © 2004 Massachusetts Medical Society. All rights reserved.

Additionally, patients with Global Initiative for Chronic Obstructive Lung Disease stages III or IV COPD have a much higher death rate (42.9 deaths per 1000 person years) than that of healthy individuals (5.4 deaths per 1000 person years; hazard ratio = 5.7).[1]

Morbidity

Patients with end-stage COPD may have to endure symptoms long term. Given the difficulty of predicting mortality in end-stage COPD, morbidity and symptom management is of prime importance.

For acute exacerbations, usual management includes antibiotics, steroids, and bilevel positive airway pressure (BiPAP) use. Almost 25% of COPD patients die within 1 year of hospitalization for an acute exacerbation. The median survival for COPD patients who have had an acute exacerbation after intensive care unit (ICU) admission is 2 years, with a 50% likelihood of further hospitalization within 6 months.[1]

Circulatory effects

COPD patients have a high risk of developing circulatory compromise that affects other organ systems. The risks of atherosclerosis and mortality are increased in COPD patients who smoke.[1]

Nutrition

In patients with advanced COPD, the increased work required to breathe increases energy expenditure and may lead to cachexia. General health status can be further compromised by a lack of exercise due to low exercise tolerance and dyspnea.

COPD patients who have a normal weight or are underweight have a significantly higher risk of death than patients who are overweight or obese.[1]

Palliative care

Assessment

A pulmonologist, intensivist, primary care physician, or palliative care physician should direct palliative care in COPD patients according to the guidelines of the American Thoracic Society or Canadian Thoracic Society. Patients should have access to an interdisciplinary palliative care team.

Comprehensive assessment involves accurately predicting the trajectory of functional decline to provide patients with early access to specialized palliative care services; performing detailed symptom assessment using validated symptom assessment tools such as the Edmonton Symptom Assessment Scale on a routine and consistent basis; screening patients for anxiety, depression, and spiritual or social distress; assessing caregiver burden in family members; evaluating patients for dyspnea (see Chapter 14) and managing it as appropriate in a palliative care setting with the goal of improving quality of life; and performing individualized diagnostic evaluations focused on determining the underlying cause of COPD and providing care accordingly.

End-of-life decision-making

Initiating end-of-life care planning should occur soon after the patient has been diagnosed with end-stage COPD. Discussions about a patient's preferences for end-of-life care should include the patient, the patient's primary health care provider, and the patient's caregivers. Patients should be given information about the potential benefits and burdens of therapy.

Other important decisions may involve the patient's preferences regarding resuscitation, intubation, mechanical ventilation, surrogate decision makers, and advance directives, which should be discussed while the patient's health is stable.[1,3,4]

Psychosocial, spiritual, and family distress

Although 37% of patients with advanced COPD are depressed, only 30% of these patients receive treatment for depression. Patients with end-stage COPD may benefit from antidepressive therapy if they have significant depressive symptoms.[1,3]

Because COPD also affects quality of life, the patient's ability to perform activities of daily living independently or without dyspnea should be addressed.

Barriers to providing palliative care

Several issues complicate or prevent the delivery of appropriate palliative care to COPD patients.

Inadequate communication between health care providers, patients, and families regarding end-of-life care, especially early in the course of the disease, can impede the delivery of appropriate palliative care.

For example, when asking oxygen-dependent COPD patients about their avoidance of discussing end-of-life care, Curtis et al.[3] found that more than 50% of patients provided responses such as "I'd rather concentrate on staying alive than talk about death" and "I'm not sure which physician will be taking care of me if I get very sick." Recent studies[4] have underscored the need for clinicians to be able to communicate openly with their COPD patients regarding end-of-life decisions and comprehensive symptom management.

Predicting the disease course in COPD patients can be challenging because of the disease's variable trajectory, thus patients with end-stage COPD often do not receive adequate palliative care services.[3]

Various tools such as the BODE index, Hansen–Flaschen criteria, and Acute Physiology and Chronic Health Evaluation IV scores can be used to predict increased mortality in COPD patients who require ICU admissions. Inadequate assessment and management of severe symptoms related to end-stage COPD can also complicate the delivery of palliative care.[1,3]

Communication

Discussions about end-of-life care can be difficult but are important aspects of the care provided to terminally ill patients and their families. Approximately 56% of terminally ill COPD patients want to know their life expectancy.

In addition, many patients with end-stage COPD report wanting to discuss the following topics with their physician:
• Diagnosis and disease progression
• Effect of treatments on symptoms, quality of life, and life expectancy
• Prognosis for survival and quality of life
• Aspects of the dying process, specifically issues regarding breathlessness or suffocation)
• Advanced planning for foreseeable medical needs and end-of-life care[3–5]

Management

Individualized treatment should be provided for patients with end-stage COPD. The underlying cause of COPD should be determined and care provided accordingly. COPD patients should be evaluated for dyspnea and cared for as appropriate in a palliative care setting with the goal of improving quality of life.

Although only smoking cessation and long-term oxygen therapy (LTOT) have been shown to improve survival in COPD patients, other interventions may be beneficial in improving the quality of life of patients with end-stage COPD.[1,5]

Pharmaceutical interventions

Pharmaceutical interventions for COPD are presented in Table 34.3. Inhaled corticosteroids have been shown to decrease mortality from all causes in COPD patients. The combination of long-acting agonists and steroids may provide a survival benefit, but this has not been tested in patients with end-stage COPD. Because they are an independent risk factor for death, oral corticosteroids should be limited to the short-term treatment of acute exacerbations in COPD patients.[1]

LTOT has been shown to prolong survival in severly hypoxemic patients (partial pressure of oxygen in arterial blood [PaO_2] <55 mmHg).[6] Moderately hypoxemic patients with pulmonary hypertension, cor pulmonale, and/or secondary polycythemia may also benefit from LTOT. In COPD patients with mild hypoxemia (PaO2 >59 mmHg), the prescription of oxygen may improve quality of life and relieve dyspnea but should be determined on an individual basis.[1]

The sensation of dyspnea can be an incapacitating and distressing symptom in end-stage COPD.[1] The use of opioid medications in the relief of dyspnea is discussed further in Chapter 14.

Nonpharmaceutical interventions

Patients with end-stage COPD may remain self-sufficient but have limitations in activities of daily living and quality of life. The use of non-pharmaceutical therapies has been shown to be effective in controlling the symptoms present in this group of patients.[7]

Nocturnal noninvasive ventilation assistance in conjunction with LTOT and daytime exercise training improves dyspnea and quality of life in COPD patients. However, larger studies are needed to identify the patients who would most benefit from this approach.[7]

Regular exercise decreases the likelihood of hospitalization and mortality in COPD patients; in particular, whole-body strengthening exercises are helpful in successfully weaning patients off chronic ventilation.[7]

Neuromuscular electrical low-voltage stimulation has been shown to increase muscular oxidative capacity in COPD patients and can be used to treat debilitated patients.[7]

Poor caloric intake and high-energy requirements often lead to malnutrition in COPD patients. COPD patients with a body mass index (BMI) <20 have lower survival and higher hospitalization rates than COPD patients

Table 34.3 Pharmaceutical interventions for COPD

Drug class	Initial dose	Indication	Caveats	Interactions	Common side effects
Short-acting β-agonists (levalbuterol)	MDI: 45 mcg/puff, 2 puffs every 4–6 hours PRN	Bronchospasm		Furosemide, haloperidol, methadone, duloxetine, moxifloxacin	Dizziness, dry mouth, nervousness
Long-acting β-agonists (salmeterol)	INH: 50 mcg every 12 hours	Bronchospasm, maintenance	Do not use for acute treatment	Carvedilol, flucanazole	Headache, sinus congestion, nervousness
Short-acting anticholinergics (ipratropium)	NEB: 500 mcg every 6– 8 hours	Bronchospasm	NEB: May mix with short-acting β-agonists	Tiotropium bromide	Cough, dry mouth, headache, nausea, nervousness
Long-acting anticholinergics (tiotropium)	INH: 1 18-mcg capsule every 24 hours	Bronchospasm, maintenance	Do not use for acute treatment; must use dosing device	Metoclopramide	Blurred vision, dry mouth, GI intolerance

Methylxanthine (theophylline)	300–400 mg/day for 3 days, then 400–600 mg/day	Bronchospasm, maintenance	Must monitor blood levels; care with reduced clearance	Tramadol, metoprolol	Temporary changes in behavior, increased urination
Inhaled glucocorticosteroids (budesonide)	180 mcg/puff, 1–2 puffs bid	Bronchospasm, maintenance	Titrate to lowest effective dose; taper to discontinuation		
Systemic glucocorticosteroids (prednisone)	60 mg/day for 7–10 days	Acute exacerbation	Short-term use only	Furosemide, fluoroquinolones	Difficulty sleeping, increased appetite, nervousness
Antibiotics	Patient- and agent-dependent	Infection	Use only for infection in acute exacerbation	Varies	Varies
Oxygen	Titrate to 90% saturation	Hypoxemia	Must demonstrate need		

Abbreviations: GI, gastrointestinal; INH, inhaler; MDI, measured-dose inhaler; NEB, nebulizer; PRN, according to circumstances.

with a BMI >20. All COPD patients should undergo a thorough nutritional assessment and be cared for accordingly.[7]

Bullectomy in patients with a bulla that is compressing functional lung tissue, and lung volume reduction surgery in patients with upper lobe disease may improve quality of life and exercise capacity.[7] However, given the frailty of patients with limited life expectancy, the risks and benefits of surgery must be weighed carefully.[7]

Summary

Palliative care in COPD patients should focus on relieving dyspnea and optimizing quality of life. LTOT and inhaled corticosteroids have shown benefit in COPD patients. Attempts should be made to improve endurance and nutritional status.

Clinical pearls

• Early and extensive communication regarding end-stage COPD and its implication for quality of life between the patient and family and the health-care provider is critical.
• Discussions about end-of-life care preferences should be initiated after a patient recovers from acute exacerbation.
• Assess the perceived effect that COPD has on the patient's quality of life.

References

1. Ambrosino, N, Simonds, A (2007). The clinical management in extremely severe COPD. *Respir Med* 101:1613–1624.
2. Celli BR, Cote CG, Marin JM, et al. (2004). The body-mass index, airflow obstruction, dyspnea, and exercise capacity index in chronic obstructive pulmonary disease. *N Engl J Med* 350(10):1005–1012.
3. Curtis JR (2008). Palliative and end-of-life care for patients with severe COPD. *Eur Respir J* Sep;32(3):796–803.
4. Goodridge DM, Marciniuk DD, Brooks D, et al. (2009). End-of-life care for persons with advanced chronic obstructive pulmonary disease: report of a national interdisciplinary consensus meeting. *Can Respir J* 16(5):e51–e53.
5. Reinke LF, Engelberg RA, Shannon SE, et al. (2008). Transitions regarding palliative and end-of-life care in severe chronic obstructive pulmonary disease or advanced cancer: themes identified by patients, families and clinicians. *J Palliat Med* 11(4):601–609.
6. Cranston JM, Crockett AJ, Moss JR, Alpers JH (2005). Domiciliary oxygen for chronic obstructive pulmonary disease. *Cochrane Database Syst Rev* 2005;4:CD001744.
7. **Clini EM, Ambrosino N (2008). Nonpharmacological treatment and relief of symptoms in COPD.** *Eur Respir J* 32:218–228.

Further reading

Global Initiative for Chronic Obstructive Lung Disease (2009). The Global Strategy for Diagnosis, Management and Prevention of COPD. Available at www.goldcopd.org
Lexi-Comp, Inc. http://online.lexi.com/crlsql/servlet/crlonline. Accessed May 2010.
Uronis HE, Currow DC, McRory DC, et al. (2008). Oxygen for relief of dyspnoea in mildly or non-hypoxaemic patients with cancer: a systematic review and meta-analysis. *Br J Cancer* 98(2):294.

Palliative care in the intensive care unit (ICU)

Rony Dev, DO

Overview

The aim of palliative care is to prevent unnecessary suffering experienced by patients facing an incurable illness. Patients admitted to the intensive care unit (ICU) often experience a high symptom burden secondary to their underlying disease and face the risk of dying. Painful invasive procedures and medical treatments not consistent with a patient's goals of care can add additional suffering for ICU patients.

In the United States, one in five deaths occurs in ICUs, which accounts for greater than 500,000 deaths annually.[1] Roughly, 5–30% of patients die while hospitalized in an ICU, which would indicate a need for integrating palliative medicine with critical care.

The goal of relieving suffering in patients with complex illnesses can coexist with the curative treatment offered in an ICU. Often, it is difficult to distinguish between critical illness and terminal illness. Offering palliative care only at the time of withholding or withdrawing treatment may diminish the benefits of physical and psychosocial support that could be provided for ICU patients and their families. When critically ill patients are not responsive to curative treatment, the goal of comforting patients could and should always be continued.

In addition to assisting with symptom management in an ICU, palliative care providers can also assess and comfort family members whose loved ones are critically ill. By taking the time to listen to the concerns of family members and answer their questions, distress in family members can be assessed and interventions offered. After a patient has died, interventions to lessen the burden of bereavement should be initiated.

Communication and end-of-life discussions

Open and regular communication is essential for adequate palliation. For critically ill patients and their families, information regarding findings, medications, and expected changes may need to be repeated several times by health-care professionals. In general, the use of graphs, question prompt lists, and recordings of consults can increase recall and satisfaction with information.

In the ICU setting, written materials including information leaflets have been shown to improve communication between health-care providers and patients. However, patient and family satisfaction depends on their understanding, which may be limited.[2]

Family conferences can facilitate communication with patients and their caregivers. Results of prospective cohort trials in the ICU setting have shown that end-of-life family conferences are associated with improvement in family satisfaction, reduction in length of stay, and increased access to palliative care without an increase in mortality.[3]

Family members rate communication skills equal to or more important than a physician's clinical skills. Studies of communication have revealed the importance of the following: assurance of non-abandonment by health-care providers, honoring patients' requests to be kept comfortable, and the health-care team's support of decisions made by families regarding treatment preferences.[4]

In addition, listening, acknowledging emotions, and explaining surrogated decision-making have been rated by families as critical to their satisfaction when their loved one is hospitalized.[5]

The VALUE mnemonic (Table 35.1) has been developed as a checklist to verify that adequate support in an end-of-life conference is provided for families of ICU patients. Survey responses from family members of 126 ICU patients in France who were randomized to receive either usual care or a communication-based intervention based on the VALUE strategy resulted in significantly decreased anxiety and depression.[3]

In addition, family members who were surveyed 3 months after the patients had died showed decreased post-traumatic stress disorder.[3]

A summary of recommendations for optimal negotiation of the goals of care is provided in Table 35.2.

Table 35.1 VALUE mnemonic

V	Value family statements
A	Acknowledge family emotions
L	Listen to the family
U	Understand the patient as a person
E	Elicit family questions

Adapted from Lautrette A, Darmon M, Megarbane B, et al. (2007). A communication strategy and brochure for relatives of patients dying in the ICU. *N Engl J Med* 356(5):469–478.

Table 35.2 Protocol to negotiate goals of care

Recommendations include the following:

• Create the proper setting.
• Clarify what the patient and family already know.
• Explore the hopes and expectations of the patient and family.
• Suggest realistic goals.
• Use empathic responses.
• Make a plan and follow through with it.

Adapted from the Education on Palliative and End-of-life Care Project.

Interdisciplinary team collaboration

In addition to effective communication with patients and their families, communication provided by and within the interdisciplinary team of clinicians, nurses, respiratory therapists, pharmacists, social workers, and spiritual care support staff needs to be clear and consistent. Mixed messages by ICU clinicians were associated with increased anxiety and depression in family members.[6]

Observational research in the ICU setting has shown that increased interdisciplinary collaboration results in decreased ICU mortality, shorter length of stay in an ICU, lower rates of ICU readmission, and minimized stress in the workplace, for nurses in particular.[7]

Do not resuscitate (DNR) orders

A DNR order is often implemented for patients with an advanced illness. It reflects a patient's preference for end-of-life care. A DNR order in place for critically ill patients is not to be confused with a patient's preference about other life-sustaining treatments, such as the administration of antibiotics, transfusion of blood products, and artificial nutrition or hydration. The establishing of goals of care consistent with patient preferences is critical for providing palliation at the end of life.

DNR orders are often not elicited by health-care professionals. Reasons for clinicians not writing a DNR order include the belief that patients are not in imminent danger of dying, the belief that the primary care physician should be responsible for obtaining the DNR, and the lack of opportunity, or reimbursement for the time, to discuss end-of-life issues.[8] In addition, fear of litigation, discomfort, and lack of training for discussing end-of-life issues can result in avoidance of writing a DNR order.

Withdrawing mechanical ventilation

The withdrawing of mechanical ventilation can cause symptom distress in patients and stress on their family. Prior to withdrawal, appropriate communication with family members is critical to ensure that discontinuation of ventilation is in the best interest of the patient's overall well-being and is consistent with their goals of care.

The patient and family should be given reassurance that discontinuation of mechanical ventilation will be supervised by a qualified clinician and that any subsequent discomfort after withdrawal will be aggressively treated.

One protocol that has been studied[9] enables an ICU team to withdraw life-supporting mechanical ventilation in a way that minimizes unnecessary suffering (Fig. 35.1). Incorporation of the protocol resulted in increased opioid and benzodiazepines use without an impact on the time to death.[9]

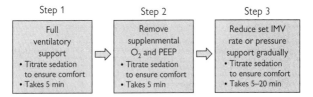

Fig. 35.1 Protocol for withdrawing mechanical ventilation. IMV, intermittent mandatory ventilation; PEEP, positive end expiratory pressure.
Adapted from Treece PD, Engelberg RA, Crowley L, et al. (2004) Evaluation of a standardized order form for the withdrawal of life support in the intensive care unit. *Crit Care Med* 32(5):1141–1148.

Symptom distress in ICU patients

Patients hospitalized in an ICU may experience an increased symptom burden that can go undetected if not appropriately assessed. Both physical and psychological symptoms can be identified by careful and thorough symptom assessment.

In one study of 50 communicating patients hospitalized in an ICU, patients expressed a high level of distress, including symptoms of pain, thirst, insomnia, anxiety, depression, hunger, and dyspnea.[10]

In a recent retrospective review of 88 palliative medicine consults (6% of 1383 ICU admissions), interventions recommend included opioid adjustment (99%), initiation of steroids (70%), withdrawal of mechanical ventilation or bilevel positive airway pressure (BIPAP), discontinuation of total parental nutrition, addition of antiemetics and antipsycotics, and discontinuation of benzodiazepines or other sedating medications. After the consultation, patients reported improved levels of pain, dyspnea, anxiety, and delirium.[11]

Symptom assessment scales for the ICU patient

In order to provide effective analgesia with minimal side effects, daily bedside symptom assessments should be incorporated into routine practice. In the ICU, patients' pain is often not assessed adequately, and when it is assessed, assessment tools are infrequently used.[12]

When patients are able to communicate, their subjective rating of discomfort should be used too titrate medications to control symptoms. Studies show that when nurses assess pain, 35–55% underrate the intensity of a patient's pain level. When assessing symptoms in patients able to communicate, a numeric pain scale between 0 and 10, a visual analog scale, or patient questionnaires may be used.

Symptom assessment can be complicated by the fact that many ICU patients are not able to communicate, since they are either intubated or too sedated. Examples of symptom assessment scales for noncommunicative patients include patient comfort, FLACC (face, legs, activity, cry, consolability), the Critical Care Pain Observation Tool (CPOT), and the Behavior Pain Scale (BPS) (facial expression, movement of upper limbs, and compliance with mechanical ventilation) (Table 35.3).[13]

In noncommunicative patients, both the BPS and CPOT have been validated and shown to be reliable; however, no scale has been incorporated as the standard pain assessment tool in the ICU setting. In one study of 230 ICU patients, incorporation of the BPS resulted in a decreased rate of severe pain as well as decrease in the duration patients were placed on mechanical ventilation.[14]

Table 35.3 Behavioral Pain Scale

Item	Description	Score
Facial expression	Relaxed	1
	Partially tightened (brow lowering)	2
	Fully tightened (eyelid closing)	3
	Grimacing	4
Upper limbs	No movement	1
	Partially bent	2
	Fully bent with finger flexion	3
	Permanently retracted	4
Compliance	Tolerating movement with ventilation	1
	Coughing but tolerating (most of the time)	2
	Fighting ventilator	3
	Unable to control ventilation	4

Scores from each of the three domains are summed, with a total score of 3 to 12.

Pain secondary to invasive procedures

In addition to the symptom burden secondary to an underlying disease, critically ill patients may undergo invasive procedures that may be painful. ICU patients often experience a high level of discomfort during endo-tracheal tube placement and suctioning, arterial and central line placement, and arterial blood sampling.

A strategy of premedicating patients prior to painful procedures should be used to diminish patient discomfort.

Sedation assessment

The provision of adequate pain control can be complicated by excessive sedation in critically ill patients. A balance between pain control and excessive sedation must be attained such that sedation should be tolerated only when its benefits outweigh the risks.

To attain a balance beneficial to patients, clinicians need to make frequent assessment of symptoms, carefully adjust opioids and sedatives while monitoring for side effects, and communicate with all members of the health-care team, with careful attention to the bedside symptom assessment made by ICU nurses.

Examples of sedation scales that have been used in the ICU include the Ramsay Sedation Scale (Table 35.4), Richmond Agitation–Sedation Scale (Table 35.5), Motor Activity Assessment Scale, Vancouver Interactive and Calmness Scale, Adaptation to Intensive Environment, Minnesota Sedation Assessment Tool, and the Confusion Assessment Method (CAM).[13]

Benzodiazepines and propofol are commonly used sedatives in the ICU setting. Benzodiazepine use, however, has been shown to be a risk factor for delirium for ICU patients, and recent studies support a reduction in reliance on benzodiazepines as a sedative.[15] The use of validated sedation scales and interruption of continuous sedation[16] with close monitoring of adverse events have shown improved clinical outcomes in ongoing clinical trials.

The sedative dexmedetomidine, an alpha-2-receptor agonist, promises to be an effective sedative for ICU patients without being associated with an increased risk for delirium,[15] but further research is needed.

Table 35.4 Ramsay sedation scale

Score	Definition
1	Anxious and agitated or restless or both
2	Cooperative, oriented, and tranquil
3	Responds to commands only
4	Brisk response to a light glabellar tap or loud auditory stimulus
5	Sluggish response to a light glabellar tap or loud auditory stimulus
6	No response to a light glabellar tap or loud auditory stimulus

Performed using a series of steps: observation of behavior (score 1 or 2), followed (if necessary) by assessment of response to voice (score 3), followed (if necessary) by assessment of response to loud auditory stimulus or light glabellar tap (score 4 to 6).

Table 35.5 Richmond Agitation–Sedation Scale

Score	Term	Description
+4	Combative	Overtly combative or violent, immediate danger to staff
+3	Very agitated	Pulls on or removes tube(s) or catheter(s) or exhibits aggressive behavior toward staff
+2	Agitated	Frequent nonpurposeful movement, patient–ventilator dyssynchrony
+1	Restless	Anxious or apprehensive but movements not aggressive or vigorous
0	Alert and calm	
−1	Drowsy	Not fully alert, but has sustained (>10 seconds) awakening, with eye contact, to voice
−2	Light sedation	Briefly (<10 seconds) awakens, with eye contact, to voice
−3	Moderate sedation	Any movement (but no eye contact) to voice
−4	Deep sedation	No response to voice, but any movement to physical stimulation
−5	Unarousable	No response to voice or physical stimulation

Performed using a series of steps: observation of behaviors (score +4 to 0), followed (if necessary) by assessment of response to voice (score −1 to −3), followed (if necessary) by assessment of response to physical stimulation such as shaking shoulder and then rubbing sternum if there is no response to shaking shoulder (score −4 to −5).

Reprinted with permission from Sessler, et al. (2002). The Richmond Agitation–Sedation Scale. *Am J Respir Crit Care Med* 166(10):1338–1344.

Delirium

Delirium, defined as a disturbance of consciousness and cognition that fluctuates over time and develops acutely (hours to days), is often unrecognized by ICU health-care providers. Prevalence of delirium in the ICU varies from 20% to 80% (see Table 35.6 for risk factors).[17] Delirium is associated with poor outcomes, including removal of Foley catheters, self-extubation, prolonged hospital stay, and even increased mortality.

Preliminary data confirming the increased risk of long-term cognitive impairment in delirious patients who survived ICU hospitalization have been brought to the attention of clinicians; however, more research is needed.

Analgesic and sedative medications are used to treat pain and anxiety in patients placed on mechanical ventilation; however, these medications have the potential to increase the likelihood of delirium.

Studies examining benzodiazepines have consistently shown an associated increased likelihood of delirium in ICU patients; however, data regarding opioids as a risk factor for delirium are less consistent. One study discovered higher opioid doses among ICU patients without delirium than with delirium.[18] Patients treated with meperidine were found to have an increased risk.

Providing adequate analgesia for ICU patients with close monitoring for signs and symptoms of delirium is warranted. Validated tools to screen for delirium in the ICU include the Intensive Care Delirium Screening Checklist (ICDSC) (Table 35.7).[19] and the Confusion Assessment Method for the ICU (CAM-ICU).[20]

Table 35.6 Risk factors for delirium in ICU patients

Host factors	Factors of critical illness	Iatrogenic factors
Age (older)	Acidosis	Immobilization
Alcoholism	Anemia	Medications (e.g., benzodiazepines)
APOE4 polymorphism	Fever, infection, sepsis	Sleep disturbances
Cognitive impairment	Hypotension	
Depression	Metabolic disturbances	
Hypertension	Respiratory disease	
Smoking	High severity of illness	
Vision/hearing impairment		

Risk factors associated with delirium in both intensive care unit (ICU) and non-ICU studies. APOE4, apolipoprotein E4.[18]

Table 35.7 The Intensive Care Delirium Screening Checklist

Checklist item	Description
Altered level of consciousness*	
A	No response
B	Response to intense and repeated stimulation
C	Response to mild or moderate stimulation
D	Normal wakefulness
E	Exaggerated response to normal stimulation
Inattentiveness	Difficulty following instructions or easily distracted
Disorientation	To time, place, or person
Hallucination-delusion-psychosis	Clinical manifestation or suggestive behavior
Psychomotor agitation or retardation	Agitation requiring the use of drugs or restraints, or slowing
Inappropriate speech or mood	Related to events or situation, or incoherent speech
Sleep–wake cycle disturbance	Sleeping <4 hours/day, waking at night, sleeping all day
Symptom fluctuation	Symptoms listed above occurring intermittently
Total score	0 to 8

* If A or B, then no other items are assessed that day.[20]

A paucity of research exists on the prevention and treatment of delirium in ICU patients. Nonpharmacological strategies in non-ICU patients include frequent reorientation, restoration of normal sleep–wake cycles, early mobilization, removal of catheters, and minimizing unnecessary visual and auditory stimuli. These are often recommend for ICU patients but are not well studied.

Specific to the ICU setting, correction of electrolyte abnormalities, treatment of underlying infections, correction of hypoxia and hypercapnia, treatment of hypoglycemia, and cautious use of opioids and sedatives are all critical to reducing the incidence of delirium.

Haloperidol is the initial recommended drug to treat delirium, resulting in a reduction of hallucinations, episodes of agitation, and unstructured thought patterns.[21] From clinical experience, the therapeutic dose of haloperidol ranges between 4 and 20 mg/daily.

Atypical antipsychotics may also be effective for the treatment of delirium; however, no placebo-controlled trials of either haloperidol or atypical antipsychotics have been conducted to help guide clinicians in the management of delirium in the ICU.

Benzodiazepines are often used to treat delirium tremens but are not recommended for treatment of delirium secondary to being a potential precipitating factor.

Conclusion

Critical care physicians and palliative care providers share a common goal of decreasing the suffering experienced by critically ill patients in the ICU and that of their family members. With careful assessment of a patient's symptom distress and aggressive medical management with both a curative intent and the goal of patient comfort, the ICU team can provide the best possible care for patients and their families.

By integrating palliative care into the intensive care setting, improving symptom management, and providing clear and timely communication with patients and their families, health-care providers can improve the overall care provided for ICU patients (see Table 35.8).

Table 35.8 Checklist for palliative care in the ICU

- Goals of care for the patient and/or family are addressed.
- Treatment is consistent with the patient's goals of care.
- Sedation assessment is done.
- Delirium screening is done.
- Symptom assessment is done.
- Pain and symptoms are adequately treated.
- Communication with the patient and/or family is carried out by the ICU team.
- Emotional and spiritual support is offered to the patient and/or family.

Clinical pearls

- Clear and timely communication with ICU patients and their families is essential for palliation.
- Excessive sedation can result in increased morbidity and mortality in ICU patients.
- Mixed messages by the healthcare team can result in increased family distress.
- Delirium is often missed in ICU patients.

References

1. Angus DC, Barnato AE, Linde-Zwirble WT, et al. (2004). Use of intensive care at the end-of-life in the United States: an epidemiologic study. *Crit Care Med* 32(3):638–643.
2. Azoulay E, Pochard F, Chevret S, et al. (2002). Impact of a family information leaflet on effectiveness of information provided to family members of intensive care unit patients: a multicenter, prospective, randomized, controlled trial. *Am J Respir Crit Care Med* 165(4):438–432.
3. Lautrette A, Darmon M, Megarbane B, et al. (2007). A communication strategy and brochure for relatives of patients dying in the ICU. *N Engl J Med* 356(5):469–478.
4. Stapleton RD, Engelberg RA, Wenrich MD, et. al. (2006). Clinician statements and family satisfaction with family conferences in the intensive care unit. *Crit Care Med* 34(6):1679–1685.
5. Curtis JR, Engelber RA, Wenrich MD, et. al. (2005). Missed opportunities during family conferences about end-of-life care in the intensive care unit. *Am J Respir Crit Care Med* 171(4):844–849.
6. Pochard F, Azoulay E, Chevret S, et al. (2001). Symptoms of anxiety and depression in family members of intensive care unit patients: ethical hypothesis regarding decision-making capacity. *Crit Care Med* 29(10):1893–1897.
7. Curtis JR, Shannon SE (2006). Transcending the silos: toward an interdisciplinary approach to end-of-life care in the ICU. *Intensive Care Med* 32(1):15–17.
8. Eliasson AH, Parker JM, Shorr AF, et. al. (1999). Impediments to writing do-not-resuscitate orders. *Arch Intern Med* 159(18):2213–2217.
9. Treece PD, Engelberg RA, Crowley L, et al. (2004). Evaluation of a standardized order form for the withdrawal of life support in the intensive care unit. *Crit Care Med* 32(5):1141–1148.
10. Nelson JE, Meier DE, Oei EJ, et. al. (2001). Self-reported experience of critically ill cancer patients receiving intensive care. *Crit Care Med* 29(2):277–282.
11. Delgado-Guay MO, Parsons HA, Li Z, et al. (2008). Symptom distress, interventions, and outcomes of intensive care unit cancer patients referred to a palliative care consult team. *Cancer* 115(2):437–445.
12. Gelinas C, Fortier M, Viens C, et al. (2004). Pain assessment and management in critically ill intubated patients: a retrospective study. *Am J Crit Care* 13:126–135.
13. Sessler CN, Grap MJ, Ramsay MA (2008). Evaluating and monitoring analgesia and sedation in the intensive care unit. *Crit Care* 12(Suppl3):S2.
14. Chanques G, Jaber S, Barbotte E, et. al. (2006). Impact of systematic evaluation of pain and agitation in an intensive care unit. *Crit Care Med* 34(6):1691–1699.
15. Pandharipande PP, Pun BT, Herr DL, et al. (2007). Effect of sedation with dexmedetomidine vs. lorazepam on acute brain dysfunction in mechanically ventilated patients: the MENDS randomized controlled trial. *JAMA* 298(22):2644–2653.
16. Kress JP, Pohlman AS, O'Connor MF, et al. (2000). Daily interruption of continuous sedative infusions in critically ill patients undergoing mechanical ventilation. *N Engl J Med* 342(20):1471–1477.
17. Girard TD, Pandharipande PP, Ely EW. (2008). Delirium in the intensive care unit. *Crit Care* 12,(Suppl 3):S3.
18. Ouimet S, Kavanagh BP, Gottfried SB, et al. (2007). Incidence, risk factors and consequences of ICU delirium. *Intensive Care Med* 33(1):66–73.
19. Bergeron N, Dubois MJ, Dumont M, et al. (2001). Intensive Care Delirium Screening Checklist: evaluation of a new screening tool. *Intensive Care Med* 27(5):859–864.
20. Ely EW, Inouye SK, Bernard GR, et al. (2001). Delirium in mechanically ventilated patients: validity and reliability of the confusion assessment method for the intensive care unit. (CAM-ICU). *JAMA* 286(21):2703–2710.
21. Jacobi J, Fraser GL, Coursin DB, et al. (2002). Clinical practice guidelines for the sustained use of sedatives and analgesics in the critically ill adult. *Crit Care Med* 30(1):119–141.

Research in terminally ill patients

Sriram Yennurajalingam, MD
Eduardo Bruera, MD

Introduction

Palliative care is an approach that aims to improve the quality of life of patients facing the problems associated with life-threatening illness. Generally, palliative care provides prevention and relief of suffering by means of early identification and assessment and control of symptoms (physical and psychological).

However, palliative care also relies on proper decision-making; good communication; addressing of family, caregiver, and spiritual issues; and a support system to help the family cope during the patient's illness and in their own bereavement.[1] These areas require a solid body of knowledge, which in turn depends on good research.

This chapter summarizes practical issues and gives a brief overview of the conducting of palliative care clinical trials.

Challenges in conducting palliative care research

Research in the palliative care clinical setting is greatly needed to address gaps in knowledge. Such research would help clinicians develop appropriate measures for assessing the symptoms and unmet needs of patients with life-limiting illness and those of their families; determine active and effective treatments; and determine efficient use of resources for patients with terminal illness.

Unfortunately, research in palliative care is limited and challenging, owing to the severity of patients' illnesses, the presence of coexisting symptoms, polypharmacy, and other logistical factors inherent to treating palliative care patients (see Box 36.1).

Conducting clinical research on patients receiving palliative care presents many challenges, including the following:

1. Patients at various stages of the disease trajectory have comorbidities that tend to confound the outcomes for a given research question tested, especially during the last months, weeks, or days of life.
2. It may be ethically challenging to investigate the effectiveness of treatment when suffering worsens.
3. Even when a patient or family member agrees to participation in a clinical trial, attrition occurs because of disease progression, transfer of the patient to a different facility, loss of patient or family interest, or the patient's death.

These factors affect not only sample homogeneity but also the sample size and the ability of the investigator to complete the clinical trial in a timely manner. Other challenges in clinical trial research include the small number of palliative care researchers and limited funding.

Box 36.1 Challenges in conducting palliative care research

- *Severity of illness:* unstable patient population (owing to unstable disease and general medical condition); limited patient and family participation (due to lack of interest or time, logistics, or perception of increased burden as a result of participation; concerns about or aversions to randomization); may result in attrition or slow accrual
- *Heterogeneous* (confounding variables): patients having various comorbidities; polypharmacy, including disease-specific treatments; complications
- Limited resources: research faculty and personnel, funding, collaboration
- Ethical concerns: use of placebo in a vulnerable population
- Complexity in attribution of treatment-related adverse events because of disease progression
- Limited consensus on prioritization, definitions, objectives, and end points in the research community (e.g., fatigue trials)

Palliative care research

Prior to embarking on new research, it is important to develop research queries. Once queries are generated, they should be prioritized.

Experience, expertise, and the practice of evidence-based medicine in palliative care are used to define and refine the questions to be asked. The process of framing a research direction can be summarized by the acronym *PICO* (problem, intervention, comparison, and outcome).[2]

The *problem* is defined as a patient population or condition that is being dealt with.

The *intervention* commonly includes treatment, diagnostic tests, prognostic factors, and exposure to risks. It is common for the intervention to be kept as simple as possible and for external extraneous variables to be minimized.

A *comparison* is defined as an alternate intervention with which to compare the intervention of interest. To give a patient a placebo when there is a proven treatment variable would be unethical. In palliative care, it is always pertinent and important to compare an intervention or treatment with the standard of care rather than with a placebo, owing to ethical considerations.

An *outcome* is a measurable study end point. For example, a logical study end point for treatment of fatigue near the very end of life would be the use of a validated tool, such as the Functional Assessment of Chronic Illness Therapy fatigue subscale.

Palliative care studies include ethnographic studies and observational studies. *Ethnographic studies* describe people through writing (e.g., case reports). *Observational studies* include descriptive, analytical, cross-sectional, and cohort studies; surveys; controlled clinical trials; and experimental studies.

Palliative care studies can also be classified into qualitative and quantitative studies. *Qualitative studies* include analysis of language, behavior, or recordings. Such studies may also include data-collecting interviews, the use of focus groups, analyses of primarily involved grounded theory, and content analysis, as well as schematic analysis.

Quantitative studies look for whether a given event regarding disease is a random event or chance event. These require statistical analysis of numerical data.

Furthermore, palliative care studies can be prospective or retrospective. A *prospective study* is designed to address a particular research question via defined eligibility criteria, statistical analysis, and evaluation of outcome in a controlled setting. A *retrospective study* is a review of previously collected patient data—for example, toxicity and patient survival.

Clinical trials are categorized by phase. A *phase I* trial focuses on safety, optimal dose, and dosing schedule or method. A *phase II* trial focuses on initial efficacy response of a therapy, effect on a particular tumor type (in cancer care), or state of disease.

Phase III trials are usually randomized, controlled studies or studies that compare experimental treatment drugs or therapy to current standards. *Phase IV* is a further evaluation of an approved strategy—for example, evaluating the long-term toxicity of a given treatment over a period of years.

Phase I clinical trial present unique challenges. They may create an ethical dilemma of therapeutic intent vs. understanding the safety of a given drug. There is also extensive use of pharmacokinetics and molecular markers or biomarkers in phase I trials, leading to a significant amount of patient burden. Use of phase I trial design in palliative care, especially in terminally ill patients with good performance status, needs to be individualized, especially with regard to ethical issues and quality of life.

Most clinical trials in palliative care are phase II, in the early stages of studying a given drug's efficacy. The major complication of a phase II trial is the use of a placebo. Placebos are important in palliative care and symptom control; in fact, the placebo effect usually ranges from 30% to 50%.[3]

At the same time, given the focus on quality of life and the need for immediate relief of symptoms, patients and their caregivers and healthcare providers are reluctant to use a placebo, as they want the patient to receive a potentially effective treatment instead of no treatment.

The other major challenges with phase II trials, as well as phase III trials, are blinding, attrition, and dropout rates. These impact both the understanding and effectiveness of a given treatment as well as the timely completion of a trial.

Protocol development

A well-written protocol is essential for the successful outcome of any research trial. A protocol that is complete and clearly defined will be successful and easy to execute. A protocol should be viewed as an instruction manual or road map that clearly defines how the study will answer a research question and how the trial is being conducted. The following elements of a protocol are important for proper execution.

The *objectives* should be consistent with the phase of the protocol.

The *background* should give information on the disease being studied. It should contain the rationale for the study, the hypothesis (the formal prediction), and an assumption of something that is observed in clinical practice and needs to be clearly defined. The background should be followed by intervention information or, in the case of a treatment trial, drug information.

The research *design* should include a well-characterized patient population to be evaluated. This should be included in the subject information, along with the setting where the treatment or trial is being conducted (for example, the hospital—outpatient or inpatient—or hospice).

The *eligibility criteria* should include the inclusion and exclusion criteria for the trial and should be followed by a well-defined treatment plan. The *treatment plan* includes the outcome measures and assessment tools used to evaluate these outcomes. The outcome measures should also include the toxicity of a given treatment.

The time points of assessment and the outcome measures should be as minimal as possible so as to reduce patient and caregiver burden. Always consider conducting some of the assessment via telephone or online, if appropriate or feasible, given the frail nature of the patient population, to avoid missing data.

This should be followed by *statistical considerations*, which should provide detailed information on how the primary and secondary outcomes would be tested and analyzed. There should also be information on interim analysis. The sample size should be set with consideration of the attrition rate, which is approximately 30% in palliative care populations.

References should be provided throughout the protocol so as to base evidence on statements made. The *appendices* should include any questionnaires and side effects of the measures used.

The most important part of the protocol is the *informed consent* document. It should clearly state the purpose of the trial; the appendices that the patient may obtain; dated information about how long a given questionnaire should take to answer; and the time, effort, and financial requirements of participating in the trial. The informed consent document should also mention clearly any potential side effects or injury.

A *protocol* should be written with all the collaborators, including the principal investigator, the mentor, if pertinent, a biostatistician, and the interdisciplinary team (which may include the bedside nurse, the social worker, and the basic scientist, if pertinent).

Before initiation of the study, it is important to have the protocol reviewed by peers, the hospital, or a scientific committee. Many institutions have an institutional review board that considers the science and patient safety before approving a trial.

It is also essential to have a study management plan that basically establishes standards that will ensure compliance with federal regulations, good clinical practice, and assurance and accountability requirements. This ensures proper conduct of the study, provides the general rules of the study and roles of the key roles of the study personnel, and provides for patient confidentiality and a monitoring and auditing plan.

The most important aspect prior to activation of the study is the meeting with the biostatistician. This meeting should also involve the principal investigator, co-investigators, collaborators, the data collection and management team, and the regulatory management team. A clear timeline of activation, implantation, and analysis of a given protocol should be documented.

An important consideration is proper training of all personnel. This includes orientation of the collaborators and proper training of the research nurse and investigators about adverse events and deviations that need to be filed in a timely manner. The data manager should enter the data in a timely fashion.

Another important consideration is financial—specifically, that reimbursement of the patient is clearly documented in the form of a contract.

Developing appropriate skills, applying ethical principles to the conduct of research, and, above all, processing good research questions with a productive protocol and study management will help improve the standards of palliative care treatment.

Recruiting and retention in clinical trials: measures to be considered to facilitate accrual and completion[3–8]

One of the most challenging aspects of conducting a successful clinical trial is accrual. Various measures have been described in the literature. Patient-related factors that facilitate enrollment include the following:

- Fear of a breach of privacy or autonomy or suspicion regarding the research itself may impede authorization.
- The research team's ability to explain the possible outcomes as potentially beneficial for future patients may trigger an altruistic tendency in the patients (a desire to create a legacy) and may prompt patients to enter the trial. Investigators should explain that the discernable benefits of participation in a clinical trial are the possibility of new treatment for a refractory symptom, the possibility of the research team adding an extra dimension of care for patients, and a meaningful task for the patient.

Measures for successful recruitment

1. Establish a study identity.[4,5]
2. Emphasize the benefits of participation.[6]
3. Minimize the burden for participants.
4. Involve the caregivers during the informed-consent process, along with the patient.
5. Provide incentive (but not through coercion).
6. Retain a control group.
7. Retain project staff and participants.
8. Offer support.
9. Be flexible.
10. Maintain tracking systems.

Ethics in palliative care research

Key factors in the ethical conduct of research in palliative care, in which participants are particularly vulnerable because of their desperate need for treatment options, must be considered:

1. The objectives of clinical trials in the terminally ill should take into consideration the possibility of minimal potential harm (including research-related distress and burden on the patient and caregiver) and a possible improvement in quality of life.
2. Informed consent for clinical trials must include understanding of the purpose of the research, any foreseeable risks, any possible benefits, any appropriate alternative procedures or treatments, confidentiality of records, participation being voluntary, ability to withdraw at any time, and that continuing care is not dependent on participation in the trial. The informed consent may sometimes need participation of caregivers. Precaution should be taken to ensure the decision-making capacity of the participant. Surrogate consent needs to be obtained in certain situations (e.g., child, delirium studies).
3. Ethical conduct of research studies is reviewed by an institutional review board or research ethics committee.

References

1. World Health Organization (2009). WHO definition of palliative care. Retrieved November 18, 2009, from http://www.who.int/cancer/palliative/definition/en/

2. NHS-Executive-Anglia-and-Oxford (1999). Asking the question: finding the evidence in evidence based health care. In: *An Open Learning Resource for the Health Care Practitioners*, Vol. 2. Luten; Chiltren Press, pp. 3–16.

3. de la Cruz M, Hui D, Parsons HA, Bruera E (2010). Placebo and nocebo effects in randomized double-blind clinical trials of agents for the therapy for fatigue in patients with advanced cancer. *Cancer* 116(3):766–774.

4. Davis LL, Broome ME, Cox RP (2002). Maximizing retention in community-based clinical trials. *J Nurs Scholarsh* 34:47–53.

5. Coday M. Boutin-Foster C, Goldman Sher T, Tennant J, Greaney ML,,Saunders SD, et al. (2005). Strategies for retaining study participants in behavioral intervention trials: retention experiences of the NIH Behavior Change Consortium. *Ann Behav Med* 29(2 Suppl.):55–65.

6. Wright JR, Whelan TJ, Schiff S, Dubois S, Crooks D, Haines PT, et al. (2004). Why cancer patients enter randomized clinical trials: exploring the factors that influence their decision. *J Clin Oncol* 22,:4312–4318.

7. White C, Hardy J (2010). What do palliative care patients and their relatives think about research in palliative care? A systematic review. *Support Care Cancer* 18(8):905–911.

8. Bruera E (2006). Practical tips for successful research in palliative care. In Bruera E, Higginson IJ, Ripamonti C, Von Gunten C (Eds.), *Textbook of Palliative Medicine*. London: Hodder Arnold, pp. 202–207.

Prevention and management: burnout in health-care providers

Mary L.S. Vachon, RN, PhD

Introduction

Several reviews of the literature[1-5] and a recent study from Japan[6] have shown that staff in hospice and palliative care experience less stress and burnout than those in other areas of health care.

The reasons for this are not clear. It may be the recognition from early in the field that there needs to be support within the system[1] and the fact that palliative care specialists do not feel as overwhelmed by work overload as colleagues in other specialties,[6] report more satisfaction with relationships with patients, families, and staff,[7] feel more confident in psychological care of patients, and feel they will have sufficient time to engage in communication with patients and families.[6]

It would be worth investigating whether palliative care staff practice more wellness strategies, as oncologists who practiced personal wellness strategies had greater well-being.[8]

This chapter will review the sources of stress associated with burnout in palliative care, protective factors that may mitigate the stress, signs and symptoms of burnout, and strategies to prevent and treat burnout.

Burnout and job engagement

Burnout is a "psychological syndrome in response to chronic interpersonal stressors on the job".[9] The three key dimensions are emotional exhaustion, cynicism and detachment from the job(depersonalization), and a sense of ineffectiveness and a lack of personal accomplishment.[9]

Burnout is a form of mental distress manifested in "normal" persons who did not suffer from prior psychopathology, who experience decreased work performance resulting from negative attitudes and behaviors.[10]

Job engagement is the opposite of burnout. Engagement is a persistent, positive-affective motivational state of fulfillment in employees that is characterized by vigor, dedication, and absorption.[11]

Engagement is associated with a sustainable workload, feelings of choice and control, appropriate recognition and reward, a supportive work community, fairness and justice, and meaningful and valued work.

Other frameworks for understanding person–job interaction

Although burnout is by far the most researched approach to understanding stress in hospice and palliative care, other concepts are also of interest. These include the following:

- *Stress*, which is "experienced when the demands from the work environment exceed the employee's ability to cope with (or control) them."[3]
- *Compassion fatigue* is almost identical to post-traumatic stress disorder, except that it applies to those emotionally affected by the trauma of another person (usually a client or family member). Compassion fatigue is also known as *secondary* or *vicarious traumatization*.[5]

Compassion fatigue shares some characteristics with burnout: depression, anxiety, hypochondria, combativeness, the sensation of being on "fast forward," and an inability to concentrate.

- *Compassion satisfaction* (CS) is satisfaction derived from the work of helping others. It may be the portrayal of efficacy. Caregivers with CS derive pleasure from helping others, such as their colleagues, and feel good about their ability to help and make a contribution.

There may be a balance between compassion fatigue and compassion satisfaction. Caregivers may experience compassion fatigue, yet they like their work because they feel positive benefits from it. They believe what they are doing is helping others and may even be redemptive.[4]

- *Countertransference* has recently been applied to end-of-life care.

In this context, countertransference is defined as "an 'abbreviation' for the totality of our responses to our work—emotional, cognitive and behavioral—whether prompted by our patients, by the dynamics incumbent to our helping relationships, or by our own inevitable life experiences."[4] Countertransference then involves

- *Alchemy* —"that space" that takes its own place in the poignant relationship between helper and patient. Through the experience both can be transformed."[4]

Who is at risk for burnout?

Burnout has been associated with the following variables:
- Younger age
- Being under age 55
  - In a large UK National Health Service study of physicians, middle-aged physicians were particularly at risk.[7]
- More responsibility for dependents, either children or elderly parents
- Being single
- Being female, although males were more at risk in a recent UK study
- Personality characteristics associated with burnout: neuroticism, lower levels of hardiness and self-esteem
- Work–home interference

Highly motivated health professionals with intense investment in their profession are also at a greater risk for the development of burnout.[4,5]

Research is much stronger on the association between burnout and a wide range of job characteristics, including chronically difficult job demands, an imbalance between high demands and low resources, and the presence of conflict (whether between people, between role demands, or between important values) than that on personal variables.[11]

What protects against burnout?

- Being religious
- Supportive spouses or partners
- The personality characteristic of hardiness—a sense of commitment, control, and challenge—helped to alleviate burnout in oncology staff and was associated with a greater sense of personal achievement.
- Both hardiness and a sense of coherence were associated with resilience in palliative care nurses. Those with a strong sense of coherence had more difficulty with change than those with a hardy personality.
- A full life outside of the work situation with time for good nutrition, exercise, a good social support system, and personal interests[4,5]

Signs and symptoms of burnout

Box 37.1 Signs and symptoms of burnout

Physical
- Fatigue
- Physical and emotional exhaustion
- Headaches
- Gastrointestinal disturbances
- Weight loss
- Sleeplessness
- Hypertension
- Myocardial infarction

Psychological
- Anxiety
- Depression
- Boredom
- Frustration
- Low morale
- Irritability
- May contribute to alcoholism and drug addiction

Occupational
- Depersonalization in relationships with colleagues, patients, or both
- Emotional exhaustion, cynicism, perceived ineffectiveness
- Job turnover
- Impaired job performance
- Deterioration in the physician–patient relationship and a decrease in the quality and quantity of care
- Increase in medical errors

Social
- Marital difficulties

A model for understanding occupational stress

Recent research on burnout has focused on the degree of match or mismatch between the person and six domains of the job environment. The greater the gap or mismatch between the person and the environment, the greater the likelihood of burnout. The greater the match or fit, the greater the likelihood of engagement with work.

Six areas of work life encompass the major organizational antecedents of burnout. These include workload, control, reward, community, fairness, and values.[9]

Burnout arises from chronic mismatches between people and their work settings in some or all of these areas. The area of values may play a central mediating role for the other areas,[9] although for individuals at risk of burnout, fairness in the work environment may be the tipping point determining whether people develop job engagement or burnout.[10]

Emotion-work variables (e.g., requirement to display or suppress emotions on the job, requirement to be emotionally empathic) account for additional variance in burnout scores over and above job stressors.[9] Table 37.1 shows the hospice/palliative care research within this model.

Factors related to burnout and job engagement in hospice and palliative care

Workload

Excessive workload exhausts the individual to the extent that recovery may be come impossible.[1–5] Emotional work is especially draining when the job requires people to display emotions inconsistent with their feelings.[9] Workload relates to the exhaustion component of burnout.[9]

Palliative care physicians had more stress from workload than colleagues in clinical and radiation oncology.[7]

Palliative care workers in rural Australia reported difficulty with being expected to work beyond normal working hours and with the lack of anonymity in a small rural community.[12]

Despite workload being a frequently reported stressor, it was not related to burnout in UK palliative care nurses.[4]

Control

Control is related to inefficacy or reduced personal accomplishment. Mismatches often indicate that individuals have insufficient control over the resources necessary to do their work or insufficient authority to pursue the work in a way that they believe is most effective.[9]

Stress also results from a lack of knowledge in interpersonal skills and a lack of communication skills and/or management skills.[1–5]

Nurses report being in situations both in the hospital and in the community where they feel responsible for alleviating the pain of a palliative care patient yet do not have a physician willing to order the medication they feel would be sufficient to control the pain.[4]

Table 37.1 Lifestyle management promoting wellness and preventing burnout

- Recognize and monitor symptoms
- Good nutrition
- Meditation
- Spiritual life
- Grieving losses, personally and as a team
- Reflective writing
- Decrease overtime work
- Exercise—aerobic, yoga, qi gong, tai chi
- Time in nature—walking, gardening
- Music—singing, listening to music, playing an instrument
- Energy work—reiki, healing touch, therapeutic touch
- Maintain sense of humor
- Balance work and home lives to allow sufficient "time off"
- Go on a retreat
- Have a good social support system—personally and professionally
- Seek consultation if symptoms are severe
- Discuss work-related stresses with others who share the same problems
- Visit counterparts in other institutions; look for new solutions to problems
- Remember the Serenity Prayer at work: God grant me the serenity to accept the things I cannot change, the wisdom to change the things I can, and the wisdom to know the difference." Sometimes work-related problems can be solved; other times, leaving the work environment and taking the wisdom gained with one is a good solution.

With earlier discharge of sicker patients, nurses with limited experience may be expected to care for seriously ill palliative care patients in their home, without access to physicians skilled in effective palliative care and symptom management.[4]

Reward

Lack of reward may be financial when individuals don't receive a salary or benefits commensurate with their achievements, or it may be social when one's hard work is ignored and not appreciated by others. The lack of intrinsic rewards (e.g., doing something of importance and doing it well) can also be a critical part of this mismatch.[9]

Australian hospice providers reported that economic pressures resulted in less staff support, competition between services for funding, inadequate funding to provide services in areas of need, lack of support for psychosocial needs including bereavement care, and experienced staff leaving palliative care.[12]

Community

Community contributes to burnout when people lose a sense of personal connection with others in the workplace.[9] Problems with colleagues have been reported in many studies.[1–5]

Our personal identity is formed and shaped as a result of our interactions with other people and is an expression of our basic genetic makeup. Therefore, we seek out and develop formal and informal social groups and networks in our private and working lives that supplement the relationships we already have within our family unit.[13] Social support from people with whom we shares praise, comfort, happiness, and humor affirms membership in a group with a shared sense of values.[3,9]

The quintessential feature of a small, well-balanced team is leadership that is shared or is rotated, depending on the issue involved.[13] In a healthy team, there is room for disagreement. However, teamwork may not be the best way to carry out palliative care. Research does not indicate that teamwork makes palliative care effective.[13]

In a study of a German palliative care team, factors crucial to successful communication were close communication, team philosophy, good interpersonal relationships, high team commitment, autonomy, and the ability to deal with death and dying. Close communication was by far the most frequently mentioned criterion for cooperation.

Team performance, good coordination of workflow, and mutual trust are the basis of efficient teamwork. Inefficient teamwork is associated with the absence of clear goals, tasks, and role delegation, as well as a lack of team commitment.[14]

Fairness

Another crucial factor is when there is not perceived fairness in the workplace. Fairness communicates respect and confirms people's self-worth. Mutual respect between people is central to a shared sense of community.[9]

For individuals at risk of burnout, fairness in the work environment may be the tipping point determining whether people develop job engagement or burnout. A lack of fairness was perceived with unrealistic expectations of the organization.[1,15]

Concerns about funding[12] and rivalries between hospices and other settings of care as well as those between different hospices have long been an issue contributing to burnout.[1–4,15]

Values

Palliative care staff often choose this line of work because it allows them to bring personal values to the workplace and encourages personal growth.[12]

Teamwork depends to a certain extent on people being able to subscribe to a *shared* set of values that reinforce the team's way of working and reduce the likelihood of clashes with personal values.[13]

Individuals need to reconcile their individual moral values with those required by or most readily identified with their professional role and with their membership of a larger moral unit, the team. There can be challenges if individuals do not agree with a strong philosophy or ethos of the team.

A team may decide to change or modify its philosophy in light of external factors, or an individual may feel that his or her personal philosophy no longer fits with that of the team.[13]

Emotion-work variables: issues of death and dying

Emotion-work variables (e.g., the requirement to display or suppress emotions on the job, requirements to be emotionally empathic) account for additional variance in burnout scores over and above job stressors.[9] The most problematic stressor reported by hospice nurses was "death and dying."

In one study, 43% of UK general practitioners respondents needed to give more time to dying patients, and around one-third had trouble coping with their own emotional responses to dying patients. These general practitioners seemed most likely to have difficulty communicating with patients who were dying and with their relatives.[4]

In a study of Japanese oncologists and palliative care physicians, insufficient confidence in the psychological care of patients was associated with physician burnout more than involvement in end-of-life care.[6] Those who were less confident in dealing with psychological care and demonstrated higher levels of emotional exhaustion were more likely to choose continuous-deep sedation for patients with refractory physical and psychological distress.

In the context of hospice and palliative work, personal closeness and distance have to be negotiated, and this can be a tightrope act. The value of hospice and palliative work lies in clinicians' closeness to patients and relatives and in the empathic, familiar, and confidential mode of dealing with each other. But this closeness and distance must be balanced continuously.[4]

The difficulty of establishing more distance to avoid too much closeness and the problems involved in this process are well illustrated in an academic palliative care unit that was having trouble retaining nurses.[16] The larger group strove "to adopt a well-organized and purposeful approach as a nurse" ($N = 12$); the second group strove "to increase the well-being of the patient" ($N = 2$). The first group's strategy significantly distanced the nurses from patients. In the second group, care appeared to be a central concern for the nurses and a main source of satisfaction.

Education in palliative care involves learning the art of building and sustaining relationships and of using the self as a primary instrument for diagnosis and treatment. This involves psychological risk-taking that may be unique in the health field,[17] as palliative care takes caregivers into emotional realms that are neither easy nor comfortable. The caregiver may be permanently changed through this encounter.[18]

At the same time, increased exposure to patients' deaths has been linked to higher reports of stress and burnout in physicians and nurses. Constantly confronting the death of others causes caregivers to repeatedly re-evaluate their own mortality and re-examine the meaning of life and death.

Constant exposure to multiple deaths and losses may leave staff with grief overload and considerable distress. However, participating in the death of some patients may also result in intense positive experiences that promote professional development.[1–4]

Grief is like a powder keg. Caregivers may not be aware that they have been challenged by grief, but the effects of grief can be explosive and can cause problems at any time. Yet caregivers are expected to carry on "as usual" once a patient has died.[4]

Coping with and avoiding burnout

While there are new findings regarding the interpersonal dynamics between the worker and other people in the workplace, yielding new insights into the sources of stress, effective interventions to prevent burnout have yet to be developed.[11]

In the model proposed by Maslach and colleagues, effective interventions to deal with burnout should be framed in terms of three dimensions: exhaustion, cynicism, and sense of inefficacy. Their interventions focus on building job engagement, rather than reducing burnout.[11]

A recent study[10] found that if staff in a university setting had either of the burnout components of emotional exhaustion or cynicism, then the perception of fairness in the work situation was the tipping point determining whether people developed burnout or job engagement. One of these signs is potentially an early warning sign of burnout.

A Cochrane review assessed the prevention of occupational stress in health-care workers,[19] concluding that there was limited evidence for the effectiveness of person- and work-directed interventions to reduce stress levels in health-care settings. Only two trials, one in oncology on attitudes and communication skills,[20] were rated as being of high quality.

Finding meaning in work–job engagement and compassion satisfaction

When caregivers to the critically ill, dying, and bereaved were interviewed and asked what enabled them to continue working in the field, the top five coping mechanisms identified were a sense of competence, control, or pleasure in one's work; team philosophy, building, and support; control over aspects of practice; lifestyle management; and a personal philosophy of illness, death, and one's role in life.

More recent studies have looked at sources of satisfaction in the work of palliative care staff. These include dealing well with patients and relatives[16] and helping patients to find meaning in suffering and death.

Palliative care has been described as a way of living.[12] Vitality, the capacity to live and develop in a way that is associated with energy, life, animation, and importance, is the core meaning of palliative care.[12] This way of living involves unity with self, being touched to the heart, and personal meaning. Crucial to the experience of palliative care is the patient and family, holistic care, and the interdisciplinary team.

In one study, palliative care providers were asked to define spirituality.[21] They responded with concepts related to integrity, wholeness, meaning, and personal journeying. For many, their spirituality was inherently relational. It might involve transcendence, was wrapped up in caring, and often manifested in small daily acts of kindness and love.

For some participants, palliative care was a spiritual calling. A collective spirituality stemming from common goals, values, and belonging had surfaced. Palliative care can take caregivers into emotional realms that are neither easy nor comfortable.[18] The caregiver and client may be permanently changed through this encounter.[18]

Meditative and reflective practices

Daily spiritual practices might mitigate physical, cognitive, and emotional forms of burnout in the workplace.[5,22] A negative correlation was found between the amount of end-of-life training received and the burnout in the physical and cognitive domains. However, training was not related to caregivers' emotional exhaustion.

The stress of palliative care and bereavement work might be ameliorated through enhanced training efforts and creative facilitation of diverse spiritual practices, such as inclusive forms of ritual recognition of loss in the workplace.[5,21,22] Developing group meditation programs and encouraging individual meditative practices are other useful strategies.

Mindfulness meditation refers to a process of developing careful attention to minute shifts in the body, mind, emotions, and environs while holding a kind, nonjudgmental attitude toward self and others. The practice of mindfulness meditation simultaneously raises caregivers' consciousness of their inner reality (physical, emotional, and cognitive) and that of the external reality with which they are interacting.

It teaches caregivers to develop a "kind, objective witnessing attitude" toward themselves and helps to develop empathy for others.[5] The practice of exquisite empathy is facilitated by clinician self-awareness, identified as the most important factor in psychologists' functioning well in the face of personal and professional stressors.[5]

Self-awareness involves both a combination of self-knowledge and development of *dual-awareness*, a stance that permits the clinician to simultaneously attend to and monitor the needs of the patient, the work environment, and his or her own subjective experience. When functioning with less self-awareness, clinicians are more likely to lose perspective, experience more stress in interactions with their work environment, experience empathy as a liability, and have a greater likelihood of compassion fatigue and burnout.

Clinicians functioning with greater self-awareness may experience greater job engagement with less stress in interactions with their work environment, experience empathy as a mutually healing connection with their patients, and derive compassion satisfaction and vicarious post-traumatic growth. Self-awareness may both enhance self-care and improve patient care and satisfaction.[5,23]

In planning interventions, it must be recognized that not all caregivers will benefit from the same approach. There must be awareness that different team members may have different ways of dealing with challenging situations such as grief.[24] Physicians and nurses may prefer different coping strategies and may have different personality structures that lead to different responses to patient deaths.

Individuals have natural propensities and aversions for minimizing grief reactions. Some caregivers are likely to talk with others about their grief, whereas others attempt to understand their grief through its depiction in literature and the arts. Some might dampen their grief with alcohol or drugs, while others use personal faith to resolve their grief.

Speck[13] speaks of valuing the people one works with and attending to the dynamic processes that develop as a way of fostering mutual respect and achieving the desired outcome for the work of the team.

Meditation and reflective practice interventions

Recently developed interventions reflect approaches that build on concepts of job engagement and compassion satisfaction, enabling caregivers to learn approaches that sustain themselves, while acknowledging and celebrating their engagement with their clients and in their work.

Such interventions include mindfulness meditation and narrative approaches. These interventions have the potential to help caregivers enrich their personal lives, enhance their involvement with patients, and avoid some of the team conflicts noted earlier as being a significant source of stress in palliative care.[4,5]

Fillion et al.[25] developed and tested a meaning-centered intervention with palliative care nurses. The intervention applied didactic and process-oriented strategies, including guided reflections, experiential exercises, and education based on themes of Viktor Frankl's logotherapy. The palliative care nurses in the experimental group reported more perceived benefits of working in palliative care after learning the intervention and at 3-month follow-up. Spiritual and emotional quality of life, however, remained the same.

Danieli[26] has adapted her group intervention, developed over three decades of working with trauma, to use with caregivers dealing with countertransference difficulties in end-of-life care. Although the intervention has been developed to be used with groups, it can also be used by individuals.

Danieli's approach has two phases: 1) deep relaxation and in-depth connecting with an end-of-life experience most meaningful to the individual and with the implications of that experience, and 2) group sharing about the consequences of their experiences with dying and death. The sharing serves to counteract individuals' potential sense of isolation and alienation in working with the dying.

Educational interventions

Communication training

Given that communication problems with patients and family members are associated with stress and burnout,[1,4,16] communication skills interventions have been tried, and some have been found to be effective.[20]

Chochinov[27] has proposed the A, B, C, and D of dignity-conserving care. Using empirical evidence, he showed that kindness, humanity, and respect, the core vales and behaviors of medical professionalism, often relegated to the "niceties" of care, embrace the true essence of medicine. These aspects of care, variably referred to as spiritual care, whole-person care, or dignity-conserving care, involve attitude, behavior, compassion, and dialogue.

Chochinov provides a core framework of dignity-conserving care to guide health-care providers in incorporating this important facet of patient care. Hospice and palliative care specialists may feel that they have already incorporated these values into their work, but there is still more work to be done in this area.

Changing models of practice

In the European Union, a model for shifting established patterns is being tried, with the goal of improving the interaction between mobile palliative care teams (PCMT) and the hospital staff with whom they interact.[28]

In this model, recognizing the full range of convictions held by persons in a hospital setting, the concept of palliative care and terminal care has been bolstered by the concept of continuous care. In continuous care, curative and palliative procedures that focus on the holistic care of patients and their family tend to be used.

"Promoting the integration of continuous care in the hospital intends to identify the challenges in integrating continuous care through an inventory and analysis of the activity of palliative care mobile teams in several countries of Europe. Competencies for PCMTs have been derived and based on these, and a pilot three phase educational programme with PCMTs undertaken and evaluated."[28]

At the San Diego Hospice, the model of care is being changed in part to cope with the nursing shortage.[29] The Shared Care Model changes the interdisciplinary process from a nurse-driven, case-management model to a team-managed, self-governing model. Responsibilities are redistributed to each team member, within their scope of practice, to more evenly share the workload and increase the interaction with patients and their families.

Unit-based intervention

LeBlanc et al.[30] did a quasi-experimental study of a team-based burnout intervention on 29 oncology units in the Netherlands. Nine wards were randomly selected to participate in the Take Care! intervention. The program consists of 6-monthly 3-hour sessions including education about the mechanisms of stress as well as feedback on the participants' work situation. This feedback was used to help participants structure their subjective feelings by providing them with relevant topics for discussion and for their plans to reduce work stress on their ward.

At the end of the first session, the job stressors to be dealt with during the training session were selected. The remaining sessions consisted of education and an action component.

During the action component, participants formed problem-solving teams. Outcomes of these sessions included the introduction of more efficient procedures for reporting on patients and for ordering supplies (quantitative demands), the appointment of staff members as "guardian angels" who would watch over team members' well-being (support), and the restructuring of weekly work meetings to enable more participation (voice) of staff members (participation in decision-making).

Results of multilevel analyses showed that staff in the experimental wards experienced significant decreases in burnout scores initially and over time. Moreover, changes in burnout levels were significantly related to changes in the perception of job characteristics over time.

Self-care and personal wellness

Of great importance to the prevention of burnout are the well-known line that one cannot give from an empty vessel and the warning that when traveling on an airplane, first put on your own oxygen mask.

The best prevention for caregiver burnout is to promote personal and professional well-being on all levels: physical, emotional, psychological, and spiritual. This must occur throughout the professional life cycle of professionals, from professional school through retirement. It is a challenge not only for individual caregivers in their own lives but also for the professions and the health-care system.

Shanafelt et al.[8] assessed the well-being and personal wellness strategies of medical oncologists in the North Central Cancer Treatment Group. Half of the respondents reported high overall well-being. Being age 50 or younger, male, and working 60 hours or less per week were associated with increased overall well-being.

"Ratings of the importance of a number of personal wellness promotion strategies differed for oncologists with high well-being compared with those without high well-being. Developing an approach/philosophy to dealing with death and end-of-life care, using recreation/hobbies/exercise, taking a positive outlook and incorporating a philosophy of balance between personal and professional life were all rated as substantially more important wellness strategies by oncologists with high well-being…. Oncologists with high overall well-being also reported greater career satisfaction."[8]

These coping strategies are similar to the top five coping strategies identified two decades ago[15]: a sense of competence, control, or pleasure in one's work; team philosophy, building, and support; control over aspects of practice; lifestyle management; and a personal philosophy of illness, death, and one's role in life.

Meier et al.[23] have proposed a model for increasing physician self-awareness, which includes identifying and working with emotions that may affect patient care. Kearney and colleagues[5] have written of the need for physicians to be "connected" in order to continue to practice end-of-life care.

Table 37.1 provides a list of lifestyle practices that promote wellness and prevent burnout.

Clinical pearls

- Research over four decades shows palliative care practitioners generally experience less stress and burnout than practitioners in other health-care settings.
- The perception of unfairness in the workplace may be the tipping point for burnout.
- Job engagement is the opposite of burnout and is characterized by a state of fulfillment, characterized by vigor, dedication, and absorption.
- Compassion satisfaction (CS) is derived from the work of helping others. It may be the portrayal of efficacy. Those with CS derive pleasure from helping others, such as their colleagues, and feel good about their ability to help and make a contribution.
- Daily spiritual or meditative practices might mitigate physical, cognitive, and emotional forms of burnout in the workplace.
- Oncologists' personal wellness-promotion strategies were associated with high levels of well-being and greater career satisfaction.

References

1. Vachon MLS (1995). Staff stress in hospice/palliative care: a review. *Palliat Med* 9:91–122.
2. Vachon MLS (2008) Stress and burnout in palliative medicine. In Walsh D, Caraceni AE, Fainsinger R, Foley K, Glare P, Lloyd-Williams M, Núñez-Olarte J, Von Roenn J, Tieman E (Eds.), *Palliative Medicine*. Philadelphia: Elsevier, 2008.
3. Vachon MLS, Sherwood C (2007). Staff stress and burnout. In Berger AM, Shuster JL, Von Roenn JH (Eds.), *Principles and Practice of Palliative Care and Supportive Oncology*, 3rd ed. Philadelphia: Lippincott Williams & Wilkins, pp. 667–686.
4. Vachon MLS, Müeller M (2009). Burnout and symptoms of stress. In Breitbart W, Chochinov HM (Eds.), *Handbook of Psychiatry in Palliative Medicine*. New York: Oxford University Press, pp. 559–625.
5. Kearney MK, Weininger RB, Vachon MLS, Mount BM, Harrison RL (2009). Self-care of physicians caring for patients at the end of life: "being connected … a key to my survival". *JAMA* 301:1155–1164.
6. Asai M, Morita T, Akechi T, et al. (2007). Burnout and psychiatric morbidity among physicians engaged in end-of-life care for cancer patients: a cross-sectional nationwide survey in Japan. *Psycho-oncology* 16:421–428.
7. Ramirez AJ, Graham J, Richards MA, Cull A, Gregory WM, Learning MS, Snashall DC, Timothy AR (1995). Burnout and psychiatric disorder among cancer clinicians. *Br J Cancer* 71:1263–1269.
8. Shanafelt TD, Novotny P, Johnson ME, Zhao X, Steensma DP, Lacy MQ, Rubin J, Sloan J (2005). The well-being and personal wellness promotion strategies of medical oncologists in the North Central Cancer Treatment Group. *Oncology* 68:23–32.
9. Maslach C, Schaufeli WB, Leiter MP (2001). Job burnout. *Annu Rev Psychol* 52:397–422.
10. Maslach C, Leiter MP (2008). Early predictors of job burnout and engagement. *J Appl Psychol* 93:498–512.
11. Maslach C (2003). Job burnout: new directions in research and intervention. *Curr Dir Psychol Sci,* 12:189–192.
12. Webster J, Kristjanson LJ (2002). "But isn't it depressing?" The vitality of palliative care. *J Palliat Care* 18:15–24.
13. Speck P (Ed.) (2006). *Teamwork in Palliative Care: Fulfilling or Frustrating?* Oxford, UK: Oxford University Press.
14. Jünger S, Pestinger M, Elsner F, Krumm N, Radbruch L (2007). Criteria for successful multiprofessional cooperation in palliative care teams. *Palliat Med* 21:1–8.
15. Vachon MLS (1987). *Occupational Stress in the Care of the Critically Ill, the Dying and the Bereaved.* New York: Hemisphere.

16. Georges JJ, Grypdonck M, De Casterle BD (2002). Being a palliative care nurse in an academic hospital: a qualitative study about nurses' perceptions of palliative care nursing. *J Clin Nurs.* 11:785–793.

17. Barnard D, Towers A, Boston P, Lambrinidou Y (2000). *Crossing Over: Narratives of Palliative Care.* New York: Oxford University Press.

18. Boston P, Towers A, Barnard D (2001). Embracing vulnerability: risk and empathy in palliative care. *J Palliat Care* 17:248–253.

19. Marine A, Ruotsalainen J, Serra C, Verbeek J (2006). Preventing occupational stress in health-care workers. *Cochr Database Syst Rev* 4:CD002892.

20. Delvaux N, Razavi D, Marchal S, Brédart A, Farvacques C, Slachmuylder JL (2004). Effects of a 105 hours psychological training program on attitudes, communication skills and occupational stress in oncology: a randomized study. *Br J Cancer* 90:106–114.

21. Sinclair S, Raffin S, Pereira J, et al. (2006). Collective soul: the spirituality of an interdisciplinary palliative care team. *Palliat Support Care* 4:13–24.

22. Holland JM, Neimeyer RA (2005). Reducing the risk of burnout in end-of-life care settings: the role of daily spiritual experiences and training. *Palliat Support Care* 3:173–181.

23. Meier DE, Back AL, Morrison RS (2001). The inner life of physicians and care of the seriously ill. *JAMA* 286:3007–3014.

24. Redinbaugh EM, Schuerger JM, Weiss L, Brufsky A, Arnold R (2001). Health care professionals' grief: a model based on occupational style and coping. *Psychooncology* 10:187–198.

25. Fillion L, Duval S, Dumont S, Gagnon P, Tremblay I, Bairati I, Breitbart WS (2009). Impact of a meaning-centered intervention on job satisfaction and on quality of life among palliative care nurses. *Psychooncology* 18(12):1300–1310.

26. Danieli Y (2006). A group intervention to process and examine countertransference near the end-of-life. In Katz RS, Johnson TA (Eds.), *When Professionals Weep: Emotional and Countertransference Responses in End-of-Life Care.* New York: Routledge, pp. 255–265.

27. Chochinov HM (2007). Dignity and the essence of medicine: the A, B, C & D of dignity-conserving care. *BMJ* 334:184–187.

27. European Commission (2004). *Promoting the Development and Integration of Palliative Care Mobile Support Teams in the Hospital.* Brussels: Directorate-General for Research Food Quality and Safety.

28. Nadicksbernd JJ, O'Mary S (2008). Shared Care Model: An Agency's Transition to Team Case Management. Paper presented at The Humber College Annual Palliative Care Meeting, Toronto.

30. LeBlanc PM, Hox JJ, Schaufeli WB, Taris TW (2007). Take care!: the evaluation of a team-based burnout intervention program for oncology care providers. *J Appl Psychol* 92:213–227.

Index

St. Joseph Medical Center
The Otto C. Brantigan Medical Library
7601 Osler Drive
Towson, Maryland 21204